THAT HIGH DESIGN OF PUREST GOLD

A Critical History of the Pharmaceutical Industry
1880–2020

THAT HIGH DESIGN OF PUREST GOLD

A Critical History of the Pharmaceutical Industry
1880–2020

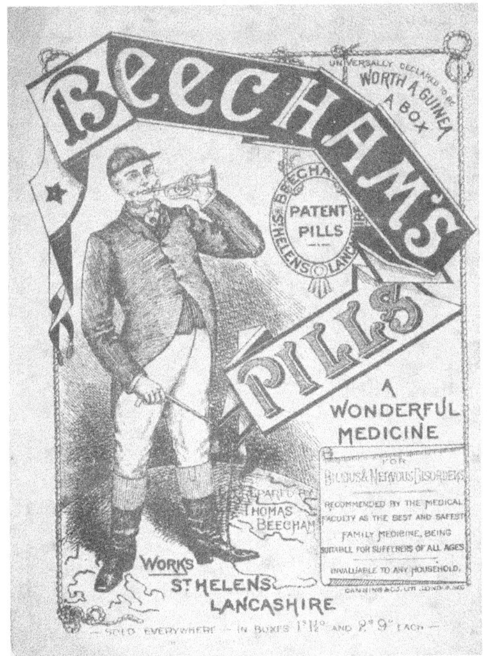

Graham Dutfield
University of Leeds, UK

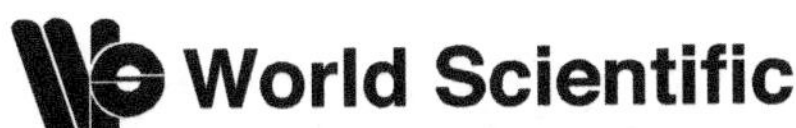

NEW JERSEY · LONDON · SINGAPORE · BEIJING · SHANGHAI · HONG KONG · TAIPEI · CHENNAI · TOKYO

Published by

World Scientific Publishing Co. Pte. Ltd.

5 Toh Tuck Link, Singapore 596224

USA office: 27 Warren Street, Suite 401-402, Hackensack, NJ 07601

UK office: 57 Shelton Street, Covent Garden, London WC2H 9HE

Library of Congress Cataloging-in-Publication Data

Names: Dutfield, Graham, author.

Title: That high design of purest gold : a critical history of the
   pharmaceutical industry, 1880 to 2020 / Graham Dutfield.

Description: Hackensack, N.J. : World Scientific, [2020] |
   Includes bibliographical references and index.

Identifiers: LCCN 2020023372 | ISBN 9789811222474 (hardcover) |
   ISBN 9789811222481 (ebook for institutions) | ISBN 9789811222498 (ebook for individuals)

Subjects: MESH: Drug Industry--history | Pharmaceutical Research--history |
   Economics, Pharmaceutical--history

Classification: LCC RA401.A3 | NLM QV 711.1 | DDC 338.4/76151--dc23

LC record available at https://lccn.loc.gov/2020023372

British Library Cataloguing-in-Publication Data

A catalogue record for this book is available from the British Library.

First published 2020 (hardcover)
Reprinted 2022 (in paperback edition)
ISBN 978-981-124-992-1 (pbk)

For any available supplementary material, please visit
https://www.worldscientific.com/worldscibooks/10.1142/11889#t=suppl

"Dutfield's book is breathtaking, a history of the pharmaceutical industry since the late nineteenth century in Germany, France, Britain, and the United States in broad-stroke relationship to the sciences that undergirded it, the patent laws that encouraged it, and the regulatory systems that have governed it. The book is salted with vignettes of the industry's principal progenitors from their emergence out of the German dyestuff industry to their engagement with human genomic data. It showcases the drugs they devised ranging from hormones to antibiotics and on to the myriad products of biotechnology. Wide-ranging in its knowledge, it is rich with reflections on multiple topics, including alternative and native medicines as well as the pharmaceutical industry and the public interest. The book is authoritative, provocative, and a compellingly accessible read — in all a tour de force."*

Daniel Kevles
Stanley Woodward Professor Emeritus of History,
History of Medicine & American Studies
Yale University

"I found Prof. Dutfield's work to be truly outstanding. So I am sure this forthcoming book will be excellent as well."

Myles Jackson
Professor of the History of Science,
Institute for Advanced Study,
Princeton University
author: *The Genealogy of a Gene: Patents, HIV/AIDS, and Race*

"The Highest Design of Pure Gold is a lively and engaging history of the pharmaceutical industry that deserves a wide readership. Dutfield deftly traces the complex process through which the industry has developed over the past 140 years in terms of scientific progress, business strategy, regulation, and intellectual property law. Filled with fascinating details and compelling stories, he brings a rare depth of knowledge to the topic and, in particular, to his analysis of intellectual property and its relationship to innovation. Dutfield also offers a measured yet penetrating critique of the industry and discusses potential remedies for the widespread problems that characterize our current drug-development system. He has provided us with a valuable contribution to an incredibly important discussion."

Joseph M Gabriel
Associate Professor of the History of Medicine,
Florida State University
author: *Medical Monopoly: Intellectual Property Rights and the Origins of the Modern Pharmaceutical Industry*

"A unique and masterful overview of the co-evolution of pharmaceuticals development and intellectual property law to the present day, over more than a century in many national contexts.

For Nicholas-Sejong Dutfield

There needs no verse to beavtifie thy praise
Or keepe in memory thy spotles name
Religion, vertve, & thy skil did raise
A threefold pillar to thy lasting fame
Thovgh poisnovs envye ever sovght to blame,
Or hyde the frvits of thy intention
Yet shall all they commend that high desygne
Of pvrest gold to make a medicine
That feele thy helpe by that thy rare invention

Tribute to Francis Anthony Doctor in Physick carved on a stone in the North Aisle of the Priory Church of St Bartholomew the Great at Smithfield, London.

Preface

This book was originally conceived as a third edition of my earlier *Intellectual Property Rights and the Life Science Industries*, editions of which came out in 2003 and 2009. However, this volume became something quite different. First, it focuses more explicitly on the pharmaceutical industry. Second, it withdraws from the earlier books' specialisation on intellectual property law, opting instead for a broader coverage and analysis over 140 years of interactions between commerce, science, regulation and law in the context of pharmaceuticals. Chapters 5–7 contain large passages of text that can be found also in the previous edition, albeit in revised and updated form. However, the rest of the book consists almost entirely of new writing.

Contents

Chapter 1

Introduction

This book is about medicines and the commercial actors that make and sell them. On the face of it, it's hard to think of anything nobler than to bring to the world a medicine that saves lives: 'that high design of purest gold', as the tribute on that ancient church in London affirms. But making medicines is a business, and it is very big business. By dint of what it sells and the profits it makes, the pharmaceutical industry wields immense power over lives and economies. How has it risen to this position of dominance? Are the interests of the industry and the public in balance? What should we admire about the industry? What should we criticise and seek to change? This book is my attempt to answer these questions.

Such an uplifting title joined to a more sceptical subtitle might seem an odd look. As we will see, one can certainly admire the industry's greatest achievements: cures for incurable diseases; drugs reducing death sentences to manageable conditions, such as the possibility now of *living with* AIDS when *dying of* AIDS used to be inevitable; and vaccines preventing people catching diseases in the first place.

Yet idealism plays very little part in the pharmaceuticals business. It may of course be very different for the scientists — the ones who deserve most of the credit for these amazing feats. The companies that employ those scientists — but be aware that a large proportion work outside of industry — strive to maximise shareholder value. That is their primary mission. CEOs good at this are handsomely rewarded with eye-watering salaries. In pursuit of such value accumulation, delivering cures may not be the best way; nor is making products accessible to all those needing them, if setting higher prices that exclude many people generates more profit. The people at the top of these companies are well aware of the financial 'dangers' of cures and price reducing competition. In the late

1990s the international pharmaceutical industry giants sought to prevent South Africa from introducing modest reforms to its patent law to improve access to medicines; reforms that were demonstrably legal under international law. The industry association representing these companies backed down presumably because they knew they were on shaky legal ground and were revealing more about their true motivations than they wanted the South African and global public, alerted to the dispute by the worldwide media attention, to know about. The point is that this instance of muscle-flexing by the industry, and one could find many others, shows how resistant it is to any serious attempts to challenge its profit maximising business model. Patients may die due to lack of access, but the business model must come first. In the United States, this muscle-flexing is given extra leverage by way of hundreds of millions of dollars every year spent on lobbying and election campaigns. It is all legal apparently, though for me the temptation to use words like 'corruption', 'influence peddling' and 'bribery' is hard to resist. That said, even with this much political influencing it seems unlikely that any US administration would have shown much respect for patents if that country had had the HIV/AIDS infection rates being faced then by South Africa. As it was, in the face of the very short-lived post 9/11 anthrax scare which affected a minuscule number of people, the US government showed very little respect for Bayer's patent rights to Cipro, deemed the most effective treatment for anthrax. Tommy Thompson, then Secretary of Health and Human Services, threatened Bayer that if they did not halve the price, he would simply acquire the drug from other sources.[1]

History certainly does not justify these hard-nosed approaches. What it does show is considerable continuity in terms of business behaviour and research priorities. This is exactly why I believe a history of an industry devoted, allegedly, to that high design of purest gold, needs to be a critical history, and not just a history. At the same time, one must avoid being tendentious. A cursory grasp of the industry's evolution might well imply that pathological behaviour is 'hard-wired' into industry culture and practice, going back to its earliest days; and that this consistency has persisted, and presumably will continue to do so, despite all of the changes taking place over the many ensuing decades including the development of ever more complex regulatory regimes. But that might go just a little too far. Despite its aggressive pursuit of profit from the start, cynicism was not always prevalent, at least not to the extent it has reached today. As regards research priorities, things seemed to change after the Second World War. Shortly after the 1953 merger of Merck with Sharp and Dohme, Henry Gadsden, the head of the company, told his researchers in a meeting that 'there are more well people than sick people. We should make products for people who are well'.[2] Examples of such products he mentioned — to the disgust of the scientists present — included a quick-tanning formula and a treatment for straightening hair. But by the normal criteria Gadsden was a highly successful business leader. Fast forwarding to the present, the first medicine to be approved by the United States FDA in 2019 was Jeuveau, an alternative to Botox for the 'disease' of frown lines. One must concede that many of the most recently approved new medicines are truly impressive therapeutic achievements, yet Jeuveau shows us that the practice does go on.

The pharmaceutical industry in its modern form has existed from about the 1880s since when it has been productive, powerful and profitable in ways that matter to us all. It is in Germany that companies resembling what we now call scientific research-based pharmaceutical companies came into existence. Now the sector is a truly global one but countries that had drug companies in the early part of the twentieth century — Switzerland, Germany, the United States and Britain — have retained that leadership for most of the time up to now. This is despite that Japan, South Korea and Israel have important international firms and are major sites for advanced biomedical research, that China, a late biomedical starter, is an emerging power, and that India has a large generics industry that can make more or less any medicine in existence. China (especially) and India are significant producers of active pharmaceutical ingredients (APIs) that they make under contract for western firms, both originator and genetic companies. The United States, despite its relatively slow start, became especially dominant after the Second World War and remains so. There is little doubt that much will change this century, including the geography of biomedical innovation and the global distribution of key firms, some of which are very likely to have started out in very different business sectors. Many may not even currently exist. But the industry's global nature will surely endure.

On the face of it, one may well ask what is *not* to love about a medicine that saves or improves people's lives? And why would we feel anything other than gratitude and respect for those responsible? Personally, I love a good story, and the discovery of new drugs is often a thrilling tale, sometimes even heroic. That's why I interrupt my narrative with such accounts, which may then be contrasted with the morally ambiguous conduct sometimes evident in the behaviour of companies which also feature in this book. There really is something noble about people who, without regard to personal gain, apply their brainpower and put in effort — whose likely outcome is failure — to invent a lifesaving medicine and then turn that invention into a product written down on thousands or even millions of prescriptions. When I saw Sir James Black speaking many years ago, a Nobel Laureate and a great biomedical scientist who shifted back and forth between academia and industry, he had none of the airs and graces one might expect of somebody who had pioneered beta-blockers and Tagamet, the first billion dollar a year medicine. He just seemed intrigued by the science of it all, and happy to have solved puzzles that had foxed other scientists, and afterwards to talk about it to students, as he did with genuine enthusiasm. Once you know the history of pharmaceuticals you will find many such people. Quite a few of them are mentioned in this book. Most of them do not win Nobel Prizes or earn enough to buy a mansion, football team, or Lear jet. But at the end of the day it is people who make new drugs, not (yet) machines or robots.

And yet, as we will see, this industry is far from being universally loved; nor does it deserve to be. Taxpayers underwrite a great deal of the scientific work, and the public sector conducts much of the underlying research underpinning drug development. Neither is necessarily a reason for criticism. But the industry has a habit of expecting to be treated as though it had invented its medicines from scratch, and solely at its own expense, and that it is therefore entitled morally to the legal and price-setting privileges of one whose achievements were attained without anybody else's help. In the United States especially the industry benefits massively from publicly funded research and the ground-breaking discoveries coming from its world-class university laboratories; yet it feels fully entitled to charge the highest prices for its medicines anywhere in the world. Another early point to make here is that the industry does not just discover, develop, and sell medicines: it also does politics, seeking to shape or change policies, laws and regulations that affect it, in their favour. Separately and collectively in the form of business associations, it is a political actor. There is much at stake in the pricing of a medicine, the conditions dictating its availability, the possibility to acquire a great number of patent and other intellectual property rights covering the product, the scope of those rights, and the shaping of regulatory pathways and checkpoints that original medicines and generic competitors must pass through to enter the market. Consequently, the industry invests lots of money in getting the legal and regulatory outcomes that it desires. In part it achieves results by persuading politicians and governments that what is good for the research-based pharmaceutical industry is good for the country. The United States government including its diplomatic missions unashamedly intervenes quite aggressively on behalf of the industry to counter foreign policies and policy reforms intended to contain or reduce pharmaceutical monopoly power and price-setting leverage. It is largely because of these activities that the industry is not immune from criticism just because Solvaldi and Glivec (or Gleevec), to give two random examples, are fabulous medicines — which they undoubtedly are.

Let us start with the absolute basics. What *is* this thing called a 'medicine'? Odd as it might sound, medicines are poisons that happen to be useful for therapeutic purposes — as opposed to for nefarious aims, such as murder. Some are therapeutic products *despite* being poisons; others *because* they are. Botulinum toxin, a bacterial product, is the most poisonous substance we know and causes botulism. But as 'Botox' it is prescribed for several muscle-related disorders and is famously a cosmetic treatment. Being toxins that people must consume to get treated, they are regulated accordingly. All new medicines and many old ones need to be treated as controlled substances for public safety. A medicine is no good if the harms it does due to toxicity outweigh the therapeutic benefits it provides. Over the years this has been the fate of many drug candidates that failed to make the grade after vast sums had been invested in their development. To make matters more complicated, a medicine can have drastically different effects on different people. It may be a miracle cure for some patients but what if it has little effect on most others and for a few it actually causes death, perhaps among the elderly, young children, people with other conditions, or those taking other medication causing adverse reactions? In hospitals a powerful painkiller like morphine gives immense relief to patients traumatised by pain. Used recreationally morphine, and its derivatives and synthetic analogues, may lead to addiction and death. Currently, the scandalous overprescribing of highly potent and addictive opioids,[3] which has led to many fatalities especially in the United States, has precipitated civil actions against companies that have overpromoted their use.[4] Context is everything in this respect, and — as we will see — in others too.

Many, perhaps most, are much less potent in their effects on people than the life saving or addictive ones. But by extending life or enhancing its quality, they are valued products for many people and beneficial for society — as long as they are accessible and respond to genuine health needs. This makes them very good for business. They may be good for business even when they are only marginally responsive to genuine needs especially if they are to be taken over an extended period. Pharmaceutical companies make these products and sell them, pursuing profit whilst navigating their way through a host of regulatory and legal norms and rules some of which they may have had a hand in designing. They are the subjects of this book.

Of course, the availability of medical treatments that work makes a massive difference to peoples' lives. Just imagine for a moment not having them. However romantically we turn to past times as golden ages, the briefest reflection on what it would be like to time-shift backwards to when there were no anaesthetics, antibiotics, vaccines and other treatments should be an effective reality check. The Age of Chivalry and the Black Death go together as closely as do the Romantic era and the slow horrible death to consumption that John Keats among countless others suffered. Most people alive today will never have to face the unspeakable agony of major surgery without anaesthetics, and in highly unsanitary conditions.

But we still have a long, long way to go. In many parts of the world, healthcare facilities are still truly grim places, unhygienic and lacking in basic facilities and equipment. In the Sudanese town of El Da'ein in

Darfur province, where I taught English in the late 1980s the stench of the town hospital was well known and very much present even to those just passing by. The high school boy I saw lying injured in a tackle playing football at the school where I worked did not survive a night there. I saw one of my Sudanese colleagues treated for hepatitis by burning him with charcoal. Whether it worked or not depends perhaps on whether he really had hepatitis but he certainly felt better the next day. At least it was cheap and it kept him away from the dreaded hospital. I treated a malaria victim in her home with my supply of chloroquine tablets, which were then still effective. Thankfully she made a full recovery.[5] As for the medicines themselves, existence and availability are two quite different things. Life in many parts of the world can still be miserable and short for many people due to the prevalence of lethal diseases. Cures may not exist, perhaps because there is insufficient profit in developing drugs for poor people to justify the investment. But it is often the case too that the medicines are simply unavailable where the sick people actually are. They may be physically present somewhere in those countries but are just too expensive due to patents, pricing that doesn't reflect ability to pay along with weak bargaining position to negotiate prices down, import tariffs, sales taxes, middlemen mark-ups, and of course sheer poverty. Sometimes they cannot be found because the market is deemed to be too small for a company to find it worth placing its products there or because pricing negotiations have broken down. And even when they *are* 'available' and affordable, they may turn out to be fakes that are of poor quality, or that contain none of the active ingredient and may include some that are lethal.

In developed countries things are not as they should be either. The United States is where many of the world's biggest drug companies originate. These businesses have developed some of the most sophisticated medical products ever conceived. Cancer death rates have been falling since peaking in 1990. However, shockingly in the last 3–4 years life expectancy rates are dropping. The US is the only developed country where this is happening. This is despite the country spending an estimated \$10,586 per capita on health in 2018, a figure that only Switzerland comes remotely close to. Out of that 12 percent goes on pharmaceuticals which amounts to well over \$1,000 per person. In contrast, again an estimate from OECD, the UK spent $4,070 per person in the same year with only $484 spent on pharmaceuticals for each person.[6]

We demand progress through constant innovation. Only sometimes do we get innovation, at least of the kind that benefits the public more than the company. Of course, medicinal knowledge has improved dramatically in many areas of health and disease and have benefited millions of people. Cancer has become more treatable. As mentioned before, AIDS was a death sentence but is now treatable; people can live with AIDS for decades, as can many people after a cancer diagnosis. People still get leprosy, but it is now curable, as is hepatitis C.

But it's a complex picture. In some other areas progress inches forward almost imperceptibly, has stalled almost completely, or may even be going backwards, as is arguably the case for certain mental health issues.[7] Moreover, while one would expect new drugs to be better than the ones they replace, often they are pretty similar in quality or substance to those we have already. Some may be deemed less good than those from previous generations.[8] Despite some major advances such as with childhood leukaemia, millions still die of cancer every year. Some of the most cutting edge products only extend the lives of terminal cancer patients (which is not to deny their importance for those patients taking them who understandably yearn to keep alive as long as medically possible — assuming pain and distress are within tolerable limits). Those of us lucky enough to expect a long life have good reason still to fear Alzheimer's when we get old. The terrifying motor neurone disease is still incurable. We remain vulnerable to new pandemics: antibiotics are working less and less well due to resistance, and only a few new ones exist to replace the ones becoming obsolete. The potential consequences of this are truly scary. Shamefully we have been aware of overprescribing and its dangers for decades. Tuberculosis is making a comeback. Over a million people a year die of it.[9] Ebola outbreaks continually flare up. Thankfully a new vaccine is available at last. Bubonic plague, one of our oldest and most devastating enemies, still kills people every year though admittedly it is rare now. When I started writing this part of the book, zika was very much in the news. As I finish it off, coronavirus is spreading around the world, making the 2011 movie *Contagion* feel like both a documentary and an unheeded warning. Borderless collaborative research and universal access to its benefits feels more important than ever. For all these reasons we should care a lot about the pharmaceutical industry and how it operates, whoever and wherever we are. We are all stakeholders whether or not we own shares.

Very few critical histories of the pharmaceutical industry have been written in book form that start from the time that companies began to make, market and sell mass-produced, standardised pharmaceutical products and continue up to the present. Even fewer are ones that treat intellectual property as being right from the start, central to the industry's behaviour, structure and general *modus operandi*, and perhaps even a defining feature. History of pharmaceutical intellectual property is not an academic subject in its own right. It is time it was, and I am hoping that this book, along with Joseph Gabriel's *Medical Monopoly*,[10] and Jeremy Greene's *Generic*,[11] two recent books which cover aspects of the same terrain from a similar general perspective, will help to establish it as one. But the present volume's account of the industry's emergence and evolution has a far broader focus than just this. It embraces the whole coevolution of the health-related life sciences and their attendant practices and technologies, business organisation and strategy, intellectual property law and management, *and* the regulation of products, technologies and practices. Taken together we might call this, as some have done in the past 'the medical-industrial complex' a term that goes back as least as far as the 1970s,[12] presumably inspired by military-industrial complex, a term coined by Dwight D. Eisenhower's speechwriters. As such, the book is a comprehensive and interdisciplinary historical record and commentary that takes us from the nineteenth century right to the twenty-first.

Coevolution and Progress

I have borrowed the word coevolution from biology. The *Encyclopaedia Britannica* defines it as 'the process of reciprocal evolutionary change that occurs between pairs of species or among groups of species as they interact with one another. The activity of each species that participates in the interaction applies selection pressure to the others.'[13] It seems self-evident to me that institutions, understood both conventionally as organisations, and in the more abstract regulatory sense, of the set of norms and rules envisaged by the Nobel Memorial Prize-winning economist Douglass

North,[14] do evolve and do so not independently but with other ones with which they relate. How the ones that this book deals with do so is a matter that merits close examination. As biological evolution is *natural* history, evolution in the sense employed in this book is also history whose purpose is to enable us to understand the present by reference to the past, and identify the source of both harmful and benign 'mutations' or dysfunctionalities.

But the book is not just about what the industry did and does given the institutional and other constraints and opportunities available to it at any time; it is also about what the industry *should* do and how one might imagine a better pharmaceutical industry by finding ways to introduce selective pressures leading to improvements of the kind that enhance its social functioning. As this book shows, there is no doubt that the industry has been responsible for a substantial number of health benefits which deserve our sincere appreciation. That's the good news. On the negative side, though, as we will see, its history *cannot* be a chronicle of continuous therapeutic progress. Science does not work that way, and neither can an industry, science-based as it is, whose *raison d'être* is to make profits — or deliver shareholder value as business executives are more likely to put it. Product regulation does not encourage progress. New drugs have to be effective to be approved, but they are not required to be *more* effective than the ones already available. And mostly they are only marginally better, if that. The pursuit of profit is not the same as the pursuit of better, even less the *achievement* of better. They may align but not necessarily, and that is the point. From a therapeutic perspective, the industry moves forward but it also goes sideways and backwards. In some health areas it doesn't appear to be moving much at all, on account either of lack of interest or because these are especially tough nuts to crack. A good example of such a 'recalcitrant' disease, albeit one of many, is lung cancer. Pharmaceutical treatments do exist but surgery remains the main medical intervention and survival depends on factors over which medical practitioners have little control.[15] These shifts back, forwards and crossways, though, are not just because that's the only way it can be. Things sometimes go wrong that don't need to. Furthermore, the industry is not self-sufficient, nor has it ever been. One thing that has not changed since the 1880s is its great reliance on science and innovation coming from other places, including universities, hospitals, tax-funded public research facilities, and charitable foundations.[16] Patient groups can also drive innovation processes. The current interest in so-called 'open innovation'[17] and 'translational research'[18] from many of the major firms is at the very least a tacit acknowledgement of this very basic fact: that they are not, and cannot be, self-sufficient. According to proponents of open innovation, business sectors whose firms typically tried to do everything in-house, and were thus practicing 'closed innovation' are now collaborating with others, sharing each other's knowledge and materials in the hope that by widening participation in this way, the speed of innovation will go up. The life science industries appear to be embracing the concept, at least going by this author's taking part in two international conference on the subject whose attendance and speakers comprised almost exclusively people from industry. But scepticism as to the novelty or radical nature of open innovation is justified. First, to suggest that pharmaceutical research and development was ever done purely in-house is simply false. The idea that companies in such a pragmatic knowledge-intensive business would opt to disengage with knowledge or techniques from outside its walls is historically false and any company insisting on behaving that way would surely not last long. This book amply bears this out. University scientists and drug companies have collaborated as far back as the nineteenth century, and at no time was this ever abnormal. Industry is arguably best at the practical end of the R&D process, but only in rare cases can any single company get that far by itself. Indeed, the discovery of Salvarsan, one of the first modern pharmaceutical products, is a perfect example of open innovation.[19] This of course suggests that open innovation — or perhaps we could more accurately call it 'networked innovation' — was pretty much there from the start. This is hardly the author's own original insight. Even in an age without the requirement for university scientists seeking funding to produce pathways to impact statements, Joseph Cooper had this to say in 1969:

> Diversity of input is needed both as to the different stages of research and development and as to different approaches to the same problem. The fundamentalist who seeks knowledge for its own sake from which may come unpredictable benefit tends mainly to find his home in academic centres, although in some measure he may also find a haven in

government and industrial laboratories. The investigator who works as part of a team pursuing a defined purpose with a practical end in view may also be supported in any of these work environments, but he tends in the main to come under the aegis of industry, where the operational incentives are directed towards practical input.[20]

Second, one must be careful not to equate the 'open' in open innovation with absence of intellectual property. There is no reduction in patent filing. Nonetheless, it is true that the industry is becoming more pro-active and strategic about research networking and knowledge management. Whether 'open innovation' is an accurate label for the various practices they are adopting to further such collaborating is a matter for debate.

As to its mode of doing business, the industry can itself obstruct social progress in terms of welfare-maximising drug development *and* provision. Might it be the case that the darker side of the industry has just as deep historical roots as the more admirable manifestations of commercial bio-medicine? Due to the high financial stakes and social welfare implications, politics cannot be left out of the story. Neither can corruption and dishonest practices. The industry has products to sell. It wants us to use them as long as they are paid. The companies' aim is to maximise profits. In pursuit of this goal, they can be ruthless. They do business; they also do politics. Indeed, the two are inseparable.

One can of course take a dim view of the industry morally but still appreciate its products, just as many North American farmers manage to appreciate Bayer/Monsanto's seeds and chemicals but still dislike the firm for the ruthless way it does its business.[21] There is no hypocrisy or contradiction between the two sentiments. Let us think again about evolution. Whether you think there are selfish genes depends on how far one agrees with Richard Dawkins's particular gene-centric view of evolution through natural selection[22] which does, incidentally, show how genetic selfishness does not exclude behavioural *unselfishness*. There is no doubt that companies are selfish pursuers of self-interest. Many scientists care deeply about patients. For all I know CEOs often do too. But business is business and the companies' mission is not really about the unfortunate patients awaiting a cure, but about making as much money as possible. To the extent that my analogy is a useful one, one might fairly ask whether this is necessarily and inherently a bad thing. Note here that I am not endorsing Gordon Gekko's view, in the 1980s movie *Wall Street*, that 'greed is good'. Neither should we feel comfortable with the CEO of Bayer's notorious but 'laudably' frank statement in 2013 regarding the compulsory license being granted on its anticancer drug Nexavar in India: 'We did not develop this medicine for Indians ... we developed it for western patients who can afford it'. (So why was he so unhappy that Indians should be able to access the drug thanks to the compulsory license — with compensation paid to his company?).

Returning to Dawkins, if he *is* right, we are the outcome of 3.6 billion years of highly successful genetic selfishness and this is something to celebrate. A lot of species, possibly the majority of those that has ever lived, have fallen by the wayside but as a species we are doing just fine — for the moment. (What we are doing to the rest of life and the biosphere is of course another matter entirely). Besides, as he has sought to show, the actions of all the world's selfish human genes do not preclude altruism and virtue. Of course, it would be better were individuals, communities, associations and companies more altruistic. But that desire, if taken too far, can lead us to utopianism that may take us the wrong way. Our record of social utopianism has been pretty catastrophic as victims of Stalin, Mao, Pol Pot, the North Korean Kim dynasty, and their gruesome ilk would confirm. The selfishness of the individual in relatively peaceful societies such as the one I am fortunate enough to inhabit is not to be denied or treated as curable by supposedly 'better' (typically dictatorial) modes of organising society, but to be allowed within limits: do not infringe the human rights of others, and do not impinge on the shared collective interests of all members of society in enjoying an acceptable degree of physical well-being and personal autonomy. Humans can do better; but we cannot do perfect. Obviously there are balances to be struck. How to do so is a philosophical question but it is also one of great importance for policymakers and of course for society as a whole who are the main stakeholders in determining what a fair society should look like, the values — whether utilitarian, communitarian, liberal or otherwise — that should guide us in determining this, and how to balance legitimate private interests, in this case the pharmaceutical industry, with social welfare.

Another lesson to be learned from the history of life on Earth is that evolution is not a story of inevitable progress. Likewise, as I said before, the pharmaceutical industry's history is not a tale of continuous improvement and it would be seriously erroneous, if not dangerous, to see it that way. Certainly, it is tempting to adopt a Whiggish view which sees history in the present context as a tale of progress leading ever onwards to a happily enlightened now. Evolution does not lead unavoidably and unidirectionally, and at all stages in between, from unsophisticated simplicity to subtle and intricate complexity. It would be as if the Palaeolithic hand axe led cumulatively and inexorably, without deviation or reversal, to today's precision tools, or Neolithic trepanning to modern brain surgery. With pharmaceuticals, things don't only get better and along a single pathway of getting-betterness; paths taken mean other paths, perhaps better ones, not taken. Some are diversions that lead us nowhere; others take us backwards. The well-known concept of path dependence explains why once one has embarked on a particular route which may turn out not to be the best one, we may be stuck with it so that turning back or switching simply does not happen even though logically it should. Some of the difficulties are the fault of the industry or the legal and regulatory system in which it operates, but not all. Suffice it to say at this point that given the financial stakes it would be naïve to suppose regressive outcomes can be entirely attributed to honest scientific error or incompetence. Where more money can be made from bad or mediocre science than from good science, the latter is unlikely to prevail.

In sum, there are at least three reasons why this is a pivotal moment for the industry, which suggests that a book like this taking critical stock of the industry from its inception to the present is timely. First, the industry has recently become truly global in ways it was not before. Trade liberalisation overseen by the World Trade Organization and promoted through an ever-increasing number of bilateral and regional trade deals, and the massive expansion of the middle class in emerging economies, promise vastly to increase pharmaceutical industry revenues across the globe. Improving scientific and technological capacity throughout the world also enables pharmaceutical research and development activities to be done in more and more areas of the world. Second, whereas until recently the industry was dominated by corporations whose lineages go back to the early days of the industry, newer firms are muscling in and becoming significant market actors. Third, non-traditional businesses especially those who control vast amounts of data in digital form or produce advanced digital technologies, such as Google and Apple, are entering the field. New and emerging technologies such as gene editing, nanotechnology, artificial intelligence and robotics have untapped medical potential. It is difficult to predict what impacts such approaches and technologies will have on the pharmaceutical industry, but they may well be profound. It is conceivable that the pharmaceutical industry as we have known it since the 1880s will no longer exist soon, to be replaced by a healthcare sector characterised by a markedly reduced centrality of the therapeutic chemical's role in its profit-driven war on ill-health however defined.

Let us turn now to the rest of the book. Part 1 ('The Nature of the Pharmaceutical Industry') seeks to flesh out the essential features of this industry, presenting our analytical approach to its evolution over a period of about 140 years up the present. As elsewhere in the book, the text is interspersed with illustrative examples and case studies. Chapter 2 seeks to explain what the pharmaceutical industry is by reference to historical context, and by differentiating between what the industry does in terms of producing, selling and making money, and what it does *not* do. The wider scientific, business, regulatory and legal setting for the emergence of this industry is crucial to any convincing account, as well as to any reliable critical assessment of its value to society. Major distinctions are those between 'modern' and 'traditional', the therapeutic chemical and the poison, and between traditional pharmacies and druggists and a new type of firm that emerged in the late nineteenth century. As we will see, the differences are not necessarily very clear cut.

My approach borrows the concept of co-evolution from biology, as set out in Chapter 2. Essentially, the industry has developed in directions that can be viewed and understood best in terms of the co-evolution of four phenomena: science, business strategy and practice, law regarding intangible property, and pharmaceutical product regulation (as well as regulation more generally). Each one of those impacts on all of the others, precipitating responses that in turn have mutual impacts.

Chapter 3 focuses on the fourth of these phenomena: regulation. This one merits special attention at this early stage of reading. This industry is not the only one that is largely based on science, or that has a business structure dominated to quite a considerable extent by long established large corporations. Nor is it the only one that is dependent on the acquisition and use of large holdings of intangible property rights. However, the way that the industry is regulated is rather specific to it. Medicines are essentially poisons used as treatments for people and thus they have massive public health implications of great interest to people and to the state. Accordingly, the regulatory frameworks under which the industry operates are, of necessity, something quite different from those of other sectors, and thus require some explanation before we delve further into the industry. Moreover, it is very hard to discuss regulation without intellectual property rights. In other words, pharmaceutical regulation is inextricably linked to trademarks, pharmaceutical test data exclusivity, which is a *quasi*-intellectual property right, and patents. Pharmaceuticals are chemicals sold under brand or generic names but comprising active ingredients whose names accord with nomenclatural norms that are understood little by most people. Thus, pharmaceutical product naming is a key element in regulation — but it is not a regulatory matter alone, also implicating trademark law. Naming serves not just to aid product identification for the benefit of patients, physicians and pharmacists but is essential to pharmaceutical business strategy.

Part 2 ('Antecedents and Origins') starts with a chapter (4) that traces changes in scientific knowledge and theories that form a background to the emergence of a modern science-based pharmaceutical industry. To the extent that the industry is, by definition, science based this discussion is necessary to understand its origins. However, it is important to underline that the emergence of what we now call biomedicine is a necessary but not a sufficient condition for the industry's rise. Chapter 5 locates the birth of the industry to late nineteenth century Germany and the synthetic dyestuff firms, some of which moved almost seamlessly into pharmaceuticals. The assertion that the dyestuff firms became the first modern pharmaceutical companies needs to be qualified a little. In their scientific approach and business practices, they do represent a genuine break with the past. But smaller natural product pharmacy companies there, in other European countries and in the United States, also underwent changes that made them what we would recognise as pharmaceutical firms rather than small manufacturing or retailing operations. Other types of firm that moved into pharmaceuticals were makers of branded secret remedies, often rather dodgy operations that 'went straight' like Beecham, and companies that started out making food supplements and crossed the line into purely medical products, such as Glaxo. But it was the dyestuff firms that put pharmaceutical discovery and making on a scientific and research-based footing.

Part 3 ('Science, Business Strategy and Growth') traces the growth of the pharmaceutical industry from the beginning of the last century, including the inter-war years and the period from the end of the Second World War to the present age of biotechnology, digitalisation, personalisation and precision medicine. During this era the industry emerged as one of the world's most important scientific research-based sectors. It was in many respects a very productive time for the industry. Admittedly, progress was initially quite slow until the mid-1930s, and decisive impacts on public health were not that great. But things improved markedly from then until, by most accounts, the 1960s. One important thing to be aware of is that through this period there was much continuity in terms of who the dominant firms were: typically, those with roots in the nineteenth century. Chapter 6 considers hormones. These are natural and synthetic medical products that proved to be profitable and that entailed a great deal of scientific learning as well as the ability to turn discoveries into medical products, something that was extremely difficult to do. Chapter 7 turns to perhaps the most prominent successes of the middle decades of the twentieth century: the anti-infective drugs, principally the antibiotics starting with penicillin. Up to the 1970s, the traditional drug discovery approach 'emphasized searches for substances — often in culture broths or biological extracts — that had desired effects on cells or organisms. The chemical composition of the active substance was identified and manufactured to yield a drug.'[23] Whether medicines were purified natural products or synthetics, nature was very much the guide. The author of that quote, Raymond Deshaies, explains the importance of this: 'This marriage of pharmacology and chemistry … launched the modern pharmaceutical industry and yielded hundreds of drugs.'[24] The hormones and antibiotics largely fit within this dominant paradigm and because they were so instrumental in the growth of the industry, this is why this book covers them in such detail. One of the main scientific weaknesses, though, was that molecular drug targets were largely unknown so the approach was bound to encounter diminishing returns.

Chapters 8 and 9 cover the period from the early 1980s up to the present. Chapter 8 focuses on advances in cellular and molecular biology and related sciences, and enhanced abilities to develop practical therapeutic applications. We will see how these transformed both the industry itself and the types of medical product becoming available. Nature is still the guide in many ways but our knowledge about it had become a great deal more sophisticated. Some of the most significant new types of product are known as biologics. These are large molecule drugs, often proteins, manufactured in living cells, and cell therapies. Chapter 8 also puts under the microscope recent trends towards personalisation of medicine through genomics and the mass production assembly, combination and analysis of digitised data not just regarding genetics but also concerning lifestyle including human behaviour, and environment. It also looks into precision medicines including small molecule drugs, and cell and gene therapies. All of this has massively transformative potential for healthcare and industry. With regard to digital and data technology, we are already seeing non-pharma businesses getting into the healthcare business on account of their advanced capacities to control and mine data. It is quite possible, for example, that the central role of the drug in healthcare may diminish, and bio-digital convergence[25] will see today's big pharma corporations transform themselves radically or else be replaced by completely different types of company entering healthcare markets with success, as businesses like Apple and Google deploying new and emerging technologies are attempting to do now. Much is at stake. Public health should improve massively and patients and the general public may find technological change to be truly empowering. The opposite is also possible with a reduction in people's autonomy and access to the best care becoming ever more a privilege for some than a right for all to enjoy. Medically speaking, one crucial therapeutic area such technologies promise to transform is that of cancer which is a hugely complex disease — or, perhaps more accurately, set of diseases. But their implications of course go much further too. Chapter 9 focuses on how intellectual property rights have been transformed during the period and seeks explanations for reforms that have taken account of science and markets and have — broadly speaking — benefited the industry by enhancing and extending market power.

Despite its impressive history and the promise — as well as early achievements — of the new and emerging technologies presented in Part 3, progress is, as with biological evolution, not a one-way street or something that is guaranteed. Non-communicable diseases, especially the complex ones like cancer, continue to be very tough nuts to crack, and drug-resistant infectious diseases we thought we had conquered for good are coming back. There have been some major achievements but millions across the world still die of cancer and other diseases every year. Responses to the return of old infectious diseases have been woefully inadequate. But this is not all that is wrong.

In one single chapter, Part 4 ('The Pharmaceutical Industry and the Public Interest') critically examines the present-day pharmaceutical industry considered in the context of history and our co-evolutionary analytical approach. It reflects on some of the lingering criticisms of the industry. In many ways the 140-year old pharmaceutical industry has been immensely successful, and has benefited the global public tremendously even if the distribution of benefits has been extremely uneven, reflective obviously of the massive income disparities. Despite this, and at the risk of sounding contradictory, the industry isn't working the way it should, and it must take a huge share of the blame. However, it would be facile to put all the blame on the industry, or to expect it to 'get better' all by itself. But whether we think the industry can be a force for good, it appears to be hampered morally by its need to generate shareholder value. Putting that point aside, though, the pharmaceutical industry sits within a legal-regulatory system comprising many interacting parts that together shape how it does its business, providing constraints here and opportunities there. Dysfunctionalities are thus not of the industry alone but implicate law, regulation and policy. Are alternative legal and policy measures necessary and feasible to make the industry more responsive to genuine health needs globally in view of present problems, and the likely scientific and business trajectories? We discuss these questions and others, and consider some possible solutions, out of which more specific measures might be considered.

****

As philosopher Jerrold Seigel rightly says, drawing for his ideas, as we all must do, on the work of others: 'What authors produce … are not "texts," but "works," which differ from texts precisely in being animated by some person's activation of language to express thoughts or beliefs.'[26] This book embodies wholly or in part the imprint of my personality — for better or for worse. There is nobody living in the world who would ever write the same book. They might be able to write a better book, but it would not be this one. Nonetheless, this book could not have been written alone on a desert island with nobody else to depend on for ideas, information, agreement and disagreement, intellectual support, love and companionship. This is the second book I have completed in a year; about both I had doubts as to whether they would ever get finished and I was not alone in that scepticism. Without Uma Suthersanen, co-author of the first one and who means so much more to me besides, nothing would be possible. I have some wonderful academic colleagues, friends and acquaintances who, whether they had anything directly to do with this book were the best possible company along what turned into quite a long journey. These include Cesar Ramirez Montes, Amrita Mukherjee and Subhajit Basu at Leeds, as well as Marc Mimler and Guido Westkamp. I am grateful to the history of science and technology scholars who admitted me into their community, especially Graeme Gooday, Greg Radick, Berris Charnley, and Stathis Arapostathis. Nicolas Rasmussen generously shared some of his work with me. I am thankful to the many people who have invited me to their conferences all over the world to speak, listen and above all to learn, and to the many scholars and civil society leaders with whom I have collaborated, and discussed and shared ideas, and without which this book would be nowhere near as good as (I hope) it is. The book may be mine alone, literally given that no research assistants were involved in any way. But my ideas were not formed in isolation. Singling out names of people is a dangerous task. But here are a few that stand out, in alphabetical order — at the risk of making this a rather ostentatious name-dropping exercise: Fred Abbott, Margo Bagley, Thiru Balasubramaniam, Henk van den Belt, Robert Bud, Julian Cockbain, Carlos Correa, Thomas Cottier, Rochelle Dreyfuss, Shubha Ghosh, Ellen t'Hoen, Daniel Kevles, Steven King, Bill Kingston, Sarah Laird, Jamie Love, Ruth Okediji, Abena Osseo-Asare, Shobita Parthasarathy, Darrell Posey and Dwijen Rangnekar (both sadly deceased), Jerry Reichman,

Hedley Rees, Pedro Roffe, Josh Sarnoff, Susan Sell, Sigrid Sterckx, Geoff Tansey, David Vaver, Rachel Wynberg, Peter Yu, and last but foremost Uma Suthersanen. I have learned much from students too, most recently from my very talented former PhD students Fifa Rahman and Adam Buick. Obviously none has the slightest responsibility for anything you will read in this book. My department at Leeds funded conference trips to such far-flung places as University of Technology Sydney and Harvard Law School where I was able to test new ideas relevant to the book before knowledgeable audiences.

It remains for me to say that in today's academic world, at least in the law part of it, book writing seems not always to be encouraged. Mainstream journal articles are what seem to count the most. Books including textbooks are considered to take up too much time to be worthwhile. I oppose this attitude with a passion. Books, whether they are made of paper or in electronic format, still matter. Indeed, I believe they matter more than any other type of publication. Few journal articles have ever inspired me in the way that a good scholarly monograph can and has done time and again. I cannot thank World Scientific enough for sharing my belief in books by publishing this one among the many others it produces, *and* for their extraordinary tolerance (and especially that of Joy Quek) as yet another submission deadline was missed.

Notes

1 To give a little more background, following soon after the September 11 attacks, there was understandable alarm that this might be a precursor to full-scale biological warfare. Consequently, the government decided to stockpile vast quantities of Bayer's ciprofloxacin (Cipro). The aim was to ensure that up to 10 million people could receive immediate treatment should the need arise.

2 Quoted in Werth (1994), 131.

3 Opioids are substances that react with the brain's opioid receptors, hence the name. They include opiates which are natural or semisynthetic derivatives from the opium poppy plant.

4 Strachan (2019).

5 One hopes there has at least been some improvement in medical facilities and treatment in the ensuing 30 years but given the Darfuri people's tribulations of recent decades that is probably too much to expect.

6   Figures from https://data.oecd.org/healthres/health-spending.htm#indicator-chart, visited 22 Apr. 2020.

7   DeGrandpre (2006); Healy (2012); Shorter (2009).

8   Ibid.

9   Altink (2015), 3.

10   Gabriel (2014).

11   Greene (2014). I should also add to these books the outstanding publications authored by Nicolas Rasmussen that you will find in the bibliography.

12   Weller (1977).

13   http://www.britannica.com/EBchecked/topic/124291/coevolution, visited 8 March 2015.

14   Institutions are not organisations but are what North refers to as 'the humanly devised constraints that structure political, economic and social interaction'. These 'consist of both informal constraints (sanctions, taboos, customs, traditions, and codes of conduct), and formal rules (constitutions, laws, property rights)'. North (1991), 97.

15   Timmermann (2014).

16   Mazzucato (2018), 70.

17   Schuhmacher *et al* (2013).

18   Fishburn (2013).

19   Hüntelmann (2013).

20   Cooper (1969), 51.

21   Pechlaner (2012).

22   Personally, I am not convinced due in part to the fuzziness of the gene concept and the possibility of other levels of life where selection also drives evolution. But I shall put my reservations aside for the sake of argument. As for whether genes are selfish at all, Dawkins is of course being metaphorical. Genes have no consciousness.

23   Deshaies (2020), 329.

24   *Ibid.*

25   According to legal scholar Shubha Ghosh, who has observed this phenomenon, 'the synthesis of biology and data analytics … is one possible future for genomic-based medicine. One example of this convergence is the $1.9 billion acquisition in February 2018, by Roche Holding of Flatiron Health, a New York-based company that has developed software to collect and aggregate data from cancer patients'. Ghosh (2020), 4.

26   Seigel (2005), 35.

Part 1

The Nature of the Pharmaceutical Industry

Chapter 2

What is the Pharmaceutical Industry?

'There is nothing which is not a poison. The right dose differentiates a poison and a remedy'

The Housekeeper's Guide; Or, Every Man His Own Doctor was published in Leeds in 1835. It contained 'many valuable Receipes and Prescriptions … for the cure of the human body'.[1] As if it posed a genuine threat to the average housekeeper, several among these were treatments for venereal disease.[2] One which particularly stands out was quicksilver dissolved in hydrochloric acid. As a book aimed at the non-medically trained public this highly toxic treatment must have been quite easy to acquire from the local chemist.

Startling as such a remedy may be to us, mercury had been in wide medical use for a long time. Somewhat earlier an English doctor, Thomas Dover (1660–1742), appropriately nicknamed 'Quicksilver', did much to promote its wider application including for such ailments as hysteria, asthma and 'the pox'.[3] Its known toxicity was no barrier to its availability and medical use for syphilis sufferers well into the twentieth century until it was replaced by Salvarsan (just as mercury years earlier had replaced guaiacum), followed by the antibiotics. It continues of course to be used in dentistry; this author's mouth contains quite a lot of it. A mercury-containing compound, thiomersal, is used today as a preservative in some vaccines and certain other health products.

If one were to define a pharmaceutical as a substance that in the right dosage is supposed to provide therapeutic effects whilst keeping harmful ones to a minimum, the use of mercury is not quite so incongruous. It is of course true that a lot of diseases are now treatable that historically were death sentences. But in a world in which many drugs are not available over the counter but require a prescription, and fatal adverse drug reactions (FADRs) cause many deaths,[4] any notion that modern medicines are toxicity-free, or that they would work just as well if they were, is profoundly wrong. This has been known for a long time. Philippus von Hohenheim, better known as Paracelsus (1493–1541), an advocate of both plants and minerals as drugs, and a revolutionary who publicly burned the classic works of Galen and Avicenna (Ibn Sina), famously wrote that 'all substances are poisons: there is nothing which is not a poison. The right dose differentiates a poison and a remedy.'[5] Similarly, according to famed experimental physiologist Claude Bernard three centuries on: '*Tous les médicaments sont, en définitive, des poisons*'.[6] Indeed, in the early days of scientific medicine, much was learned from the study of poisons and their interaction with body tissue, a preoccupation especially for those working in forensics, but that was still highly relevant to medicine.[7] François Magendie and Claude Bernard were among those doing such research, on arrow poisons for instance. (See Chapter 4 for more on Magendie and Bernard). Doubtless the potent toxicity of many medicines unnerves many people, and this is entirely understandable. Chemotherapy can be an utterly miserable experience. But whether opting for 'natural' remedies and the extreme minimalism of homeopathy is a good idea is another matter which this book does not attempt to prove one way or the other.

Nowadays we talk about the 'therapeutic window' and the importance of establishing dosage regimens that keep levels of the drug consumed inside that window, where the patient gets enough of the drug to benefit but within acceptable toxicity limits. A major part of the problem is that many drugs were, and continue to be, rather blunt instruments whose selectivity of action is lacking and whose effects vary among different people, sometimes quite substantially. Anti-cancer drugs are a case in point. Although targeted therapies are becoming more available, the traditional chemotherapies attack all actively dividing cells. This would be fine if cancer cells were the only ones quickly and continuously dividing, but some normal cell types do as well. Damage to those causes unpleasant side-effects.[8] Currently, much effort is being made to optimise dosage regimens for individual patients as 'just right' can vary between individuals for reasons requiring further research to uncover. The rapidly increasing amounts of genomic and other molecular data on human genetic variability being gathered and analysed promise to help here.

Unintended deaths by treatment are of course tragic and shocking. But if all medicines with toxicity were banned one wonders if any would be left. Arguably pure water is nearest to an entirely non-toxic substance that we ever actually consume, though water intoxication (or water poisoning) is a potentially fatal albeit rare medical condition.[9] It is vital to life and well-being but, like the air we breathe, it cures you of nothing but the physical effects of its own absence. The stringent regulatory oversight that medicines are subjected to is recognition of this. Pharmaceutical scientists are well aware that potent toxins and metals can have genuine therapeutic applications, as are the regulators who approve their use, and those doing cancer research know this better than most: mustard gas,[10] platinum,[11] silver[12] and lithium[13] are examples likely to surprise many readers. It is intriguing to consider that mercury has been used in other medical systems, including in China, India and Tibet, often in the form of mercury sulphide. It has been used to treat venerable disease in Tibet from at least as far back as the eighteenth century.[14] In Tibetan medicine, mercury is known to be toxic but can supposedly be rendered therapeutically harmless through certain processing methods.[15] Practitioners of rasashastra, a branch of Ayurveda, also use processed mercury.[16] The substance is mentioned in at least one ancient Chinese pharmacopoeia.[17] The famous Persian physicians Rhazes and Avicenna had a great interest in the medical uses of mercury. It is possible they were influenced by India but Aristotle's theory of the elements may have guided them to mercury too. This is very plausible; after all, the history of ancient medicine, as of contemporary traditional medicine, is very much an entangled one. As practical testers of their own ideas, they both appear to have been sufficiently aware of its toxicity to advocate its use only externally in the form of ointment.[18] Paracelsus, who like others had a deep interest in alchemy also advocated use of mercury which was essential to a medical theory he devised that rejected Galen wholesale while adopting an alchemical version of Aristotelian elements theory.[19] Who used it first for syphilis and where is something we may never find out. Besides, what is a poison and what is a treatment is also a matter of context. Mustard gas, curare and warfarin had lethal effects on First World War infantrymen, rainforest monkeys and rats but they turned out to be lifesavers for cancer victims, patients in surgery and those with thrombosis. Note that the mechanisms by which they kill are identical to the ones that cure.

In 1909, a chemical initially named compound 606 was synthesised and patented by the great German scientist, Paul Ehrlich, (who we will hear more about in the chapter after next) and then found by his Japanese assistant Sahachiro Hata to work against the parasite causing syphilis. Identified as arsphenamine and marketed by Hoechst under the trade name Salvarsan, it was the first effective treatment for syphilis. As such it was one of the original pharmaceutical products of the kind being sold today. The shift from mercury to Salvarsan marks a transformation over the intervening period from the plying of often useless, and sometimes lethal, drugs made by pharmacists to modern pharmaceuticals most of which actually do work, despite themselves being toxic. As the prefix of its chemical name suggests, Salvarsan is arsenic based.

Warfarin is an instructive and entertaining illustration of how the difference between a drug and a poison is often not so different from the one between a flower and a weed. It largely depends on whether it's in the right or wrong place, and whether there's the right amount or too much. Warfarin shows also how observations of natural phenomena apparently unrelated to human health — in fact to livestock *ill*-health — may eventually lead to an important new pharmaceutical product. As it happens, the product in question *did* originate in a weed!

Warfarin: A livestock disease agent, rat poison, and a medicine

Warfarin is a university invention named after the Wisconsin Alumni Research Foundation (commonly abbreviated as WARF), which owned the patents and licensed them to industry. The pathway to warfarin's discovery began with investigations undertaken to find out why cattle in North Dakota, USA, and Alberta, Canada, in the 1920s were suffering severe internal haemorrhages from diminished ability of the blood to clot. This was linked to their consumption of stored sweet clover hay. While often fatal, the hay did not cause permanent bodily harm in that full recovery from 'sweet clover disease' was often attained when the afflicted livestock were

(Continued)

given blood transfusions and simply not fed the spoiled clover. By 1931, it was known that the loss of coagubility was linked to a reduced activity or presence of prothrombin, one of the substances involved in blood clotting.

Karl Paul Link, a biochemist at University of Wisconsin, started work on this topic in 1933. One afternoon in February of that year he was visited by a Wisconsin farmer called Ed Carlson, who had travelled for 190 miles through a blizzard, according to Link's own account, with 'a dead heifer, a milk can containing blood completely destitute of clotting capacity, and about 100 pounds of spoiled sweet clover — the only hay he had to feed his cattle.'[20] Extracting and purifying the haemorrhagic agent was a six-year effort involving Link and several of his colleagues and PhD students including Harold Campbell, Charles Huebner and Mark Stahmann. 'Finally in the dimness of dawn on June 28, 1939, after working all night, Campbell saw on a microscope slide what turned out to be crystalline Dicumarol. Two hours later he had collected about 6.0 mg. of it'.[21] This achievement was followed by the isolation of 1,800 mg. by Stahmann with Miyoshi Ikawa, after which Huebner determined the substance's chemical structure as 3,3′-methylene-bis (4-hydroxy-coumarin). In April 1940, Huebner synthesised it.

The substance was marketed for human therapeutic use under the name Dicumarol, but it was considered rather unsafe. This was largely due to initial unwillingness to accept the finding of Link's team that vitamin K, which in the human body is involved in prothrombin manufacture and is chemically related to Dicumarol,[22] is an effective antidote in cases of excessive bleeding by patients taking the drug. By 1942, Link's team had synthesised over 100 related chemicals, and these were waiting to be tested. While recuperating from illness in late 1945 and early 1946, Link did some reading on rodent control. In his entertaining account, Link prepares us for what came next:

Now brace yourselves, for I propose to shift from a 'cow poison' that had become a drug of substantial clinical usefulness, to a 'rat poison' converted to a drug, which has I believe most of the desirable features that can be expected from an anticoagulant to be given primarily via the oral route.[23]

Two convenient-to-make derivatives showed powerful and uniform activity in rats and dogs. One of these, numbered 42, came on the market in 1948 as a rat-killer, and turned out to be a hugely successful product. It was named warfarin by Link after the Wisconsin Alumni Research Foundation with the added 'arin' from coumarin, the natural product from which it was derived.

(Continued)

(*Continued*)

There the story might have ended. Link believed that warfarin should be tried out on humans, but clinicians were understandably sceptical that a powerful rat poison could be either safe or effective as a treatment for humans. Link may never have got the chance to test out his theory if it had not been for his learning in April 1951 of an army conscript who had attempted suicide with warfarin. Link describes what happened:

The inductee had followed the multiple dose directions on the package. It became clear to him that warfarin was not an efficient agent 'to shuffle off this 'mortal coil.' It allowed too much time for thinking — so he went to the hospital with a fully developed case of hemorrhagic 'sweet clover disease.' He was treated per the directions — blood transfusion and large doses of Vitamin K — and made an uneventful recovery.[24]

The outcome was a potent, fast acting and easy to deliver anticoagulant product, warfarin sodium, marketed as Coumadin, which achieved celebrity status after it was given to a sick President Eisenhower in 1955. It is still commonly used today. Such are the long and winding roads that drug discovery processes sometimes follow. While several people were involved in different parts of the story, Karl Link was by far the most important actor, seeing the discovery process to its conclusion from a cow disease to a rat poison, and finally to an important pharmaceutical product.[25]

In some ways, things have changed less than we think. For one thing, not all those early remedies were useless or else lethal; nor are today's all useful and safe, apparently. Charlatanry and the ignorance and gullibility they profit from were still common in the 1830s, as they seem to be today,[26] but reasoned voices attacking quacks and crooked apothecaries for their bogus and dangerous remedies, including mercury, long existed too. For another, just glance through a magazine, look at today's newspaper front pages, surf the web, or take a walk through your local high street. Has there ever been a time when so much money was made from treatments for perfectly healthy people as today, many of which are no more efficacious than mercury albeit probably less harmful? It seems unlikely. Most weeks a cure for cancer, Alzheimer's or whatever disease the readership is thought that week to be worrying most about is announced on the front pages of a tabloid newspaper due to something or other shown by a recent laboratory study. If you feel as fit as a fiddle but are anxious about your health or that of your equally well children, the chances are that someone somewhere is making money out of you. And that anxiety is strongly encouraged. So we have still not wised up entirely to charlatanry, trendiness and other forms of manipulation or self-deception, or to the skilful marketing of bogus health fixes, sometimes by celebrities, that really do us little good and may even cause harm.

Nowadays, the direct to public marketing of drugs *as well as of medical conditions themselves*, and even the promotion of anxiety about health, has helped lead to a situation whereby lots of medicines are being taken by people who simply do not need them or else could derive the same benefits through modest changes to lifestyle. This is largely a consequence of two phenomena that you might argue are social in nature but have massive regulatory and commercial repercussions given the health implications and the vast amounts of money potentially to be made. The first is 'medicalisation', whereby the most minor deviations from some ideal standard of health that are hard for many people to attain at any stage of their lives — but who could still end up having perfectly normal lifespans with few substantial health problems along the way — require medical intervention. This is all part of a general tendency, which marketeers and advertisers of a whole range of products and services know is highly effective, to make people feel unduly anxious about their health, as if unwellness is a normal human condition that requires some kind of intervention needing to be purchased. One aspect of this trend is to create an impression that we suffer from medical conditions that require pharmaceutical (or other) responses.

This leads to the second, 'pharmaceuticalisation', by which that response takes the form of a drug, perhaps one to be taken for an indefinite period. Even 'normally' healthy people must contend with risk factors whose mitigation may require some intervention that is intrusive to them but delivers value to industry.[27] Thus in a sense we are, supposedly, all inherently ill however fine we actually feel. Being ill, or at least at serious risk of getting ill, is not just normal but universal: to be human *is* to be ill.[28] In principle mitigating risk of harm is a good thing. But there is so much money to be made from hypochondria and fuelling it through marketing and by other means. Diet, lifestyle, environment and genetics are all relevant, but what is easier: changing your food choices, going jogging, learning to meditate, moving home from the polluted city to the country-side, or taking a pill once or twice a day? The question answers itself.

Although the pharmaceutical industry is far from being the only guilty partner, disease-mongering, or 'the selling of sickness that widens the boundaries of illness and grows the markets for those who sell and deliver treatments',[29] is certainly good for business. Ritalin is an excellent example, as are Viagra and generic sildenafil, as we will see later.

Pharmaceuticalisation has not been left unchallenged. Limited health-care funds encourage a reduction in prescribing 'unnecessary' drugs. Preventive measures are frequently promoted, and the need for non-drug-related interventions is well undersood by public health professionals around the world including those who have worked very hard, and success-fully, to bring down malaria infection rates. Research has shown that most of the recent reduction in Africa is attributable not to the drugs but to insecticide-treated mosquito nets.[30] Nonetheless, regulatory systems tend not to be well equipped to challenge pharmaceuticalisation especially the United States due to direct to consumer marketing and the lack of pressure to limit spending on pharmaceutical products. None of this should be taken to treat pharmaceuticalisation as an entirely negative phenomenon, of benefit exclusively to industry: there are probably instances where a pill really could be the most convenient and effective response to well-being issues currently un- or under-pharmaceuticalised.[31]

Ritalin: A case of pharmaceuticalisation?

Ritalin (methylphenidate) is routinely given to children in the United States with the willing consent of parents. Specifically, it is prescribed for children afflicted with so-called Attention Deficit Hyperactivity Disorder (ADHD). Like many mental health afflictions ADHD was not known to exist till comparatively recently, at least insofar as it had not been named as such. As the philosopher of science John Dupré puts it with incisiveness, and (probably justified) sarcasm:

I do not find it surprising that many children now, and in the past, have had difficulty paying attention in schools. What I worry about is the basis for the con-clusion that there is something disordered in the heads of these children which is appropriately treated with psychotropic and addictive drugs. Schools are, after all,

(*Continued*)

often boring… The fact that powerful drugs can alleviate the manifestations of the syndrome shows very little. One can easily imagine, for instance, that threats of violence would concentrate the minds of recalcitrant students. But this hardly shows that they are suffering from corporal punishment deficiency syndrome.[32]

Handing out Ritalin to children is so commonly done despite one authoritative scientific study published in 1995 having this to say: 'Cocaine, which is one of the most reinforcing and addictive of the abused drugs, has pharmacological actions that are very similar to those of methylphenidate, which is the most commonly prescribed psychotropic medication for children in the United States.'[33] Given that Ritalin is also used for purely recreational purposes, it is far from clear why cocaine is banned from sale and unavailable to patients whereas Ritalin is deemed to be so widely acceptable for both adults and children. Admittedly it is probably less addictive given it takes longer than cocaine to clear from the brain, and there are those who genuinely find it helpful. But one must remember that these brains tend to be those of children.

Finally, it is only fair to mention that the pharmaceutical industry is not the only beneficiary of pharmaceuticalisation, at least in those countries where this is no public health service employing physicians. In the US context, 'it's not only pharmaceutical corporations that benefit materially from disease legitimization. Any disease, if recognized and validated by both the medical community and third-party players, ensures physicians an enormous number of billable hours. And while the legitimization of the disease ensures the billable hours, the mechanism of legitimization determines who gets those hours.'[34]

Viagra: Branding a product *and* a disease

Viagra's 1998 entry into the market was accompanied by media attention on a scale barely precedented for any medicine let alone one that doesn't actually save lives. Viagra swiftly became a global social phenomenon, turning a highly embarrassing and upsetting personal condition rarely talked about into a recognised medical problem susceptible to a pharmaceutical solution, one that people could hardly stop talking about. In doing so Viagra helped extend the boundaries of medicalization.

What was Viagra for? Aphrodisiacs are not medicines. Consequently, Erectile Dysfunction (ED) had to be 'invented' and mainstreamed medically

(*Continued*)

(*Continued*)

in order for sildenafil to become the prescription medicine Viagra rather than a recreational drug like ecstasy. It is worthy of note here that the ED concept is both mechanical and reductionist. It really gets to the point, that it's the penis that needs fixing. In contrast, women have the rather blander and less specific Female Sexual Dysfunction (or female sexual arousal dysfunction under the WHO-ICD) which singles out no specific organ or body part. Pfizer did not invent ED as such, but it invested huge sums in promoting the medicalisation of the condition, one previously thought either to be too trivial or inherently personal to 'deserve' its own drug. This of course suited many men who could point to their 'condition' as a medical problem that they should not be blamed for. Keeping control over use of 'Viagra' in the marketplace helped prevent it becoming a genericised synonym of 'aphrodisiac', something that was assisted by Pfizer's own educational programme to enhance public awareness of ED as a condition.

Now that the product is available over the counter in many countries and generic sildenafil can be purchased, how do rival companies market their version? Apparently, they also do it by selling the disease just as Pfizer has been doing all along. Some months before this book was finished, this author, travelling by taxi through central London spotted a red double decker bus emblazoned with an ad showing the head of a hirsute young gentleman apparently in an awestruck state next to the phrases 'MORE MORE PHWOAR' and below it in smaller type 'Erectile dysfunction has a simple solution'. To the right of this rather cheery visage apparently in the act of uttering that very expression is the word 'Manual' and a website URL (manual.co/ED) whose front page begins with the slogan 'Hard Should Be Easy', and makes reference to 'a little blue helper'. In similarly jocular fashion, an image of the plain brown packaging used to mail the product shows it decorated — on the inside — with the phrase 'You've got male'. Splashed over the front of the inner container is a design mostly comprising the word 'Yes' three times, once spelt 'Yessss' — an allusion to Sally's notorious fake orgasm in the *When Harry Met Sally* movie. The owner of the site which is authorised by the British Medicines and Healthcare products Regulatory Agency is Menwell Ltd. Subject to an online medical consultation, the website provides for "free and discrete shipping" of generic sildenafil. What is perhaps most striking about the website is less the very corny humour, presumably intended to mitigate the psychological discomfort men might feel about buying the product, but that it continues to sell the drug by selling the 'disease'.

Of course, it would be silly to deny that tremendous progress has been made, much of the groundwork for future progress being laid between when *The Housekeeper's Guide* was published and what people my grandparents' age called The Great War. The pharmaceutical science that emerged in the nineteenth century saw the start of a replacement of knowledge about *materia medica,* a term commonly used in the Roman Empire that lasted till very recently,[35] by what became known as pharmacology.[36] Physiology, immunology, bacteriology and synthetic chemistry became scientific and professional disciplines. In terms of medicines five innovations came to the fore. First, the identification and isolation of single plant-based active ingredients, such as alkaloids, often of exotic origin, and their preparation in purified form.[37] Second, the discovery of infectious disease agents, and the production of vaccines and antitoxins to prevent infection by them and in some cases cure them.[38] Third, the formulation of theories that, when combined with the experimental sciences, provided direction, reason and insight making practical therapeutic discovery more likely to happen. Fourth, the laboratory synthesis of therapeutic chemicals, including copies of ones known to exist in nature, and those that were novel. Fifth, the modification and optimisation of these molecules and their industrial mass production in standardised tablet and other forms for delivery to patients. The pharmaceutical industry had little to do with the first three of these.

Admittedly, building on these early advances to achieve anything like the vast array of treatments available today took several more decades. Only rarely is translating the findings and theories of pioneering scientists an overnight process, and late nineteenth century medical science, or perhaps more correctly 'the medical sciences', typified such lengthy time-lags. Indeed, two leading science historians, Viviane Quirke and Jean-Paul Gaudillière, have claimed that 'biomedicine was only truly "invented" after the Second World War'.[39] This seems rather late (see below), but even by a less strict definition biomedicine did not emerge hand in hand with the modern pharmaceutical industry but came in some time, and possibly by several decades, later.

A Tale of Progress?

Triumphantly charting medical advances over the years is not the main purpose of the book, though, important to my narrative (and of course to the lives of real people) as they are. Nor is pouring cold water on these advances or treating the industry as an enemy of progress. The book *is* about pharmaceuticals, but it primarily investigates — contextually and critically — the evolution and growth of the pharmaceutical *industry* from its origins in pharmacy shops, branded medicine and food extracts retailers,[40] chemical wholesalers, some of which were already quite old, and the German synthetic dyestuff-making firms, to today's global behemoths many of which have lineages going directly back to those very same shops and manufacturers. Old firms like Bayer, Merck and Pfizer remain world leading. Whether we wish to praise or bury the industry it is important that we understand this historical evolution.

We will see how progress in understanding the human body, disease agents and chemistry was harnessed in the service of an emergent industrial sector which did have a prior existence but in nothing like the form which began to take shape, largely in 1880s Germany when firms expanded from dyes to drugs. From there I trace the industry's evolution up to the present day highlighting the co-evolution of science, business growth, organisation and strategy, law, and regulation. As in its beginnings, this industry continues to be characterised not just by what it produces and sells but also by *how* it develops its products *and* how it uses intellectual property rights to market them and gain economic power within the constraints and opportunities of pharmaceutical regulation. This book, then, tells the story of an industry that emerged in the late nineteenth century to become one of the most important and profitable commercial sectors in the modern economy.

What unites the early industry and the one of today, and separates both from the time before, apart from the fact that some of the original firms still exist today, is that pharmaceutical products over the 140 or so years of the industry's existence have typically been pure single molecules, usually small in terms of molecular weight, that react with the human body to cause a therapeutic effect. Typically, a medicine works by binding to a protein such as an enzyme or receptor and inducing, modifying or disrupting chemical activity in human or foreign cells (in the case of infectious diseases).[41] It may produce harmful side-effects unexpected even after years of testing. On the other hand, there may be positive side-effects leading to the use of the active ingredient for other health problems. Nowadays, some pharmaceuticals are themselves proteins (e.g. insulin, monoclonal antibodies, etc.). Historically speaking, which type of protein was bound to and why a therapeutic effect ensued was generally unknown, as were the reasons why some people suffered from side-effects while others were unaffected. Aspirin typifies this. It was only in the 1970s that people learned how it works, more than seven decades after it came onto the market. Even today, there is often much that is unknown about how specific pharmaceuticals interact with the body and what the basis for the therapeutic effect actually is. That said, scientifically today's massively expanded diversity of cellular drug targets and the addition of protein drugs ('biopharmaceuticals' or 'biologics') produced through genetic technologies[42] would have astounded our scientific forebears of three to four generations back. But generally speaking, the above innovations still form the basis for much of what is done today: biologics form a growing share of the market but new pharmaceutical products continue largely to be synthetic chemicals, which are either completely *de novo* or are modelled on ones made earlier or on those found in plants and plant products among other natural sources. Some pharmaceuticals are still extracted directly from plants, some of which — but by no means all — were previously used medicinally.

Biomedicine, Tradition, and Colonialism

The pharmaceutical industry discovers or copies, develops, makes and sells pharmaceutical products, primarily drugs and vaccines. But what is a pharmaceutical? In the modern era, it can best be defined thus:

> A pharmaceutical is a manufacture comprising a defined chemical agent that is administered to a human for an intended therapeutic or other physiological response but is not a food or a cosmetic.[43]

Whether we know how pharmaceuticals work, we do at least know what they are and what they are for. The traditional medicinal antecedents of these products, to the extent that such antecedents exist, are completely different. As we will see below, the same goes for the traditional and other medicines and medical treatments used today.

The 'not food' part of the definition might read oddly, though. Drugs and foods used to overlap considerably. In the modern age, foods and beverages were often marketed with health claims. For example, coca cola was once advertised as a temperance drink containing 'valuable tonic and nerve stimulant properties', serving as a brain tonic and 'cure for all nervous affections' including headache, neuralgia, hysteria and melancholy. I remember from childhood the advertising slogan for Guiness: 'Looks good, tastes good. And by golly it does you good'. And with functional foods and food supplement products[44] such as vitamins, they still overlap to a degree. Grey areas cannot be swept away so easily. Indeed, the UK Medical and Healthcare products Regulatory Agency (MHRA) acknowledges so-called 'borderline products', including food supplements, biocides, cosmetic products and medical devices, where it is not a simple matter to distinguish what side of the medicinal product/ non-medicine divide that certain health-related goods should be placed. But there is a world of a difference between captopril and capsicum. In no sense is the former a food even though it is swallowed.

Before going further, note that I avoided the word 'disease' in the definition. Indeed, this is as good a time as any to clarify the differences between a disease, a disorder, a condition, and a syndrome. Definitions abound, universal ones not so much, and there is a certain amount of overlap between them. But here goes. A disease is a type of illness leading to a negative health outcome such as pain, physiological dysfunction, structural damage to the body or death, or all or some of these, and having certain shared characteristics aiding the isolation of the disease as a named phenomenon. It is caused by external factors such as an infective agent, or internal ones such as abnormal cell reproduction leading to cancer, the immune system engaging in friendly fire (auto-immune diseases), or impaired insulin production resulting in diabetes. A disorder is a harmful disruption to normal functioning caused by a disease. A syndrome is a disease or a disorder that has one or more specific symptoms. A condition is not caused by a disease. It can be the same as a syndrome or a disorder, but it does not necessarily make one ill. Arguably, it can include pregnancy, a state which may be very much desired by the person experiencing it, but which tends to require medical intervention to ensure it proceeds as it should.

Before the nineteenth century much if not most of the healthcare available in the world was *traditional*, at least insofar as it had nothing to do with the practices and procedures nowadays we call biomedicine, defined in a prominent US medical dictionary in 1922, when it was quite a new word, as 'clinical medicine based on the principles of physiology and biochemistry'[45] of which the use of pure chemical substances as drugs is an integral component. The innovations there were tended to be branded medicines whose ingredients were kept secret rather than disclosed on the labels or in patent documents (despite being referred to as 'patent medicines'). They have tended to be dismissed as quack medicines which may largely be right; but they were certainly popular, and one presumes there must have been lots of repeat customers.[46]

The humoral system of Hippocrates and Galen formed the theoretical underpinning for most medical interventions. Much of the rest of the world, including China, and the Middle East and India where there were well-documented exchanges of ideas and materials between people there and the Greeks, had humoral systems as well, as they still do.[47] It has to be said that much of European medicine up to this time seems to have been worthless if not positively dangerous. Physicians were educated academically but with no clinical training. Nosologies (disease classificatory systems) such as they were offered little useful guidance. As explained by one eminent historian, 'diagnosis consisted in establishing which of these humours was out of line, and therapy in taking steps to restore the balance, either by blood-letting (by venesection, scarification or applying leeches) or by subjecting the patient to a course of purges and emetics' followed by 'the prescription of plasters, ointments or potions'.[48] For many afflictions, surgeons, doctors, apothecaries and hospitals were people and places to be avoided at all costs. The best known English physician of the seventeenth century, Thomas Sydenham 'thought that it would have been better for many patients if the art of physic had never been invented, remarking that many poor people owed their lives to their inability to afford conventional treatment'.[49] The same is likely to have been true for many other parts of the world.

This bleak view notwithstanding, we should not be entirely negative about the state of learning. From the Renaissance onwards, there was a return to the wisdom of the Ancients. But that was not all. In time, people realised the Ancients did not know all that was knowable. If the Ancients did not know America existed, or had not invented the printing press, gunpowder and the compass, as Francis Bacon pointed out in 1620 (and which all came from China), what else did they not know or get right? It followed that people of the day had much to contribute to an ever-increasing fount of human wisdom. Much was discovered about human anatomy that was definitely unknown in past times. (Eventually this led to the idea of progress, but that's another story.) Andreas Vesalius (1514–1564), a huge admirer of Arab medicine,[50] was especially prominent in this respect. Schools of medicine were established from the Middle Ages onwards, for example the University of Padua where Vesalius studied and taught, and William Harvey also studied. Great artists like Da Vinci who were eager to perfect their depictions of the human form took great interest in the features and functions of the human body and its parts. His anatomical drawings, despite errors were generally very accurate. Medical thinking was hardly static. One of Sydenham's own innovations was to see diseases as 'real entities rather than imbalances of an individual's humours'.[51] This helped to advance the art of disease classification. In time, what we now call the early modern era emerged.

Traditional medicine of the past surely had efficacies not solely attributable to placebo effects.[52] It seems a little unfair to single out for criticism 'traditional' or premodern medicine of the time, of Europe or of any other part of the world, and its inability to cope with epidemics and other disease outbreaks if we fail also to note the questionable (to put it at its most mild) contribution of Europeans to global health in the early modern and Enlightenment eras. Diseases exported by Europeans to the Americas and the Pacific especially decimated local populations in staggeringly vast numbers, surely outweighing any positive impacts for a very long time indeed.

Traditional medicines are very much in use today and of course bear the effects of interactions, sometimes minimal other times much greater, with biomedicine. Typically, they consist of processed or unprocessed single or mixed natural products of plant, animal or mineral origin, administered orally or topically in solid or liquid form. Whole plants may be used, or else plant or animal parts or their products. Unlike pharmaceuticals they are not single chemicals obtained through industrial processes. The notion of the *active principle*, that is, the specific compound having the therapeutic effect, was, and remains, alien to traditional healers whose treatments are inherently *impure* allowing for the possibility of synergisms between the various ingredients and for customised treatments for individuals. Further, their usage was, and still is, justified on the basis of theories of health, sickness, well-being and efficacy, as well as cultural and spiritual values, which most modern medical practitioners and pharmaceutical scientists find impossible to accept.[53] They became subject to a very different regulatory system and, where available, tend to be sold over the counter by retailers.

To see how the modern emerged in part out of tradition, but also separately alongside it, we must turn to the nineteenth century, an era which saw massive advances in our knowledge about health, sickness, human anatomy and biology. Our Victorian-age forebears are owed our thanks also for safe and pain-free operations and for the knowledge that good hygiene, including underground sewage disposal systems and clean water, saves lives. From the 1880s scientists began to crack the problem of how to harness chemistry to other emerging scientific disciplines and practices to solve hitherto intractable health problems on a more regular and systematic basis.

Arguably, the theory and practice of biomedicine — I would suggest alongside industrial capitalism — made the emergence of the pharmaceutical industry almost inevitable. As physician and medical historian Jeremy Greene puts it:

> In contrast to the physiological approach of earlier Hippocratic models of disease — in which every sick person became sick and received treatment in a unique way — biomedical sciences of the late nineteenth and early twentieth century posited an ontological understanding of diseases as specific entities knowable outside of individual cases.[54]

Greene goes on to explain the universalistic aspects of this change in thinking which in turn implies market opportunities for firms able to exploit its scientific implications once chemistry, physiology and microscopy have become sufficiently advanced:

> If specific pathogens caused the same disease in different patients, it followed that specific treatments could cure those same diseases in different patients. Part of the power of biomedical categories … is their apparent universality: diseases and cures abstracted from local context and understood on a microscopic level, should in theory work everywhere, should in theory be the same everywhere.

However, things did not change overnight for the majority of doctors and patients: well into the twentieth century, the number of non-traditional drugs available for doctors to prescribe was still pretty limited.[55] In hindsight we should not be surprised by this gradualism or the inability to more abruptly shake off the legacy of the past. Indeed this legacy remains a presence albeit one largely hidden from view. However extreme the material, theoretical and epistemological differences might appear, there is no perfect traditional and modern divide marking out two quite separate worlds. And nor was there from the moment that Europeans began to ply the oceans in search of new lands, valued commodities and trading opportunities. One might assume that European colonials and traders, with their ever-growing superiority complex had nothing but disdain for local *materia medica*, but this was not necessarily the case. From the early modern era to the Enlightenment and beyond, Europeans collected, documented, traded across the world and imported into Europe medicinal plants from the East and the New World.[56]

Perhaps the earliest example of a detailed treatise on medicinal plants imported into Europe from the Western Hemisphere is Nicolás Monardes 'Historia medicinal de las cosas que se traen de nuestras Indias Occidentales' ('Medical study of the products imported from our West Indian possessions'), published in the 1570s and translated shortly after into several European languages. Monardes' work did much to popularise use of imported medicinal plants in Europe including tobacco, for which he was an enthusiastic advocate, sassafras and sarsaparilla. By that time, guaiacum had already come into wide use as a treatment for syphilis, though it is not clear that it was used medicinally before it was brought to Europe.

Use of guaiacum for syphilis was heavily promoted by the powerful German mercantile family the Fuggers who had an import monopoly on it.[57] Its efficacy was partially justified on the basis that its New World origin matched the disease it was held to cure. Interest in guaiacum did in fact diminish over time as the realisation struck that it did not actually work.[58] Syphilis did not come from America in any case.

The great international trading companies founded at the start of this age such as the Dutch East India Company were instrumental in these botanic transfers,[59] as was its British counterpart with its network of botanical stations with Kew Gardens at its apex.[60] Late eighteenth century introductions to the European pharmacopoeia coming from the New World included Jesuit's bark (quinine) and ipecacuanha.[61] American plants also reached Muslim regions and Portuguese possessions and trading posts in Asia, and in the other direction westwards to the Philippines. Apart from trading companies, merchants and Jesuits were also involved in moving these plants around the world. Other plants during the age of European exploration and colonisation came into Europe from Asia and Africa. These included foods as well as drugs. Spices from the East not only flavoured otherwise tasteless or disgusting food, but possessing humoral effects were included in the *materia medica*. This is why, surprisingly perhaps, '*the history of spices is in part the prehistory of the pharmaceutical industry.*'[62] Global bioprospecting efforts, often enabled by the scourge of slavery,[63] provided a large proportion of the drugs available to Europe in the later colonial era. Of the 175 plants in the 1885 British pharmacopoeia, 40 percent were of European origin, 25 percent each were from Asia and the Americas, 9 percent were African, and 1 percent was from Australia.[64] That the late nineteenth century establishing of ethnobotany as a respectable scientific pursuit coincided with the apogee of imperialism as well as of pseudo-scientific racism and social Darwinism is certainly intriguing suggesting that the widespread presumption of inherent European superiority to the natives was not without contradiction. There was much to be learned from people regarded as backward and primitive, whether or not it followed that they should therefore be treated humanely.

What was the attraction of these plants coming from distant lands? It is frequently claimed that their exotic origins and names, as well as the colourful stories concerning their sources, the local uses of them, and the means by which they were 'discovered' by Europeans gave them much of their appeal. According to one recent historical work, their uses by native populations was likely to have been a factor in their popularity during the late seventeenth century, though we cannot be sure how important this was. In some ways this sounds all rather modern:

> The epistemic or social value attached to 'indigenous knowledge' in the second half of the eighteenth century remains little understood, to be sure, but there is evidence to suggest that in this period the appeal of 'Indian cures' could be relied on to advertise, popularise and sell American remedies in Mexico City, Munich and Paris alike. The Enlightenment's demand that science be applied, economic and vernacular accorded novel significance to the knowledge not only of Europe's rustics, its peasants and artisans, but also to that of 'illiterate knowers' outside Europe — from Arctic shamans and Finnish rune-singers to American Indians. Physicians and sufferers alike placed their best hope for novel remedies in 'natural men' by the end of the eighteenth century, in those society-less, uncultured creatures closer to nature than those who claimed civilisation and, later, modernity for themselves. The unmediated experiences of the pristine and the primitive, their peculiar intimacy with the environment, rendered them keepers of absolute truths about both nature's toxins and cures.[65]

This sounds familiar because 'traditional knowledge' has attained a new respectability since the 1980s as if indigenous peoples know things that the rest of us have forgotten (or perhaps never knew in the first place). On the other hand, some of these remedies fitted neatly into existing *materia medica* and treatment practices because in certain senses they were *not* exotic. Their use may have been compatible with humoral approaches to sickness and health, or else they were related biologically to already known plants. In some cases, as trade expanded and populations moved on a greater scale, so did disease. A treatment used for a disease in one part of the world was perhaps presumed often to work for the same affliction in very distant places. What also has present-day echoes is the way that governments today, meeting in international forums,[66] increasingly argue that the pharmaceutical value of traditional knowledge, such as it is,[67] should be reflected in a fair exchange of benefits. And yet, beyond the rhetoric, objectively fair and workable schemes to ensure benefits flow back to the holders of the knowledge are still rare. Meanwhile, lip service tends to be paid to the same peoples' basic rights to land and to being treated humanely at both individual and collective levels.

In addition to material, recipes in the form of written texts also crossed seas and continents, and not in one direction only. From Europe to China and the Islamic world between them, medical recipes were of two kinds: formulas and prescriptions. How are these different? 'The formula contains the standard way of preparing a medication — that is, its recipe as laid down by an authoritative text. The prescription, in contrast, is a medication for an actual patient, usually contained within a practitioner's case records.'[68] From the seventeenth century, Jesuits translated medical texts from Chinese into Latin and French and vice versa. In 1693, quinine provided by Jesuits was used to treat the emperor of China.[69]

Medical historian Abena Osseo-Asare hints at an intriguing correlation between high colonialism and modern pharmaceutical development, one that is worth closer inspection: 'The rise of pharmaceutical chemistry in Europe at the end of the nineteenth century dovetailed with the wars of imperial expansion in Africa.'[70] The 1880s are the decade when British and French colonial land-grabbing had reached its highest point and new imperial nations like Germany and Belgium had just joined the global contest for territory, the United States following a decade later taking Cuba, Puerto Rico and the Philippines from the Spanish.[71] The Dutch and the Portuguese were hardy inactive either. The infamous Berlin Conference which carved up Africa for division among the European powers was concluded in 1885, truly a low point for European 'civilisation', the same decade as the dyestuff industry's pharmaceutical turn and the appearance of Antifebrin, Antipyrin, Pyramidon and Sulfonal. Admittedly none of these was for a tropical disease. Nonetheless, that the industry emerged simultaneously with the Europeans' scramble for Africa and domination of much of the world is certainly interesting. Did colonialism stimulate expansion of the industry at just the right time, or have some other significance that merits consideration? Or were there triggering events or phenomena that were common to both?

Running empires required plenty of manpower and, in a reverse direction to today's population movements, European moved in quite large numbers to the tropics, getting exposed to the same diseases as the native people. Economic and political interests are of course very important in determining where government support and private investment are directed in terms of pharmaceutical research and development. Colonialism certainly did affect which diseases should be studied, hence the interest in finding cures for tropical diseases and other ailments especially common in the colonies such as malaria, trypanosomiasis (sleeping sickness), yellow fever and plague. Numerous schools of tropical medicine were opened in Britain, Germany, other European colonial nations, and the United States.[72]

In today's world, where there is much concern about neglected tropical diseases, this might suggest that colonialism was good for global public health and a stimulus to industrial growth. But this would not be a defensible view. How could it be given the massive population collapses in the Americas and other parts of the world when the Europeans came? But one should not deny some positive consequences from the rise of the medical sciences and their diffusion around the world. This is not to say that they were anywhere near sufficient to outweigh the immense harms caused over the course of the era of European colonisations starting in 1492 and only quite recently ended. Nor did the European 'civilising mission' of which the spread of scientific medicine was one part have its own negative consequences in its far too wholesale disparagement of the indigenous cultures. As Roy Porter put it rather starkly, 'the good that western medicine did was marginal and incidental.'[73] Obviously that is far less true today. The global scourge of smallpox has been eradicated, to give one example, child mortality rates have fallen, and life expectancies have gotten longer albeit with persisting inequalities between and within different countries that may in some ways even be increasing. Some of this is surely attributable to biomedicine. However, the qualified success of the access to medicines movement of recent years testifies to 'marginal and incremental' remaining as a persisting feature of the good being done in some areas of public health. This is really not good enough.

That imperialism stimulated the growth of the industry, if not its initial emergence, is plausible. The colonies were sources of plants and ethnobotanical information, and markets for products. In addition, the colonies served effectively as scientific laboratories including for medical doctors.[74] Medical research facilities were also established in the colonies.[75] Disease-ridden areas ('White man's graves') like West and Central Africa needed to be made safer for Europeans. Soldiers and administrators of course went to the tropics in their thousands but so did scientists, including medical scientists like Robert Koch,[76] Ronald Ross, Patrick Manson, Walter Reed, and Pasteur's student Alexandre Yersin, discoverer of the bacillus causing bubonic plague.[77] Koch illustrates this turn from local to global health problems. He was among the first to offer actual preventative and curative treatments with such wide distribution, and the industry soon followed in his footsteps. Admittedly, the motive behind his travels was largely to work on problems affecting people in Europe. Paul Ehrlich was not so peripatetic, but he made contributions to tropical medicine, testing chemicals against trypanasomiasis (sleeping sickness), many supplied by Cassella and Company Dye Works; the type of medical science-industry collaboration for drug discovery that is now commonplace.[78] Treatments he sought to develop were not solely for national use but for international distribution. But imperialism, significant as it was in certain respects, seems not to have been a decisive and direct factor in the industry's emergence and probably played quite a small role in its growth. Tropical medicine was in fact largely a government and military preoccupation. It is important though to say that the period from the late nineteenth century to the First World War saw vast international movements of populations, including emigrants leaving Europe for the Americas, indentured labourers going from colony to colony, soldiers travelling *en masse* from one military engagement to another, and the colonial administrators and sundry hangers-on such as traders and missionaries, some of whom admittedly did dedicate themselves to providing healthcare to the native people. There were also wars and whenever there is a war there is a demand for medicines. After Waterloo, much of Europe enjoyed more than a half century of peace. Europeans certainly fought but it was mostly on other continents. Travel can be a killer — Rupert Brooke died before he could even get to a battlefield — but war and its aftermath is especially lethal. For obvious reasons the First World War stands out here. Where people went germs followed, where people were injured and died, germs proliferated, and then post-war things did not necessarily improve. Epidemics became global, perhaps the most devastating being the influenza pandemic that broke out in 1918. Health did become a shared global concern as it remains today. International sanitary and medical congresses started to take place from the 1850s and the International Red Cross was founded in 1863, also the same decade the first Geneva Convention was signed.[79]

What is true of the past is partly true also of the present. Even in recent years, plant and microbial chemicals remain the primary source of at least a quarter of new medicines being approved and even if these may never have been used medicinally (or as food flavourings), a substantial proportion certainly had. This is obviously a reduced share compared to the past, and it is probably going down. Nature may still be the best chemist, but screening natural products just to isolate, purify and test a single compound out of a potentially vast number in a given extract sample is a complex matter. Moreover, there are potentially serious supply difficulties with rare species or if access is restricted.[80] Unsurprisingly, many medicinal chemists much prefer to work with the synthetic chemicals in their compound libraries,[81] and also with less exotic substances such as those already inside the human body, seen as an increasingly vital source of valuable data and molecules such as antibodies. Despite all this, with greater opportunities now to overcome the technical barriers, there are renewed calls to return to our biodiverse world, including to rainforest and coral ecosystems, and some have answered.[82]

To name a few drugs in the modern pharmacopoeia sourced from traditional medicine, reserpine, the vinca alkaloids, and the opiates spring to mind. Recent additions include artemisinin, arsenic trioxide, and nicosan. Artemesinin's antimalarial activity was documented in fourth-century China. In the 1960s, Chinese scientists headed by You–You Tu of the Institute of Chinese Materia Medica conducted research into medicinal plants, and in 1972 found a substance they named qing-haosu in the leaves of the *Artemisia annua* (wormwood) plant.[83] Structurally modified qinghaosu, known internationally as artemesinin, used in combination with other products, is now the most effective anti-malarial available. The Nobel Prize she was awarded in 2015 is not only a tribute to her work but may be seen too as an affirmation by the scientific community's elite that some traditional medicine *does* have biomedical value. Arsenic trioxide, a treatment for leukaemia among a host of non-medical applications, and marketed under the name Trisenox, also comes from Chinese Traditional Medicine.[84]

Nicosan is a sickle-cell disorder treatment from Nigeria, the plant-based 'recipe' for which was disclosed by a Nigerian traditional healer, the Rev. P.R. Ogunyale, who is actually named as a co-inventor on the more than 40 patents on nicosan granted worldwide.[85] Nicosan was granted orphan drug investigational status in the United States and Europe, and has been approved in Nigeria, though currently it is not being produced. Pharmaceutical scientists *can* and *do* learn from shamans and healers even if not usually directly or even consciously. A recent historical work on plant-based medicine in colonial and post-colonial Africa convincingly asserts that 'herbal medicine and pharmaceutical chemistry have mutually supportive, simultaneous histories up to the present.'[86] Indeed, the author, the aforementioned Osseo-Asare, goes so far as to claim that biomedicine and African traditional healing 'were, in fact, actually adapted from one another.' This is highly debateable, but it is certainly more in step with the now accepted view in academia that the former imperial nations of Western Europe have been shaped far more by their encounters with the people, societies and the biodiversity of their former colonies than traditional histories that tended to be Eurocentric (or Anglocentric) and positivistic were able to admit to.[87] As the historian Richard Drayton puts it, 'what we may call the sciences of collection and comparison — among which we may include botany, zoology, and geology — depended on Europeans becoming exposed to the planet's physical and organic diversity, and often to the scientific traditions of non-European people.'[88] In turn, as he argues, 'the sciences shaped the pattern of imperial expansion'. A major consequence of this is that new economies came to arise 'on the basis of the discovery of the raw materials for food, medicines, dyes, and perfumes.'[89] There is no question that the emergence of fine industrial chemistry would come to play its part.

This encounter between European chemistry and non-European scientific traditions had long-term repercussions in various different ways right up to the present. Thus, both India and China, and probably other places too, are seeing two types of hybridisation: (a) *scientifically* in terms of describing, formulating, making, testing, evaluating, commercialising and regulating, in the ways that therapeutic claims are justified, and also of the growing centrality of 'the drug' in healthcare, and (b) *socially* in a growing turn to professionalisation.[90] This is not necessarily beneficial for poor people.[91] It has been claimed that in India at least, this development, which French historian of science Jean-Paul Gaudillière considers to be redolent of a similar process involving pharmacists that took place in Europe during the early decades of the twentieth century, continues to be plant centred rather than reliant on molecular chemistry. Accordingly, he denies that Ayurveda is becoming 'biomedicalised'.[92] Nonetheless, western biomedical practices seem increasingly to be impacting on *traditional* medicine as the latter's patient base expands globally. As the former aims to become more personalised (see Chapter 8), traditional medicines as they enter mainstream markets increasingly target generalised use. Thus, one must distinguish between traditional remedies and traditional knowledge-*derived* treatments, the latter being traditional-modern hybrids. For example, crofelemer (currently marketed as Mytesi) is a recent US Food and Drug Administration (FDA)-approved botanical medicine for non-infectious diarrhoea caused by certain anti-HIV drugs. Developed by Napo Pharmaceuticals, a US company named after a tributary of the Amazon, it is a laboratory produced, but not synthetic, substance containing active compounds isolated from the latex of the sangre de grado (*Croton lechleri*) tree used by indigenous peoples in South America as a treatment for various ailments including diarrhoea and has in fact been known to Europeans for centuries. Building upon the traditional knowledge to develop crofelemer required the contributions of formally trained scientists and the availability of well-equipped laboratory facilities.[93] Indeed, some modern pharmacologists have persuasively advocated the re-investigation of old herbal medicines no longer in use to reassess their efficacy as mixtures or to seek new therapeutically active single ingredients.[94] Some historical pharmacologists have begun to do so.[95] It remains to be seen whether they will come up with some treatments to benefit today's patients. The very existence of the discipline of ethnopharmacology[96] with its own journal, founded in 1979, underlines the argument being made here, that biomedicine and ethnobiology can and do interact — as they should.[97] Nowadays, there is a consensus that such cross-cultural exchanges should be subject to fair procedures of consent and benefit sharing, at least where ethnobiological knowledge and the plants used are current rather than merely historical.

Traditional knowledge has not gone away, but nor does it remain unchanged.[98] Indeed, the word 'tradition' is arguably misleading and problematic *especially* for medical systems that are founded upon official texts. Chinese medicine, for example, was not 'traditional' until it was named as such a few decades ago largely for political reasons. Traditional Chinese Medicine (TCM) co-evolved with western biomedicine accommodating such central elements as the germ theory of disease.[99] As for experiment and 'trying things out' in a systematic way these are not the sole preserve of the white-coated laboratory scientists; many traditional healers (and farmers) do it too. A much-cited figure from the World Health Organization is 80 percent for the proportion of the developing country population that relies on traditional medicine to meet its primary healthcare needs. What this implies for the quality of public health requires thorough debate. The fact remains that Chinese 'traditional' medicine is still highly popular as are the classical traditional Indian systems such as Ayurveda, Siddha and Unani Tibb, the latter being a hybrid 'system' with fundamental elements traceable to cultures west of India stretching as far as Greece. Indeed, 'Unani' is Arabic for Ionian.[100] These are well documented and the systems themselves are officially sanctioned and professionalised, with their own recognised training facilities and registered practitioners. However, despite their historical roots going back a very long time, they are not closed to outside influences, whether epistemologically or institutionally, including engagement with biomedicine. Patents are granted on inventions relating to them, which at least testifies to their capacity for innovativeness or at least for others to use them as a springboard for their own innovations.

Isolated indigenous peoples in places like the Amazon possess localised knowledge of flora and ecosystems enabling them to meet many of their healthcare concerns. Again, it is unlikely that all of the biota they exploit or the knowledge they apply are entirely local or have ever been. Although uncontacted groups still exist in the Amazon,[101] most human societies do not stay rooted to one spot over centuries *and* over a substantial period turn their backs on the world outside their own little part of it. One interesting aspect of traditional medicine is the way that often similar treatments for similar ailments are used by ethnic groups in distant regions of the world. Thus the apparent oddity of the rosy periwinkle being used as a treatment for diabetes in both the Philippines and in Jamaica.[102] Similarly, researchers have shown that species of the *Fabaceae* family of plants are used as antimalarials in the Upper Negro region of the Amazon, Ghana and in coastal Kenya.[103] Is there far less isolation and conservatism among 'traditional' groups than we tend to assume, and sharing of knowledge among disparate groups is more common than supposed? Or are these cases of different people facing similar health threats identifying similar treatments in the plant world quite independently of each other? If so, one could refer to this phenomenon as 'convergent therapeutics'. It would be interesting to know how common it might be.

By coining this phrase, I am suggesting an analogy with convergent evolution, whereby similar biological features evolve separately in species whose common lineages diverged millions of years before these features came into existence. This certainly does not explain all of evolution but there is no question that life on Earth in different places is capable quite independently of evolving the same advantageous traits. A good example is the camera eye possessed both by octopuses and vertebrates. Their relationship is far too distant for a common ancestor to have passed on the same similarly-designed organ to them both. So the camera eye must have evolved more than once quite separately. In the same way perhaps similar theories of sickness, health and well-being, as well as the modes of treatment deployed among geographically distant populations are arrived at independently. That is to say, not as a consequence of any past direct contact, or indirect contact through the circulation of goods, knowledge and information that inevitably take place when humans interact on a global scale but do not necessarily meet. Assuming this is a real phenomenon how much similarity can be explained in this way? Most of it, or just a small proportion? Of course we are now talking about cultural evolution rather than biological evolution which is why this is just an analogy. Having said this, humans are as much a part of nature as any other living organism and our interactions with the rest of nature shape us as we shape the living world around us. But further discussion of this specific matter falls out of the scope of this book. Anyway, whether similarities in plant uses for therapeutic purposes across vast geographical expanses can be explained by contact or by purely independent discovery, wide and sustained use of a particular treatment for the same illness does imply a strong possibility of some degree of efficacy — though we cannot simply assume this without close investigation.

What Do We Really Mean When We Talk of the Pharmaceutical Industry?

The answer is not in fact as obvious as one might suppose. Making and administering health products for material rewards is hardly recent. The ancients had their own purveyors of remedies. Archaeologists have found drugs in tablet form that had been made as early as the second century BC.[104] Most probably some of their concoctions worked, as do some of today's traditional medicines, however seemingly implausible the theory justifying them. This is not counterintuitive. As the great historian of ideas Arthur O. Lovejoy put it, 'as many historic examples show — the utility of a belief and its validity are independent variables; and erroneous hypotheses are often avenues to truth'.[105] But to say there was no pharmaceutical industry in 1850 but that there was one before that century's end, which is what I *am* saying, means we simply need an answer. Clearly *something* happened in that period.

Actually, several things had to happen for this industry to emerge. To suggest the industry broke with the past in being inherently *professionally*[106] science based may well form part of the answer but it raises difficulties, not least because the science was not at first being done in the corporate labs but in other institutions such as public and private experimental research facilities, universities and hospitals funded by the state, by public subscription or by wealthy philanthropists. Of course, much is still done in these places. One might concede that the German synthetic dyestuff firms were science based pretty much from the start and remained so as they turned to making drugs. Moreover, the new products may have been largely science based, in the sense that the latest scientific knowledge was an underlying factor enabling their discovery, description and application. But it does not follow that the businesses that made, patented and sold them were themselves science based to the extent of it being a defining feature.

The pharmaceutical industry *did* break with the past, and it did so in three ways. First, it took advantage of advances in chemistry, physiology, toxicology, cell biology and disease theory all of which improved tremendously during the nineteenth century thanks to individuals like François Magendie, Claude Bernard, Louis Pasteur, Robert Koch and Paul Ehrlich, among numerous other laboratory-based scientists working largely in France, Germany and Britain (see Chapter 4). Note that companies during these early stages played no more than minor supporting roles. Indeed, a major caveat is in order here: except for Germany where links between university scientists and industry were closest,[107] the emergent pharmaceutical industry took time to absorb fully the best human sciences coming out of university and hospital laboratories, which themselves did not get immediate results beyond the vaccines and antitoxins for common infectious diseases being quite rapidly developed in the late nineteenth century. The dominant firms certainly did depend on fine chemistry and good laboratory techniques, but the influence and, especially, the impact of the other sciences mostly came later. It might be that the industry came about when it did, not because of these obviously significant developments in chemistry and the human sciences but as a result of new opportunities to organise businesses on a bigger scale thanks to massive late nineteenth century improvements in transportation and communications including trains, steamships and the telephone as well as the replacement of steam power by electricity.[108] Indeed, the period from around 1870 to the First World War was one of tremendous innovation in a broad range of fields[109] whose global reach was possibly without precedent in human history, including perhaps the present age with all the current talk of third and — perhaps rather prematurely — of fourth industrial revolutions.[110] This new industry could be seen as being part of that innovation 'wave' but it is probably more accurate to say that the technological achievements of that period provided a springboard for the industry whose scientific character became more evident sometime after.

Second, there was a shift from science, including medical science, as being a rather individualistic, amateurish and curiosity driven pursuit, to a profession. Wealthy gentlemen-scientists like Charles Darwin were dying out. Salaried professional scientists working at science academies, universities and increasingly in companies played a major role not just in discovery but also in the sometimes quite routine laboratory work that commercially oriented chemistry required. This was part of a much wider transformation in industrial organisation heralded by the second industrial revolution, which was pioneered largely by Germany and the United States rather than by Britain and France, and which was characterised by three phenomena. One of these is the emergence of corporate in-house research and development. Another is the professionalisation of science manifested in the previously mentioned replacement of amateur scientists and individual inventors by well-trained academic and employee scientists, corporate research managers and business strategists, as drivers of innovation.[111,112] In chemistry this shift came fast in Germany. Indeed, it happened while the modern German state was coming into existence. The third is the industrial application of the scientific knowledge coming out of laboratories manned by this new scientific-worker class assisted by emerging capacities to mass-produce identical standardised high-quality products. This changed radically the context in which inventing was, and was said to be, done. It favoured more collective — and potentially anonymous — conceptions of the inventive act, and a diminished autonomy for inventors. This is something that affected patent law, and in Germany it did so almost immediately.

This leads to the third new development, one whose importance cannot be overstated: the availability of relatively secure and well-defined property rights: *intellectual* property rights, enabling their strategic acquisition and use. Patent law, trademark law, the administration of the legal rights provided under these laws, and the management of them by industry, were all taking their modern forms around the time the industry came into existence. Arguably, this development reflected and reinforced the above two developments.

Patents are legal rights over inventions deemed as such on account of the description in the application documentation fulfilling tests of novelty, inventive step or non-obviousness, and industrial application or utility. They are *novel* inventions in the sense that the object or process that is claimed was not known to exist previously. An invention may comprise anything from a new open-close device on a coffee lid[113] to a life-saving drug. Thus, the social and economic implications of a patent range from inconsequential or mildly convenient, to utterly transformative with the lives of millions at stake. Increasingly, patents were coming under the ownership not of the inventors but of the companies employing them and to whom they were assigned.[114] Accordingly, patents were ceasing to be personal property, at least in any general sense. Instead, they were changing into a class of business asset used by firms for two ends. The first of these was to actively and strategically control information and industrial processes and products embodying this information or made through these processes. The second was to negotiate access to the valuable information, processes and products of others through the licensing or purchase of patents (or the companies possessing them).

Notwithstanding its occasional appearance beforehand, the business practice of using patents and trademarks together to secure and perpetuate market power has been a key feature of the industry from the start, and its advantages are almost self-evident. Obviously, patents on money-spinning drugs are extremely valuable to a company, which can suffer severe profit losses when they expire. It is often said that patents are monopolies and that is why they are so valuable to their owners. They can indeed help secure considerable market power to owners, but it is not strictly true in the market sense. The scope of patents is limited to what they add to the state of our scientific and technical knowledge, they have exclusions and exceptions to rights, they are limited in duration, and they can be revoked — which was the fate of Bayer's British patent on the active ingredient of Aspirin.

Trademark law is what helps to make branding work for sellers, manufacturers and distributors. Let us consider branding now, and then we will look at trademarks and why they are so important to this industry. The meaning of 'brand' has evolved over the years from a mark (as well as the instrument used to make the mark) on a good conveying information as to ownership such as on a cow or sheep, or origin such as a company, craftsperson or a place, to the goods or services themselves. Indeed, the application of the word has expanded so that brand means not just the signs, but those things that are signified by them. Beyoncé is a brand, as is Apple Computers thanks to its 'cool' products, Real Madrid as Europe's most successful, and regal sounding, football club, and Switzerland as the home of fine watches, chocolate, private banking, spectacular mountain scenery, cows with bells round their necks, and its people's supposed devotion to efficiency and punctuality.

'Branding' is not a term of legal art. According to the *Oxford Advanced Learner's Dictionary*, it means 'the activity of giving a particular name and image to goods and services so that people will be attracted to them and want to buy them'. For businesses, branding can be an effective marketing approach to product differentiation in markets containing goods that are identical, similar, or are otherwise readily substitutable. As such, branding to differentiate products to attract buyers to one's own can have the biggest market impacts not by communicating an objective truth that the branded product is better in quality than its rivals where it would be quite easy for the buyer to know this independently, but where there are no quality differences or where the superior features would otherwise be hard to discern. Indeed, the branded product could be of inferior quality but is nonetheless widely deemed as more desirable in which case the branding strategy has worked very well indeed.

Clearly there is some overlap with the scope of trademark law. But the two are not the same. Trademarks are certainly relevant to branding, and are extremely useful for companies pursuing branding strategy. Essentially, brands are about identity and trademarks aim to signify or represent that identity. Thus, whereas branding strategy is highly dependent on registered trademarks, brands can exist independently, as they do for example in markets for illegal drugs.[115] There is no essential one-to-one relationship between a brand and a trademark, or indeed between either of these and a commodity. In this book I take 'commodity' to mean a type of good that is the same in terms of what it is irrespective of whoever makes or sells it. For instance acetyl salicylic acid is a commodity, whereas goods containing this active ingredient but sold under different names (Alka-Seltzer for example) are products.

Trademarks are distinctive signs capable of being represented in graphical form which communicate information to consumers about a product such as their trade origin and characteristics. A trademark can be protected legally for an eternity subject, in many countries, to payment of renewal fees and to keeping the mark in use. And just like patents, as a 'piece' of property, it can be bought, sold and licensed for others to use. According to World Trade Organization law, which most of the world's nations must adhere to, such signs may include 'personal names, letters, numerals, figurative elements and combinations of colours as well as any combination of such signs'. Nowadays, some countries allow shapes and sounds to be protected under trademark law. Typically, such signs comprise words, phrases, representational images or abstract designs, separately or in combination, that are used on products, product packaging or in advertising material. These products do not have to be new. Indeed, much of the value of the mark lies in its ability to distinguish a good from other similar ones made or sold by competitors that might otherwise be substitutable. Often, the most valuable marks are those used with products that *lack* novelty or else are very similar, if not identical, to goods already on the market. If the mark attracts customers willing to pay a higher price than similar equivalent products it is a valuable asset. This was understood by the pharmaceutical industry from the beginning. When companies file a patent on a drug, they need to make the case that it had no prior existence until they brought it into the world. Trademarks make no such claim. The sign may be new but the product itself does not have to be. Of course, all invented drugs are exposed to the possibility of competition once patents expire and this is where trademarks become especially important. The patent monopoly is at an end and the market falls open for others to enter with their own version of the product hitherto protected by the patent. Branded medicine retailers did of course already exist. But the combined and strategic use of trademarks alongside patents, enabled by the modernisation of intellectual property laws taking place over the course of the nineteenth and early twentieth centuries,[116] was largely a new thing.

We should not be surprised by the industry's huge reliance on trademarks which continues to this day as their subject matter scope and market functions keep on expanding. Indeed, it is arguably a defining feature. The value of a brand can be highly sustainable over time, but this is not to be taken for granted. Meaning and association changes over time and affects value. A serial killer in court wearing a jacket bearing a famous mark could well tarnish the brand. But the image of a mark can change in ways that may also enhance its value. And at some point, the value may fall to such an extent that a company will decide to terminate the brand by discontinuing its use or selling it off.

It is not just the naming of products that involves high financial stakes. There is also the naming of disease. This is a regulatory matter, which becomes especially important when health conditions are identified, given a name, and treated as being ones susceptible to a pharmaceutical response. Industry itself is not in a position to name diseases as such. But it stands to take advantage of an emerging or popularly accepted 'disease' category. We need to consider this later. Suffice it to say that of all types of disease mental health afflictions are a particularly tricky and highly contentious matter. The identification, naming and official recognition of such conditions has led to some to suggest the possibility that in a sense they are 'invented' categories of ill health that are brought into existence by the coinage of a name. As mentioned, industry does not categorise medical afflictions including mental health ones. That is the role of medical experts who are supposed to be objective without conflicts of interest. But we have seen already with Ritalin and Viagra how industry benefits and in fact goes so far as to promote medical conditions for which *their* product is *the* treatment.

From a historical perspective, the availability of patent protection for medical inventions is not something that the pharmaceutical industry has been able to take for granted. For one thing, many European countries for many decades were highly reluctant to extend patent protection for the benefit of private interests having control over people's lives. Thus prohibitions were placed on the patenting of both medicines and foods. Secondly, despite all the investment and sophisticated scientific expertise devoted to medical research outputs that can improve people's lives, the patentability of the various types of pharmaceutical 'solutions' developed remains uncertain. This requires a detailed discussion. While patent attorneys nowadays see no logical reason for drugs *not* to be patentable, much hangs on meanings, analogies, perceptions and assumptions that are open to challenge. Words, phrases and other signs that can be registered can convey rich meaning with power, just as they may be deployed for their purposive vagueness. Either way they do not always mean what people may suppose, or else they can mean what people want them to mean for their own ends. The impression they can leave on people's minds may have impacts well beyond the imprint left on the minds of any individual speaker, writer, listener or reader.

This is not an airy-fairy issue. It matters a lot. How scientists describe and present their achievements can have major implications in terms of legal rights. At this point, I will just focus on one core aspect of the debate on patenting in the biomedical field. Throughout this book you will frequently encounter the words 'synthesise', 'synthetic' and 'synthesis', and the term 'synthetic chemistry'. Conventionally, the idea of synthesising something is seen as a highly creative act and one deserving of a patent on the basis that as a synthetic substance it is a wholly human-made thing that results from the application of extraordinary skill or insight. The distinguished Australian Nobel prizewinning chemist Sir John Cornforth eloquently demystified the art of synthesis in a 1992 lecture.[117] Obviously no slouch in his abilities in the synthetic chemistry department, he nonetheless took pains to keep things in proportion, suggesting a modern definition of synthesis as 'the intentional construction of molecules by means of chemical reactions.' What synthesis does *not* mean, he said, is 'making new compositions of matter'. Perhaps purposely, but possibly accidentally, he was using a term in American patent law, 'composition of matter' being mentioned in the statute as a type of invention. As he put it,

> it happens that Nature and especially living Nature has exhibited to the chemist a very large variety of molecules. They are there, they are not new; but if we can make them from something else we say that we have synthesized them. And sometimes we proudly call our synthesis a total synthesis. Briefly, we are then claiming that, if we were given adequate supplies of all the chemical elements composing our compound, we could make a specimen of the compound totally derived from the matter supplied. In practice, nobody ever executes a total synthesis and few of the raw materials used have in fact been made from their elements.

Cornforth went on to point out that 'synthesis of compounds from elements is not peculiar to human beings', and that 'the rejection of competition, or even help, from other organisms in the execution of chemical synthesis is another nineteenth-century legacy.' He is of course not being disrespectful towards his fellow synthetic chemists or belittling their achievements. Indeed, he describes as 'epic' the ground-breaking 1972 synthesis of vitamin B_{12} by Woodward and Eschenmoser. But it is as well to be aware that chemical synthesis, at least in its modern sense, is a creative mimicry of nature — perhaps as artistic as it is scientific — which arguably gives nature far less credit than it deserves and humans rather too much.[118] Nonetheless, patents, as we will see, are embedded in the world of commerce more than of science (or for that matter art) and such subtleties are likely to get lost in translation. In fact, they have to for much of life science patenting to be viable.

Another example: Jacques Loeb, a US based German scientist of the late nineteenth and early twentieth centuries, was the subject of one of the most startling headlines in the history of newspapers (surely!), announcing his successful experiment in developing a sea urchin from an unfertilised egg and thereby inventing animal cloning[119]:

Creation of Life. Startling Discovery of Prof. Loeb. Lower Animals Produced by Chemical Means. Process May Apply to Human Species. Immaculate Conception Explained.[120]

A founding father of both genetic engineering and synthetic biology, albeit hardly a household name nowadays, Loeb inadvertently used what would become European patent law language in defining the ambitions of his scientific approach. This was in 1903: 'We cannot allow any barrier to stand in the path of our complete control and thereby understanding of the life phenomena. I believe that anyone will reach the same view who considers *the control of natural phenomena as the essential problem of scientific research.*'[121] This chimes with a recent statement made by the European Patent Office Enlarged Board of Appeal, which incidentally — and highly conveniently — favours quite an expansive view of the concept of invention:

Human intervention, to bring about a result by using the forces of nature, pertains to the core of what an invention is understood to be. Like national laws, the EPC does not define the term 'invention' but the definition that was given many years ago in the 'Red Dove' ('Rote Taube') decision of the German Federal Court of Justice ... set a standard which still holds good today and can be said to be in conformity with the concept of 'invention' within the meaning of the EPC.

In that decision … the … Court … defined the term 'invention' as requiring a technical teaching. The term technical teaching was characterised as 'a teaching to methodically utilize controllable natural forces to achieve a causal, perceivable result.'[122]

Let us ponder what the two scientists were saying here and search for some meaning that may or may not have been intended but which is capable of having legal repercussions. In doing so we must first understand that 'invention' can be used to refer both to a creative thought process leading to a result, and to the result itself. Cornforth does not state a point of view about the patent system and neither does Loeb. But one is left with some intriguing thoughts. A chemical newly made in the lab is certainly a composition of matter (how can anything made of atoms not be?), as is a mixture of such substances. But how might it not be novel? Here things are less clear. If Cornforth is alluding to the 'things' made in the lab, he would be suggesting that the things, that is, the synthetic chemicals, lack the novelty to be patentable, at least insofar as nature has anticipated these chemicals by having made them already. But arguably he is saying something a little different: that there is nothing novel in what the scientist does, because there is nothing in chemical synthesis that is novel. And if there is nothing novel about what she does, there is nothing novel either about the result. This is because it is a matter of making molecules, albeit in a different way from what happens in nature, and with a continuing reliance on natural products and processes to do most of the work. In other words, the scientist is doing nothing creative but is relying on nature's bits and pieces and the natural forces that transform these parts into a whole. Where this leaves the patentability of synthetic chemicals that are *not* copies of, or closely derived from, naturally occurring ones, is less than clear. Perhaps these could be new compositions of matter, but one can read Cornforth both to accept and to deny this possibility.

The law has in fact been grappling with this question since the late nineteenth century and the United States and Europe continue to have a different view on this. In much of the European continent, the patentability of chemicals was confirmed only quite recently. While public interest considerations and industry demands were often behind the prohibition, it is possible that more conceptual grounds were sometimes applied such as those proffered by the turn of the twentieth century German legal philosopher, Josef Köhler. Köhler denied chemicals could be inventions 'on the basis of the theoretical possibility that one day these synthetically chemicals might also be found in nature'.[123] He further argued that 'the tendency of chemical substances to combine with each other reflects an inherent, natural disposition, so that man's contribution consists not so much in the creation of a new compound as in the removal of the obstacles that block its formation.'[124] The fact that Germany did not allow patent claims on chemicals until the late 1960s, almost a century after infant industry protectionist and anti-monopoly arguments against such patenting had ceased to be credible, suggests these arguments would have been convenient and thus may have been influential. It also implies that in much of continental Europe, the chemicals-to-microbes-to-plants-to-animals analogical shifts may have more shaky foundations than some might suppose, an issue we will return to later in the book. However, there does not appear any likelihood of reverting to the ban on chemicals era. Patenting of chemical products is so much embedded in the ways that companies do business that it is difficult to imagine a reversal.

Returning to Loeb, the very close similarity between his statement made in 1903, and the definition of invention in the 1969 German Red Dove case cited with approval by the European Patent Office in 2010, might just be a coincidence signifying little of substance. And yet, viewing acts of creativity in terms of controlling nature and harnessing its forces to practical ends is perhaps necessary in order that one can view living things and natural occurring substances as human artefacts and therefore as inventions. The question remaining is that of how much human intervention in natural forces is required, and in what form, to convert a natural product into an artificial one.

This might all seem rather unimportant if not esoteric. In fact this discussion raises an interesting issue. Is the patent system inherently receptive towards scientific achievements in the biological sciences having therapeutic or commercial application? In other words, is the patent system bound to become ever more inclusive to accommodate the expanding scientific 'frontier'? In reality, logic, language and legal reasoning make nothing inevitable. History reveals no guaranteed alignment between the scope of patentable subject matter and what commercially oriented scientists do in biology and in the medical sciences for which they or their employees would like to acquire intellectual property protection. Recent case law in the United States, which has for the time being reversed previously permitted claims on such subject matters as isolated human DNA and methods of optimising individual medical treatments, makes this very evident (see Chapter 9). Neither is pharmaceutical regulatory reform necessarily in favour of powerful commercial interests. This book takes nothing for granted in this respect: neither alignment nor non-alignment can be assumed, nor that powerful organised interest groups will necessarily get what they want in terms of securing their preferred levels of patent protection or product (or other) regulation. We will look into intellectual property law reforms and court judgements that are relevant to the pharmaceutical industry. We will also consider how the novelty, inventiveness and industrial application criteria have been applied, as well as the scale of limitations and exceptions to the legal monopoly provided by patents.

Conclusion

In summing up what has been said in this chapter, to say what the pharmaceutical industry is from tracing its history back to its supposed origins, or from a set of essential business, legal, regulatory, or even epistemological characteristics is far from easy. Choosing one approach over the other will only take us so far. This chapter did not attempt to provide a definitive answer. What we can say is that to focus alone on the key firms, the science behind the products, or on the products themselves would paint an incomplete picture of the industry. We need to engage also with the business sector as a whole *and* with the underlying legal and regulatory regimes as these evolve and exist at any particular time. These regimes may or may not be designed with the industry in mind. Whether they are or not, regulation has a massive effect on the business models and decisions of individual firms and the structure of the industry as a whole, as we will see in the next chapter.

Notes

1   Anon (1835).
2   Until the end of that decade, gonorrhoea and syphilis were widely believed to be the same disease.
3   Morton (1968).
4   3 percent of all deaths in a recent Swedish study, making it the seventh most common cause of death in that country. Wester *et al.* (2008).
5   In the original German: '*Alle Ding sind Gift, und nichts ist ohne Gift; allein die dosis machts, dass ein Ding kein Gift sei.*' Paracelsus (1538).
6   Bernard (1872), 72.
7   Betomeu-Sánchez (2012).
8   This is not to suggest, though, that precision therapies are necessarily devoid of unpleasant side-effects either.
9   Lee and Noronha (2016).
10   Conant (2020); Goodman *et al.* (1946); 126–32; Mukherjee (2011), 89–91; Stockwell (2011), 48–53.
11   Cisplatin, first approved in the late 1970s, was first of a class of platinum-containing cancer treatments.
12   Silver nanoparticles have a wide range of health applications including, but not confined to, various cancers (Wei *et al.* (2015)). Silver also has known antibacterial effects (Baraniuk 2020).
13   For biopolar disorder.
14   Gerke (2015).
15   Dolma (2013); Czaja (2013).
16   Prakash (2013).
17   Farrar and Williams (1977).
18   Pereira (1836), 422.
19   Long (2001), 162–4.
20   Link (1959), 98.
21   *Ibid.*, 100.
22   Kresge *et al.* (2005); Last (2002), 4.
23   Link *op. cit.*, 103.
24   Link *op. cit.*, 105.
25   Unsurprisingly, his name is on all of the key patents relating to Dicumarol and warfarin. Perhaps the two most fundamental patents were: (1) US Patent no. 2,601,204 ('Process of lowering blood prothrombin level and lengthening clotting time with methylene-bis-hydroxy coumarin'), issued on 17 June 1952.

This was a continuation of an application filed originally in October 1941. Campbell, Stahmann, Huebner and Link were named as inventors. (2) US Patent no. 2,345,635 ('Di-esters of 3,3′-methylenebis (4-hydroxy coumarin) and process of making them'), issued on 4 April 1944. This was filed originally in April 1942. Stahmann and Link were the inventors.

26   Goldacre (2008).

27   Dumit (2012).

28   Alternative and complementary sectors can be like this too. Chiropractic, for example, was once sold to me in this kind of way: not feeling backache did not mean I did not require treatment on my back, besides which I would gain numerous other health advantages which I was presumably suffering a lack of. That was my first and last chiropractic session.

29   Moynihan and Henry (2006), 425.

30   Bhatt *et al.* (2015).

31   E.g. see Earp and Savulescu (2020).

32   Dupré (2001), 14–5. For similar sentiments: Smith (2012). Also, Sutcliffe (2015).

33   Volkow *et al.* (1995), 456. Quoted in DeGrandpre (2006), 4.

34   Graham (2011), 183.

35   *De Materia Medica* is the name of a book written in the first century by the Greek physician Dioscorides. This is the source of the term.

36   Porter (1997), 448.

37   Burgen (1996); Lesch (1981).

38   Gradmann (2009); Porter (1997) *op. cit.*, 431–48.

39   Quirke and Gaudillière (2008), 441.

40   For example, Beecham and Glaxo. See Corley (2011).

41   Stockwell (2011), 6–8.

42   For an excellent critical study covering the latter 'revolution', see Rasmussen (2014); also Hoffman and Furcht (2014).

43   A contraceptive pill is a pharmaceutical product even though it is not a therapy unless pregnancy is known to be a threat to the health of the woman taking it. Otherwise, stopping normal ovulation to prevent pregnancy achieves a desired physiological result but not a therapeutic one. Pregnancy is not a disorder.

44   Weiner and Will (2015).

45   Quirke and Gaudillière *op. cit.*, 445. It acquired common usage, though, from the end of the Second World War.

46   Mackintosh (2016), 542.

47   For example, in Ayurveda, individual body types ('prakriti) are classified on the basis of 'a combination of three mystical humors: windy, bilious, and

phlegmatic.' Pulla (2014). Another good example is Unani Tibb which is largely derived from Greek medicine and currently practiced in India, Pakistan and Bangladesh and among the South Asian diaspora.

48 Thomas (1971), 10.

49 *Ibid.*, 17.

50 Brotton (2002), 196.

51 Knight (2014), 183.

52 For example, see Moerman (1970). The author firmly concludes from his research that 'native American medical ethnobotany was not "only placebo medicine"'.

53 *Nature* (Editorial) (2007). For a heartfelt but excessive denunciation of traditional medicines from a contemporary medical practitioner: Tallis (2004), 132–9. One might counter this position with the argument that to denounce traditional medicine by selecting the most inhumane or futile practices is no different from using the thalidomide scandal or the use of prisoners of war in cruel medical experiments, as was done in the Second World War, as proof that there is something inherently rotten in the state of biomedicine. As regards old or traditional medicinal mixtures, recent research supports the view that therapeutic effects where they exist may not depend on an active principle in the form of a specific compound. Rather, it's the synergy itself that does the job. Understanding why every ingredient must be included is likely to be very hard to establish. For an example, see Furner-Pardoe *et al.* (2020).

54 Greene (2014) *op. cit.*, 12.

55 Le Fanu (1999), 206.

56 Voeks and Greene (2018).

57 Brotton (2002) *op. cit.*, 193.

58 Gänger (2015).

59 Cook (2007).

60 Brockway (1979), 188.

61 Bynum (1994), 18; for an excellent and comprehensive coverage, see Gänger (2015) *op. cit.*

62 Arikha (2007), 300 (emphasis added).

63 Indeed, several well-known repositories still used by researchers today contain specimens whose acquisition was enabled by slavery. Kean (2019).

64 Osseo-Asare (2008), 271.

65 Gänger (2015) *op. cit.*, 56–7. [References deleted from quote.]

66 Such as the Conference of the Parties to the Convention on Biological Diversity, and the World Intellectual Property Organization's

Intergovernmental Committee on Intellectual Property and Genetic Resources, Traditional Knowledge and Folklore.

67   According to leading ethnobiologists, the potential value of traditional knowedge as a stock of health information is probably substantial Plotkin (1993, 2000). However, a preparation made by a shaman for a particular condition does not translate well into biomedical science. Consequently, much less traditional knowledge has been recontextualised, however tangentially, into pharmaceutical products than many people assume. Dutfield and Suthersanen (2019).

68   Hanson and Pomata (2017), 3.

69   *Ibid.*, 6.

70   Osseo-Asare (2008), *op. cit.*, 269.

71   *Ibid.*, 269.

72   Bynum (2006), 239.

73   Porter (1997) *op. cit.*, 482.

74   Tilley (2011). See also Amster (2013).

75   Chakrabarti (2012).

76   Gradmann (2010).

77   For an intriguing biographical novel on Yersin's life: Deville (2013).

78   Neill (2012).

79   Bynum (2006) *op. cit.*, 221–8.

80   Supply difficulties are hardly a new challenge. The 1677 edition of the *Pharmacopoeia Londinensis* contained such hard to source, or else unpalatable, remedies as 'the fat of a man, the horn of a unicorn, and moss growing on a human skull.' Chapman-Huston and Cripps (1954), 17.

81   Cordes (2014), 71–2; Stockwell (2011) op cit., 10–12.

82   De Luca *et al.* (2012); Harvey *et al.* (2015); Ma and Wang (2009).

83   Liao (2009); Rao, Zhang and Li (2016); Tou (2016).

84   Normile (2015), 265.

85   For example, United States Patent no. 5,800,819: ('Piper guineense, pterocarpus osun, eugenia caryophyllata, and sorghum bicolor extracts for treating sickle cell disease'). Like the other nicosan patents, this was assigned to the National Institute for Pharmaceutical Research and Development of the Nigerian Federal Ministry of Science and Technology.

86   Osseo-Asare (2014).

87   Drayton (2000), xiv.

88   *Ibid.*, xiv–v.

89   *Ibid.*, xv.

90 Gaudillière (2014); Pordié and Gaudillière (2013); Lei (2014).
91 Hofer (2018).
92 Gaudillière (2014) *op. cit.*
93 King and Chaturvedi (2012).
94 Adams *et al.* (2009).
95 Everett and Gabra (2014).
96 On the origin of 'ethnopharmacology', see Heinrich and Casselman (2018). The word appears to have been coined in the late 1960s in the context of research on psychoactive drugs. Application of the term has expanded considerable since then.
97 An editorial in the very first issue of the journal defines ethnopharmacology as: 'a multi-disciplinary area of research, concerned with the observation, description, and experimental investigation of indigenous drugs and their biological activities'. Rivier and Bruhn (1979).
98 Hsu (2001); Pordié and Gaudillière (2013).
99 Lei *op. cit.*
100 Arikha, *op. cit.*, 303.
101 Lawler (2012); Wallace (2011).
102 Dutfield (2004), 47.
103 Frausin *et al.* (2015).
104 Giachi *et al.* (2013).
105 Lovejoy *op. cit.*, 333.
106 I say 'professionally' to indicate that professional scientists as a class of people emerged at this time and these were the ones doing the work. The question of what is and is not science is not one that this book seeks to shed light on.
107 Porter *op. cit.*, 450.
108 Chandler Jr. (2005).
109 Smil (2005).
110 To think one lives in a unique historical era of unprecedented change has obvious appeal but is quite difficult to think about objectively. That said, the present age does seem to be unusually innovative given the diversity of emerging technologies and their apparently quite rapid advance. *See* NRF Al-Rodhan (2011).
111 'Most historians agree that the modern scientist first came into being in the German-speaking lands, before a unified Germany was created under Bismarck.' Bynum (1994), 95.
112 Gispen (1989); McClelland (1991); Warner (1984).

113   For example, United States Patent no. 7,731,047, granted in June 2010 for a 'reclosable container lid with sliding element'.

114   Dutfield (2013); Fisk (2009); Maestrejuan (2012).

115   'Among the drugs found in Hoffman's apartment were several packets stamped with the ace of hearts, as well as the ace of spades, authorities say. *Both are said to be brand names for heroin which street dealers employ.* Philip Seymour Hoffman: '70 bags of heroin' in dead actor's home. *BBC News* website, 3 Feb. 2014.

116   Sherman and Bently (1999).

117   Cornforth (1993). All quotes below are from this paper.

118   I hesitate to go too far here. 'Synthesis' is a word whose usage over the past two centuries defies the coinage of any single or static meaning. Jackson (2012).

119   Ball (2011), 138. He managed also to clone a frog but unfortunately Loeb let it die due to his failure to realise the implications of frogs being amphibians: he let it drown.

120   This was in an 1899 issue of the Boston Herald, and is quoted in Ball *op. cit.*, 137.

121   Quote in Pauly (1987), 114 (emphasis added).

122   G 0001/08 (Tomatoes/STATE OF ISRAEL). Decision of the Enlarged Board of Appeal of 9 December 2010.

123   Quoted in Van den Belt (2009), 1301–40.

124   *Ibid.*

Chapter 3

Regulating Corporate Medicine

How is the industry regulated and for what purposes? Why is regulation necessary? What drives regulatory change? This chapter seeks to answer these questions. The pharmaceutical industry is both highly profitable and heavily regulated and has been for a long time. Having separate regulatory regimes is a large part of what makes the industry a distinct business sector. It has long been understood that regulation is not just a state activity according to which government agencies craft rules for others to follow and punish them when there are breaches. Regulation is informed by scientific and other knowledge arising from the state regulatory institutions and companies, universities, the organised professions, and other institutions involved in drug discovery, development, manufacture, and public health practice and policy. The private sector including manufacturers and suppliers, professional associations, experts, international and intergovernmental organisations, and other organised entities such as civil society organisations, business organisations, patient groups, think tanks, individuals, and courts can all play important roles. These stakeholder actors may be independent or operate in open (or closed) alliance with others. They can shape the regulations, and even write them. They may have a role in monitoring regulations, enforcing them, and in reforming them.

What is Pharmaceutical Regulation? And how does Regulation Interact and Co-evolve with Science, Business and Law?

There are four main areas of pharmaceutical-related regulation: (1) Product regulations concerning safety, efficacy, naming and marketing rights; (2) Manufacturing quality standards; (3) Disease classification;

and (4) Access including pricing and payment. Intellectual property rights and regulation are neither separate nor unrelated to one another. How intellectual property rights *should* relate to regulation has always been highly contested, which is hardly surprising given the stakes involved. It is possible to argue that intellectual property law is itself regulation.[1]

Product regulation

Let us start with the fundamental question of how regulation draws boundaries between pharmaceuticals and other products that are also health related. Not all health products to be ingested in some way or another are pharmaceuticals. Different types of business sell different types of product and they are treated differently by the regulators, for understandable reasons. Thus, product regulation serves to separate the pharmaceuticals and herbal remedies, traditional or otherwise, (and in some cases homeopathic ones), by imposing very different testing and marketing authorisation procedures. The latter are subject to far more lenient and far less costly regulations. For example, in the United Kingdom, by way of the *The Human Medicines Regulations 2012*, authorised medicinal products are either prescription only or for general sale (i.e. available over the counter). But all types of medicine must be authorised for public use, whether by a marketing authorisation for a conventional pharmaceutical, a certification of registration for a homeopathic medicine, or by a traditional herbal registration. For pharmaceuticals, general requirements for marketing authorisation include the following:

(a) pharmaceutical (physico-chemical, biological or microbiological) tests;
(b) pre-clinical (toxicological and pharmacological) tests; and
(c) clinical trials.

For homeopathic medicines, a substantial amount of scientific data including on efficacy must be submitted, but clinical trials are not required.

Consequently, registration is a far less cumbersome and expensive process. This is controversial given the widespread scepticism that homeopathy works — or indeed could possibly work. Admittedly homeopathic medicines are unlikely to do any harm in themselves given their lack of bioactive content. That said, taking homeopathic treatments in place of allopathic ones that demonstrably work and for life-threatening diseases is, at least in this author's opinion, ill advised.

Traditional herbal medicines also require results of pre-clinical tests, which homeopathic ones do not, but again no clinical trials are required. Similarly, under the EU's *Traditional Herbal Medicines Products Directive* (2004/24/EC), with which the Regulations must be consistent (at this time of writing), these must prove safety and quality. They can be registered only for minor conditions (so not for cancer, for example), and efficacy need not be proven: rather the effect of use should be 'plausible' on the basis of long use and experience — at least 30 years of continuous use, or 15 years in the EU. Obviously, this makes it much easier, quicker and cheaper to attain authorisation for herbal remedies than for pharmaceuticals. Unsurprisingly, these two commercial sectors operate separately.

There is an unavoidable epistemological dimension to this discussion. As we saw, traditional remedies remain in use and are popular in many parts of the world. But in addition, we have alternative and complementary medicinal preparations that may not be *traditional* as such, like homeopathic ones whose origins go back to 1790s Germany and which were in fact based on an approach that was *in opposition to* traditional European medical notions rooted in ancient Greece and Rome.[2] Other alternative and complementary treatments while typically having ancient roots are no longer traditional as such. Philosopher of science Keekok Lee makes an elaborate case that 'modern medicine is atomistic, reductionist, mechanistic as well as technology-oriented' and that this is a consequence of 'the philosophical worldview from which it follows' founded on scientific materialism and what I would call the 'organism-as-machine' perspective.[3] *If that is true of scientific medicine it is true also of the pharmaceutical industry.* The eminent philosopher of science Jerry Ravetz had this to say concerning the emergence of mechanical philosophy and its lingering implications for the moral integrity of science including its proper limits:

> With the rise to dominance of the 'mechanical philosophy', or more correctly with the dehumanization and disenchantment of Nature for the educated common sense of European civilization, the expected powers of scientific knowledge were reduced, and hence also the responsibilities of men of science. The association of natural science with 'progress', first with that of the intellect in the eighteenth century, and then with industry in the nineteenth, removed any fears concerning the applications of science from the traditions of self-awareness within science.[4]

Alternative and complementary medical systems, then, stand in epistemological and moral opposition to mechanism in the health sphere, most significantly perhaps in their claims to efficacy, safety and virtuousness. It is by dint of this opposition and their subjection to separate regulatory regimes that they are to be found outside of the pharmaceutical industry. As such, they help clarify what the industry is by what it is not. These anti-mechanists include practitioners and users of aromatherapy, the aforementioned homeopathy, acupuncture and cupping, but there are others.[5] They are counter-establishment and in opposition to the mainstream and while to a greater or lesser extent are rooted in tradition, whether European, Indian, Chinese, Middle-eastern or otherwise, they are not traditional as such having become modernised, professionalised, and described in ways aimed at lending them respectability. One might suppose that homeopathy is neither traditional nor exotic in origin, at least for a European. However, the European Union's rather peculiar 30-year rule for traditionality,[6] ironically equalling one 'modern' generation for which we might thank biomedicine, rather muddies the waters. It would not exclude many homeopathic treatments. Then again, if time alone is the measure of traditionality, it would not exclude most biomedical goods from being traditional either! Producers and retailers of alternative and complementary medicines operate alongside the pharmaceutical industry and interactions between these firms and the industry are uncommon. Ironically, the British retailer Boots sells such alternative and complementary medicines despite having also been a pharmaceutical company until quite recently, one of its most famous inventions being ibuprofen.

I do not think I need to get too involved in the debate on the validity of these systems, or on whether or not they deliver positive health outcomes. Suffice it to say that my deep scepticism is not tantamount to a blanket dismissal. The pharmaceutical industry almost certainly does not have a monopoly on treatments that work (not that I have ever had much use for alternative and complementary medicines). Exposing liars, charlatans, quacks and snake-oil salespeople, and their celebrity followers, can of course be great fun.[7] While people within the alternative and complementary medicines scene are frequently the targets, it is important to understand that the industry and the biomedical profession have far too many of them too.[8] The latter are harder for most of us to detect because bullshit communicated in the language of science tends to come across as good sense, whereas Gwyneth Paltrow's company's treatments and irresponsible lifestyle advice — most notoriously her vaginal eggs and steaming of the same organ using boiled water — should really fool nobody (though apparently people are still taken in to the extent that her company is highly profitable).

Another type of market impacting regulations specific to the pharmaceutical industry also relating to boundary setting is the separation of originator products from equivalent follow-on products for the purposes of marketing authorisation. Recent decades have seen the rise of an industry subsector whose market power is in large part a creature of regulation. Consider the United States first. In the 1980s, the pharmaceutical industry became the focus of transformative legislative activity in the form of the 1984 *Drug Price Competition and Patent Term Restoration Act* (usually referred to as 'the Hatch-Waxman Act'). Powerful as the research-based sector was, and experienced as it was in lobbying members of Congress, it finally had an effective competitor on Capitol Hill in the form of the generic manufacturers. These latter firms' intellectual property-related interests were of course quite different, and they had become sufficiently well-organized to ensure that any legislation affecting them would not stunt their growth.

For the research-based firms, the Act allowed patent term extensions of up to five years to compensate for the restriction on the effective protection term because of the time needed to acquire the FDA's marketing approval. There was of course some justification for this. It was taking increasingly long periods of time for the FDA to approve new chemical entities for sale, and this was reducing the effective period of market exclusivity. But the fact that the agrochemical industry, whose products also took a great deal of time and expense to get approved for sale, was unable to acquire a similar privilege is a testament to the political influence of the pharmaceutical companies.

As for the generic firms, the Act meant that they would only need to file a so-called Abbreviated New Drug Application (ANDA) with the FDA, rather than go through extensive clinical trials to demonstrate the safety and efficacy of their version of the soon to go off-patent drug. This meant that approval could take as little as three months. Second, the legislation incorporated the so-called 'Bolar exemption', which meant that certain acts performed before the expiry date of the patent that would normally infringe it were allowed as long as they were related to seeking FDA approval and did not constitute commercial use. The Bolar exemption was named after a court case involving Hoffman LaRoche and a generic producer called Bolar. Since a World Trade Organization dispute settlement panel upheld Canada's Bolar (or 'regulatory review') provision in 2000,[9] (but not its rule allowing also the manufacture and storage of the medicine with intention to sell), the same measure is now being incorporated into the patent laws of a growing number of countries, including the European Union which ironically was the source of the complaint against Canada.

Alfred Engelberg, formerly of the Generic Pharmaceutical Industrial Association (GPIA) described the legislative process which led to the Act as 'a congressionally supervised negotiation between the generic and brand-name pharmaceutical industries in which the parties were compelled to reach a compromise by the legislature'.[10] In this negotiation the respective sections of the industry were represented by the Pharmaceutical Manufacturers Association (PMA, now PhRMA) and the GPIA. According to Engelberg, the Act did not advance the interests of either side of the pharmaceutical industry, or of the public: 'patent-term extensions and the Bolar exemption are self-cancelling provisions, which, taken together, have no effect on the length of the exclusive marketing period of most drugs. The patent certification procedures are being abused by both sides and produce no public benefit that would not otherwise occur.'[11] When we consider that as many as 19 per cent of prescription drugs sold in the USA that year were generics, it was no surprise that the generics sector had become more influential and that the research-based firms in consequence had to compromise. Since then, the competition facing companies whose drugs have just gone off patent has increased considerably despite their increasingly creative lifecycle management strategies. By 1996, thanks in large part to the Hatch-Waxman Act, the generics sector of the industry had increased its share to 43 per cent.[12]

Despite the assertiveness of the generics sector and their rather different interests, the self-styled research-based firms are as influential as ever in the corridors of power. Their interests are represented by an army of Washington-based lobbyists, and they are generous donors to the electoral campaigns of parties and politicians. However, there is a growing number of pressure groups that seek to counter this influence. In spite of their relative lack of financial muscle, some of these groups carry out very impressive research and include some sophisticated and effective activists, such as Knowledge Ecology International and Public Citizen.

Licensing regimes are clearly significant in their market effects, affecting as they do who is permitted to manufacture, supply and sell medical products, and what needs to be done to fulfil the conditions for being officially registered. If official authorisation is required for manufacturing, importing, supplying and marketing, trade in medicines is not open in the sense that anybody can go ahead and do these things without the government's permission.

This is even more the case for a growing number of countries, where generic competition is restrained through a tie-up between patent status and the decision of regulators to grant marketing approval of a generic. Such a phenomenon is typically referred to as 'linkage'. 'Linkage regulations tie generic drug availability to existing drug patents by connecting approval to the resolution of patent validity or infringement.'[13] The authors from which that quote comes also note that linkage is being exported worldwide by means of free trade agreements. Accordingly, the drug regulators' marketing approval of a generic drug increasingly requires that the active ingredient not be under patent.

This is a problem because it denies the opportunity for a generic competitor willing to accept the risk of litigation from entering a market. It might be the case that the competitor believes the patent will not stand up in court. At least a few of the many patents granted every year will have been awarded in error or with excessively broad claims, so denial of the opportunity to have them tested in a court of law does seem unfortunate.

How does linkage work in practice? In the United States, the Food and Drug Administration's Approved Drug Products with Therapeutic Equivalence Evaluations publication (commonly known as the Orange Book) which contains the names of all medicines approved as safe and effective also lists patents that claim a drug or a method of using it and other exclusivities including their submission and expiry dates. Sellers of original medicines can take legal action against a generic producer for patent infringement before the latter company's product has entered the market. But the latter can contest the validity of an unexpired patent and place on the market a product they consider is not claimed by a patent. They can do this by submitting with their application for approval a certification that in their opinion and to the best of their knowledge, an Orange Book-listed patent on the medicine is invalid, unenforceable, or will not be infringed by their product. The first generic company to submit an application with such a paragraph IV certification will be eligible to enjoy the benefit of generic drug exclusively for 180 days. But if the patent owner does file an infringement suit within 45 days, the FDA approval of the generic product is delayed for 30 months.

Thus, a generic company *can* get approval to enter a market occupied solely by a patented product by formally claiming the patent has no effect vis-a-vis the competing product. But as mentioned, this still leaves it open for the patent holders to challenge the generic company applying for approval. Alternatively, the two firms can settle out of court. So-called reverse payment settlements (or 'pay-for-delay' as they are sometimes called), which are largely a United States phenomenon, refer to financial incentives being paid to — rather than by — would-be infringers in exchange for agreement by the latter *not* to enter the market. Such settlements would appear not to be in the public interest if patients and public health institutions and services are in this way potentially being denied the benefits of price-lowering competition on the basis of patents or patent claims whose validity may not stand up in court. In a 2013 Supreme Court case,[14] it was ruled that such settlements are not immune from antitrust legislation and the attention of the Federal Trade Commission even where the monopoly powers of the patent holder are no greater than are provided by the exclusionary rights of a valid patent. However, they are not presumptively unlawful either. It really depends on whether the settlement in question has anticompetitive effects or not, and this requires an analysis of each agreement. The Court opted not to provide a detailed structure for such an analysis.[15] In Europe, the European Commission opposes reverse payment settlements on the basis that they breach EU competition rules prohibiting acts incompatible with the internal market.[16] In September 2016, the General Court of the Court of Justice of the European Union found that Lundbeck had illegally colluded with four generics firms enabling the company to prevent price-reducing competition, breaching Article 101 of the *Treaty on the Functioning of the European Union*, which forms part of that treaty's rules on competition in the EU's internal market.[17] However, it remains to be seen how national authorities might view such deals.[18] In India, Bayer's effort to restrain the drug controller from approving a generic version of its drug Nexavar failed in the Supreme Court after the Delhi High Court's earlier dismissal of Bayer's petition which was partly on the basis of there being no intent by parliament that India should establish a linkage system. Therefore, the court held, it would be incorrect to read such meaning into the relevant statutory law.[19,20]

The somewhat complicated system operating in the US may be contrasted with Europe where the decision to grant marketing authorisation is made without any consideration as to the patent status of any related product. Patent linkage requirements are expressly prohibited. This is preferable. There is a strong possibility that not all patents have claims strong enough to survive validity challenges. Moreover, increasingly large numbers of follow-on patents protecting a particular medicinal product may be 'captured' by a linkage regime, and these can already cause substantial and undue delays to generic market entry at the cost of consumers.

Whether linkage as a policy change has net negative consequences or not, though, depends on the situation prior to its introduction. In the United States, prior to the 1984 legislation reliance on originator medicines' test data for approval of a generic drug was not possible. To enter the market all companies seeking to place *all* their medicines on the market, both original products and generics, had to conduct their own trials for safety and efficacy, the latter requirement being introduced by the 1962 *Kefauver Harris Amendment* to the *Federal Food, Drug, and Cosmetic Act*. This was initially quite a small barrier to market entry.[21] The costs entailed were much lower than they are today. But the barrier got higher in time as the rigour the FDA demanded got higher. So, data exclusivity (as discussed below), and regulatory linkage arguably made the situation better in the sense of facilitating generics industry growth. On the other hand, the introduction of similar linkage regulations in Canada which already had a strong generics sector that had benefited from the regular grant of compulsory licenses had the opposite effect.[22] Market entry was already quite easy so linkage had a delaying effect with no balancing measures to mitigate its impact. Having said all that, there is evidence that test data exclusivity in the United States, by itself, does delay generic market entry in some cases. And delays are likely to be greater in jurisdictions that provide lengthier exclusivity durations, such as the EU, Japan and Canada.[23]

There is of course another market in drugs: in the ones that are illegal or highly controlled. The illegal drugs trade is massively lucrative, makes fortunes, employs many people, and fuels violent crime. The notorious Pablo Escobar is said to have made $30 billion from the cocaine trade. Why some drugs are illegal and some are authorised pharmaceuticals is an intriguing matter that is far from being clear-cut, at times defying logic.[24]

Heroin, trademarked by Bayer, but now generic, was once sold legally to the public. However, under its simplified chemical name of diamorphine[25] it is still administered to hospital patients in some countries. This 'heroin' is produced from opium acquired from legal sources. Likewise, cocaine used to be legal but is now banned. It is of course widely used albeit not for medical purposes. Cocaine actually kills fewer people than paracetamol, which is very cheap and easy to get. That said, for the benefit of a little instant gratification the drug damages noses, causes lethal effects on the thickness of people's wallets, finances civil wars and extreme violence, and supports the luxurious lifestyles of some extremely vicious people. And addiction is terrible for one's state of mind. For all these reasons it is best avoided as is heroin, and controlling or banning both of them seems like a reasonable course of action all things considered. (Reasoned arguments have been made by some public health experts for legalisation of some such currently banned substances but I shall leave this highly emotive debate for others.)

But how consistent are we really? Many people have suffered addiction to Valium, but while in many countries it is available only on prescription, the fact is that it is not banned. So the illegality of drugs like heroin and cocaine cannot just be because they are addictive, dangerous, or liable to be misused. In fact, bans are often a consequence of 'moral panics', frequently led by the popular press whose only genuine interest is to sell newspapers. Often such ban-the-whatever campaigns are neither rational nor consistent. Especially problematic is the assumption that the same drug has identical effects on people across different cultures and that misuse by some should necessarily be dealt with also by preventing proper use by others in some faraway place. Some 'addictive' drugs freely used within a specific socio-cultural or spiritual context may not be associated with addiction problems to any great extent, whereas they lead to major social problems among other groups. For example, hallucinogenic substances like ayahuasca may perform important functions in some societies that are by no means negative. In South America chewing coca leaves provides harmless relief for people inhabiting the highlands of the Peruvian and Bolivian Andes where the air is thin. Should the indigenous peoples of these countries be denied access because of addiction problems among young people in faraway countries like the United States or Britain? One might add here that an unfortunate consequence of the war on narcotics is that many hospitals around the world lack access to supplies of morphine meaning that many patients suffer undue pain.

Nor do we do the consistent thing of banning all drugs that are devoid of medical benefits, whilst allowing those that do have benefits. Tobacco is undeniably dangerous and has no health benefits (except perhaps for mild stress relief for which far less harmful treatments are readily available). But it is legal everywhere — possibly because governments have their own tobacco-related addiction: to the revenues gained from taxing cigarettes. Marijuana has genuine medicinal uses and is not particularly addictive or dangerous, but it remains illegal in many parts of the world though things seem to be changing here.

Further discussion falls a little outside the scope of this book but it is as well to be aware that regulatory distinctions are drawn between safe *and* effective pharmaceuticals and substances which may be safe *or* effective, but are not both; as they are between modern biomedical products on one side, and alternative, complementary and traditional drugs. However, distinguishing between approved medicines and banned substances while purportedly made on the basis of sound science, good policy, and societal consensus may be done in ways that are not clear, objective or consistent.

Drug approval regulation has evolved in line with the growth of the sector, the business strategies employed, and intellectual property law. It hardly needs to be said that product regulation has massive market effects. In the beginning medicines were of course barely regulated at all and they were treated no differently from foods and beverages. In the nineteenth century some countries passed legislation protecting the public from dangerously poisonous and adulterated health products. Regulation of pharmaceutical medicines over time became increasingly strict, befitting their dual nature as both poisons and cures, but also taking into account that, as potentially life-saving products, public availability is very important too as is the encouragement of innovation. That the Greek word from which 'pharmaceutical' derives, *pharmakon* (φάρμακον), also has this ambiguous meaning feels quite appropriate. Few people now would dispute the need to require new medicines to undergo up to several years of extensive testing before allowing marketing approval. Regulation influences our attitudes towards pharmaceutical products, enhancing our trust in them. It also shapes the structure of the industry, serving as a barrier to entry. Moreover, the cost of demonstrating safety and efficacy, which for original medicines typically requires toxicity testing and extensive and highly expensive clinical trials, the conduct of and results of which require the production of vast amounts of documentation, 'justifies' the setting of high prices and the tendency towards aggressive marketing and intellectual property management strategy. Regulations concerning use of this documentation by drug regulations to approve original drugs and subsequent competing ones have themselves evolved into a *quasi*-intellectual property right which again has market impacts.

It is trite to say I cannot make a chemical composition in my kitchen or garden shed for 'the pox' or whatever, and try to sell it as 'Professor Dutfield's Amazing Anti-Pox Salts', and then tout the product to pharmacies to supply it, to doctors to prescribe it, or to the public directly at a market stall. The fact is that there was a time in the past when I could have done just that. Indeed, many did so and the industry evolved in part out of such dodgy operations. These were the worst of the so-called 'patent medicines', which we consider below. It is highly unlikely my equipment would be state of the art, besides which hygiene standards in my kitchen may be good enough for my family and two dogs but not really for making drugs for public consumption including perhaps for the very ill.[26] As the industry evolved, the freedom to enter the market in such a way has become ever more constrained. You need to prove your health claims are valid and the medicine is safe to use. Nowadays national and regional official drug regulators require all manufacturing of approved medicines, whether originator drugs or generic copies, to meet acceptable quality standards. Your facilities must be inspected to ensure that these standards are met.

It is easy to see why this change is a good thing. Who would wish to return to a time of legitimate products competing with useless ones made in unhygienic conditions for diseases that do not exist, and sold under deceptive names? Product regulation is not just about approval for this or that drug to be placed on the market. The most import aspect of product regulation is the indication for which it is approved. It is as much about the information including labels and guidelines for use of the product as it is about the product itself. The product obviously needs to be tested for safety and efficacy before it can be marketed. But toxicity alone is not a bar to approval. Indeed, the drug may cause serious harm, even death, to some people. But the drug can still be available if its benefits are deemed to outweigh its harms and warnings and counter-indications are provided in the packaging or instructions inserted inside. This underlines the importance of submitting all findings from the testing and clinical trials including negative ones such as that the drug is ineffective or harmful to children, pregnant women, the elderly or people taking another medicine at the same time resulting in harm when the two are taken simultaneously. Withholding relevant information, which companies are sometimes tempted to do, can lead to criminal investigation and possible prosecution if it results in the prescribing of drugs to vulnerable patients.

Much can of course be learned from toxicity testing and clinical trials. But clinical effectiveness is hard to prove from randomised controlled trials alone. One might assume that efficacy and effectiveness are the same thing, but they are not. An efficacious drug is one that *can* work as shown for example in artificial circumstances such as in a randomised trial. An effective drug is one that *does* work overall for sick people in normal circumstances.[27] An efficient drug is one that is worth the price. All effective drugs must be efficacious, but not all the latter are effective.[28] Even effective drugs are not necessarily efficient, although determining efficiency in a climate of limited budgets and rationing is hardly straightforward for health economists, though there are generally accepted methodologies. This leads us to the role of physicians and other healthcare workers. Valuable healthcare innovation does not end with the development and approval of a new medicine. Pre-market clinical trials simply don't tell you everything you need to know under real conditions, hence the need for postmarketing surveillance, sometimes referred to as phase four clinical trials, of which pharmacovigilance is a key aspect. Physicians and other healthcare workers responsible for delivering treatments directly to patients acquire medically valuable knowledge and experience on effectiveness that can be of benefit not just to the people they actually treat, but to the wider group of patients undergoing the same treatment. Physicians will be first to know what works and how well, what doesn't and for what kind of patient,[29] what can happen when a patient is on more than one medication, as well as what side effects ensue and their impacts on the patient. Obviously, patients themselves are important sources of information.

How did we get here? Does pharmaceutical regulation evolve incrementally, in occasional giant leaps, or are both types of change relevant to what has happened since the 1880s? Some commentators highlight the effects of health disasters such as sulphanilamide in the United States in the 1930s and thalidomide in Europe in the late 1950s and early 1960s. Accordingly, cumulative regulatory evolution, if there is any, is interrupted by sudden radical reforms where governments are compelled to respond to a disaster that existing regimes had failed to prevent. Others more susceptible to the well-known regulatory capture model tend to assume that the best organised and most economically powerful interests tend to get regulatory regimes and changes to them that suit their interests irrespective of what the public wants or needs. Regulatory capture is a real phenomenon, being most likely when industry and regulatory institutions share the same ideology, one that suits industry. It is certainly true that health disasters have driven radical change. But it would go too far to suggest that people need to die before regulation gets overhauled. Consumer deaths have undoubtedly been impactful in terms of regulatory reform, even if they haven't always been. Of course, given that these are toxic products, the industry can hardly be against regulation *per se*, but what it can try to do is help to shape them. This book's co-evolutionary approach treats regulatory regimes, which as this chapter shows, are not just about health and safety, as dynamic and shaped by markets, the interests that businesses pursue politically which are of course about making money, science, and law, as these are shaped by regulation.

In the early days, pharmaceutical regulation did evolve incrementally, and was initially and for quite a long time regulated alongside foods and beverages and with rather a light touch by today's standards. Typically, regulatory processes comprised bringing together specialised government agencies with health professionals and their representative associations but not necessarily industry. Sometimes new regulations and reforms came in response to new innovations such as new classes of drugs coming onstream, or incidents including public health scandals.

In Britain, a parliamentary select committee report of 1914[30] summarised the situation in several countries concerning the sale and marketing of proprietary and patent medicines, that is, those that may be sold directly to the public. German regulations excluded certain medicines from open sale, providing a list of medicines that could only be sold in pharmacies and that required medical prescription. Austria required that proprietary medicine be officially authorised for sale first, and that their contents be known. France also banned secret remedies. Italy required all proprietary medicines to be submitted with all relevant information to the interior ministry. Packaging should provide information which needed to be true and without grossly exaggerating as to the medicine's contents and benefits. However, these rules were apparently enforced without much rigor. The United States had laws against the sale and marketing of fraudulent treatments including for 'misbranding'.

As for Britain, the above committee confessed to some confusion as to the law and its administration, particularly their piecemeal aspects. It took a very dim view of the effectiveness of this regulatory regime such as it was. It identified the sale and advertisement of proprietary and patent medicines as being the subject of numerous laws covering stamp duties, pharmacies, poisons, merchandising, sale of foods and drugs, indecent advertising and larceny. Two statutory bodies with important roles to play were the General Medical Council which published the British Pharmacopoeia, and the Pharmaceutical Society which had regulatory powers over substances containing poisons including their listing in the official schedule. Departments of state with some jurisdiction over proprietary and patent medicines comprised the Privy Council, the Home Office, the Local Government Board, and the Patent Office. With regard to the latter the report noted as follows:

> The Comptroller-General [i.e. head of the Patent Office] informed us that 312 patents granted to 1912 for medicines and medicinal preparations are in force. There are very few patents of the remedies to which our enquiry was specially directed, as a patent cannot be secured without (a) proof of usefulness and novelty, and (b) disclosure of formula.[31]

The Committee identified two main classes of proprietary remedies: secret and non-secret. The latter were either: (1) 'proprietary preparations', that is, legitimate drugs produced synthetically or extracted from crude compounds and properly tested and manufactured, and typically patented or sold under registered names; (2) 'remedies owing their value to skilful combination' whose active ingredients are not new; and (3) 'non-secret drugs with secret excipients' protected as trade secrets. Generally speaking, such non-secret drugs would not be the target for the necessary regulatory reform. The secret remedies were quite another matter. The types identified by the Committee comprised 'simple house-hold remedies', 'dangerous remedies, and drugs for improper purposes', 'fraudulent remedies', and 'remedies making grossly exaggerated claims'. Apparently, many such treatments were imported from the United States where a tightening of the law had restricted their domestic sale. However, the British-made Beecham's Pills were also cited for hinting at the laxative's use for inducing abortion.

However, reform was very slow in coming, with a number of bills failing to get passed into law. For much of the nineteenth century political orthodoxy tended to take a dim view of the idea of state regulation. *Laissez faire* lost some of its hold over the political establishment in the later decades of that century but the pharmaceutical trade was still largely successful in keeping the state at bay.[32] This apparently persisted well into the twentieth century. Unscrupulous drug makers continued to sell secret remedies of dubious quality and publicised by dishonest advertising.[33] Eventually laws were passed to prevent sale and advertising for certain diseases. From 1917 medicines for venereal diseases had to be prescribed by medical practitioners. In 1939 a similar law was passed for cancer. Further laws passed in the 1940s and 50s extended such controls over treatments for various diseases and types of medicine including tuberculosis and the antibiotics.

However, radical changes also took place. Sometimes these were indeed in response to avoidable tragedies. The 1937 tragedy in which 76 people in the USA were killed by a medicine called Elixir of Sulfanilamide led to new rules in that country requiring medicines to be tested for safety prior to sale that were adopted subsequently by other countries. In other times regulations were imposed to ban or suppress the use and/or advertising of drugs seen as being widely misused such as cocaine and opium, or deemed as immoral such as abortifacients. That for a long time many drugs have been made unavailable for self-medication but instead require a prescription is of course as things should be.

Since the last decades of the twentieth century, the pharmaceutical industry has had to deal with increasingly stringent safety and efficacy regulations requiring the production of vast amounts of data acquired through not just toxicity studies but randomised double-blind clinical trials. Randomised clinical trials were pioneered shortly after the Second

World War by the British Medical Research Council and the US Public Health Service, both to test streptomycin for tuberculosis. During the late 1960s and early 1970s, they became mandatory in the United Kingdom and the United States for all new products including for all therapeutic claims.[34]

Even so, change in some countries was surprisingly late. Although drug regulations in Prussia go back to the beginning of the nineteenth century, up to 1962 West Germany did not require drugs to be tested prior to receiving marketing authorisation. However, the rules brought in that year were still not particularly demanding. Modern-day drug approval procedures requiring testing for efficacy and safety were not introduced in that country until administrative and legal reforms in 1976 and 1978 largely in response to the infamous Contergan/thalidomide tragedy. The tragedy was manifested as a massive spike in worldwide incidences of a terrible affliction called phocolemia, in which people are born with severe limb deformities. In time the phenomenon was linked to pregnant women taking a sleeping pill drug called thalidomide (marketed as Contergan) to relieve morning sickness. Even then, West Germany, where it was available over the counter from 1957 to 1961, despite being so affected by thalidomide's awful consequences, was surprisingly slow to respond. After some modest regulatory steps forward, the country finally brought in rigorous approval procedures fifteen years after the manufacturer Grünenthal had withdrawn this highly lucrative product from the market. The United States, with its by then relatively strong regulatory requirements — which it subsequently strengthened further — largely escaped the disaster. The UK and several other countries did not.

In the United Kingdom, the 1968 *Medicines Act* set up a licensing regime and required the authority in reviewing applications from prospective product licence holders 'in particular' to 'take into consideration'

(a) the safety of medicinal products of each description to which the application relates;
(b) the efficacy of medicinal products of each such description for the purposes for which the products are proposed to be administered; and

(c) the quality of medicinal products of each such description, according to the specification and the method or proposed method of manufacture of the products, and the provisions proposed for securing that the products as sold or supplied will be of that quality.

Does the public benefit from this much heavier dose of regulation? And, is such regulation an unambiguous loss for industry, or are there gains? In fact, the answers to both — which in fact cannot be completely separated — are a little more nuanced that we might initially suppose.

Objective, large-scale and rigorous *in vivo* testing seems like an inherently good thing, without downsides. For those still living with the horrific limb deformities resulting from their mothers taking thalidomide, this is surely a no-brainer. As with Big Data today, large datasets from testing can identify patterns and marginal differences that would otherwise be unnoticeable, and that might, for example, guide decisions on what claims and warnings prescribers and patients need to know about. They can also presumably eliminate bias through the generation of reliable statistical data.

On the other hand, such testing challenges, and perhaps undermines, the judgement of physicians treating individual patients, and represents a shift in power from doctors to corporations who are responsible for carrying out or sponsoring the trials. The benefits and disbenefits of generalised treatment regimens based on statistical interpretations of clinical trial data are especially challenging for chronic conditions where results are likely to be long term and perhaps ambiguous and less than wholly conclusive. The prescribed medicines may well be effective for many people but provide little or no discernible benefit for individual patients placed on a treatment regimen that doctors are expected to comply with, perhaps against their better judgement in specific cases. This begs the question of whether clinical trials are conducted with a view to optimising healthcare solutions for patients, or are primarily geared towards profit-making where the two may be in conflict. As Joseph Dumit has shown, 'the real issue is that clinical trials are driven by the need to grow the market in medicine and that this is a very different goal for a clinical trial than arriving at the best therapy for people.'[35]

This takes us towards the second question (but without entirely leaving the first). Stringent regulation is clearly a challenge for industry and may in fact lead to suboptimal outcomes for both patients *and* the industry. Apart from the huge compliance costs, it is possible that several drugs that could have provided substantial benefits for patients in spite of their side-effects were weeded out that ought not to have been. Walter Sneader, a medical historian, has suggested that if current safety standards had been applied to Aspirin and paracetamol, they might well not have been approved.[36] But regulators have been criticised both for being not just too tough, but also too lax although apparently laxity may be a function of clinical trials. *Efficacy* as demonstrated in clinical may not translate with precision into *effectiveness* in real world situations — hence the need for post marketing surveillance to identify adverse drug reactions. Drugs have turned out to be dangerous for some people after marketing approval had been granted, and subsequently had to be withdrawn even though they were beneficial for others.

But are there any ways one could claim the industry has gained from them? One can argue that pharmaceutical regulations' consequences for the industry have also been positive especially for established firms with deeper pockets and experience of navigating the regulatory pathways that small and emerging companies cannot match. Accordingly, they form a serious barrier to entry. Smaller firms will most likely opt to license their promising but untested drug candidates. Meanwhile marketing approval for general use on the basis of the clinical trial findings as interpreted, including for chronic conditions that could be treated by means other than ingesting a pharmaceutical, helps turn promising drugs including ones sufficiently different from existing ones to fall outside the scope of patents, but that may not necessarily be improvements, into blockbusters. One interesting unintended consequence, identified among others by medical historian Viviane Quirke as being positive, at least for the British industry, is that — of necessity — it encouraged broadening the scope of biomedical research and technology adoption in unprecedented ways, integrating

> biological disciplines such as biochemistry, pharmacology, and toxicology, and of physical methods and instrumentation, especially

high-performance chromatography, mass spectrometry, and nuclear magnetic resonance, thus transforming the organization and practice of pharmaceutical R&D.[37]

One regulatory area to focus on — which we will consider later in the chapter — concerns the naming of chemicals and products. This area is very specific, goes back to industry's beginnings, has always had a huge influence on how it does its business, and can thus be seen as part of what makes the industry special and unique. There are two aspects to consider. First, we have the framework of rules concerning the naming of chemicals and products which partially operates in conjunction with trademark law (and to a lesser but still very important extent, patent law). These have enormous repercussions for business strategy, industrial structure, research and development decisions, and the interests of the public. Second, we must consider the way that product regulation enabling differentiation between different types of therapeutic entity effectively sets boundaries both within and around the industry and thus helps to define not just the pharmaceutical product but also the pharmaceutical company *and* the industry itself.

Product regulation as it became stronger had major impacts on the structure of the industry, catalysing a divergence according to the types of product that companies tended to concentrate on. The first group comprised those companies specialising in developing and selling original prescription-only single-compound 'ethical' drugs.[38] These became the ones responsible for all new medicines. Of course, these were the biggest and most profitable firms, and also the most select. The second was formed of those making generic copies of the same medicines. The third included those dealing mainly in consumer products — typically-branded — sold over the counter. The three-way split was hardly a neat one; indeed, nor is it now, and not just because such firms were not necessarily independent of one another. Some companies making ethical drugs often continued to market cheap branded medicines, like headache pills, and other household products. Beecham, for example, continued to sell Beechams Powders which in fact are available today. As in the past, indeed going back to the industry's beginning, there are companies whose role is to manufacture active ingredients on behalf of the above types of company. This is rather similar to some of today's big pharma companies that were founded to supply pharmacies rather than to make pharmaceutical products *per se*. Nowadays, many of these are located in China and India.

Manufacturing quality standards

In my brief discussion about the imaginary 'Professor Dutfield's Amazing Anti-Pox Salts', I mentioned manufacturing standards not being regulated in the past. Regulation is not just about *what* medicines can be made for public consumption; *how* they are made matters enormously too. Thankfully things have changed over the years. Testing medicines for which approval is sought is not just about safety and efficacy of the active ingredient, or bioequivalence of the generic substitute. At national level, countries have Good Manufacturing Practice (GMP) regulations which drug makers must comply with. Poor practices can lead to contamination, mixing up of products and false labelling whether through negligence or any other reason, hence the need for strictly binding rules.

In the European Union, the legal basis for GMP as regards medicines for human use is *Commission Directive 2003/94/EC of 8 October 2003 laying down the principles and guidelines of good manufacturing practice in respect of medicinal products for human use and investigational medicinal products for human use*. There is a separate directive for medicines for veterinary use. Eudralex Volume 4, entitled *The rules governing medicinal products in the European Union*, is a lengthy document that provides guidance on how to put into practice the principles and guidelines set out in the two directives, and its strictures apply to medicines manufactured in the EU region and those made elsewhere but authorised in Europe. It is a 'living document' in the sense that it is subject to revision and amendment as deemed necessary. In the United States, the legal basis is the *Food, Drug, and Cosmetic Act* (FD&C Act), of which Chapter V covers drugs and medical devices. These rules are interpreted by the relevant sections of the Code of Federal Regulations. The FDA carries out inspections of manufacturing facilities worldwide, as does its European counterpart, the European Medicines Agency (EMA),[39] who have recently started working together with a number of national regulatory agencies and the World Health Organization on joint inspections and information sharing.

Despite this, there have been scandals and these have involved some of the best-known international corporations, such as GlaxoSmithKline and Abbott, and not just generic firms in countries like India (most notoriously Ranbaxy) and China that tend to attract more suspicion anyway.[40]

Disease classification

It hardly needs to be stated that just as nomenclatural systems are required for pharmaceuticals, there are sound public health reasons also to classify diseases, disorders, conditions and syndromes some of which fall beyond the scope of this book. But who does the classifying? These are done by way of diagnostic manuals developed and updated by medical specialists. International cooperation in disease classification began in the 1890s with the development of a system based on French scientist Jacques Bertillon's statistical work on causes of death in France. This evolved into the periodically updated International Classification of Diseases and Related Health Problems (ICD) that the World Health Organization took over in 1948 and which most countries adopt to a greater or less extent. The latest version, ICD-11, was adopted by the World Health Assembly in 2019 and is now available for national implementation. Alongside ICD are two other WHO classification systems, the International Classification for Functioning Disability and Health (ICF), and the International Classification for Health Interventions which is under development. There are several other systems derived from the ICD and the ICF. One very important complementary national system is the American Psychiatric Association's Diagnostic and Statistical Manual of Mental Disorders (DSM), first published in 1952 but into its fifth revision. The DSM is highly influential internationally, and not just in the United States.

There are high stakes in disease classification, or nosology to use the scientific name for this. The phenomenon of 'lumping and splitting', a term often attributed to Charles Darwin, very much applies to nosology. Of the two, splitting tends to be more common in recent years as we seek ever increasing specificity, not just through more traditional procedures for identifying and naming diseases but applying data-driven and molecular methods, among other novel approaches for stratifying diseases that have much in common in order to benefit individual patients and groups with more specific personalised medical interventions.[41]

Cancer is commonly regarded as a disease all of its own, and we all yearn desperately for some amazing substance that can cure all cancer. But we are of course nowhere near to having such a thing, and it may not be a feasible aspiration anyway. Cancer is really a family of diseases with highly varied causes and characteristics, and just as pharmaceutical treatments are increasingly specific to the type of cancer, classification of cancers involves the ongoing identification of types and subtypes. Consider leukaemia for example. 100 years ago, diseases of the blood were largely undifferentiated, and then in time leukaemia and lymphoma emerged as separate diseases. There are now around 40 types of the former and over fifty of the latter, to which one can add numerous subtypes of both.[42] Lumping or splitting debates are particularly fraught in the general field of mental health problems, psychiatric disorders, and behavioural and developmental deviations from the normal. There is a wealth of literature on this matter.

On the one hand, some have argued that more lumping might be desirable. It has been noted that an unfortunate consequence of splitting is medicalisation and pharmaceuticalisation, at least in the case of anxiety disorders.[43] The point is that more and more members of the general population for whom a more generalised categorisation would exclude them from the need for treatment, can be 'captured' by one or more specific categories and thereby deemed to be unwell and in need of treatment that may in fact be unnecessary or even harmful — albeit profitable for industry. They may also quite possibly be less effective than medicines developed long before such specialised disorders were 'discovered', a concern that has arisen with undue lumping as we will see now.

The leads us to a further criticism of the industry, which is that it exploits the situation by the practice of the so-called 'disease mongering' phenomenon mentioned in Chapter 2. In an economic sense, prioritising research in these ways is perfectly rational, whether or not it is entirely admirable. As we saw in Chapter 2, the marketing of Ritalin, Viagra and a recent generic version are blatant instances of disease-mongering.

But lumping can have socially suboptimal consequences as well. In at least one case it has allegedly led to the development of medicines for specific treatment that are of lower quality than earlier generations of drugs for mental health issues. This happened in the United States when the authorities in 1980 merged melancholia, a condition long recognised in Europe based as it was on humoral theory,[44] and non-melancholia into a single category: major depression. The consequence was the elimination from the pharmacopoeia of many old medicines that were perfectly effective and the approval of a class of drugs whose performance, despite their massive use, appears to have been grossly overrated: the SSRIs, or selective serotonin reuptake inhibitors. To make matters worse, these medicines are based on a theory ('the serotonin theory') that is allegedly false.[45] Medical historian Edward Shorter expresses what happened in very stark terms:

> the rise of the SSRIs fit hand in glove with this new unitary concept of depression: a single drug class for a single depression, as opposed to the many agents that had thrived before for a complexly layered notion of mood disorders. This Prozac-style drug class went on to drive all the competing drug classes, many of them more effective, from the stage. Thus the story ends in the triumph of a manifestly less effective class of drugs for a kind of illness, major depression, that was, essentially, a political artefact born of academic infighting.[46]

Naming of disease (as of other things of course, like names of medical products), has massive ramifications for business. But naming is also an ontological matter. Exploring the relationship between classification and objective truth is necessary though at the extremes one can end up either with an unhelpful conservatism or, at the other extreme, with either a refusal to accept the veracity or worth of any classificatory system, or else some bizarre arguments. As to the latter, to give one well-known example, it is absurd to deny the evidence that Pharaoh Rameses II died of tuberculosis, as Bruno Latour provocatively did for no other reason than that the microbial disease agent was unknown and unnamed until 1882.[47] We might call this the fallacy of the false anachronism. It implies also a failure to distinguish between discovery (revealing what is there) and invention (coming up with something that, ostensibly, is not) where such a distinction is very clearly warranted. Similarly, naming a certain internal secretion 'insulin' did not suddenly bring it into existence because a name had been coined for it or a concentrated form was placed in a glass container to treat diabetics for the first time. Try convincing a diabetic that insulin is socially constructed: that it did not exist until Banting and his colleagues isolated it and gave it to patients, therefore diabetics would not have needed it previously because you cannot suffer from being deficient in a non-existent substance when others are not suffering due to having this fictional thing in their bodies. It is true that in the early stages of discovery the name for something may be applied in an unclear and inaccurate fashion, embracing not just the 'right' substance but others that exist naturally in the same place which may or may not be closely related chemically. Arguably this is what happened with adrenaline (see Chapter 6). But the existence of something is independent of humans knowing they are there and giving them a name. Admittedly, things many people believe to exist and give a name to turn out not to — fairies for example. The history of medicine supports this counter-argument. There have been many 'things', physical and abstract that were thought to exist but were later proven not to. Moreover, human-devised classification systems are social constructs to a greater or lesser extent. So, if Latour seeks to shake us from our complacency, he may be playing a useful role. But diabetes, insulin, tuberculosis and the microbe that causes it and the drugs that treat it exist beyond any reasonable doubt.

Access including pricing and payment

In the United States, pharmaceutical companies face few restraints on their freedom to set prices of prescription medicines; or to advertise directly to the general public which is subject to light touch regulation officially under FDA oversight, and leads to a tendency to overprescribe, including the more expensive brand name medicines requested by patients. Reportedly, 'the average television viewer in the United States ... watches as many as nine drug advertisements per day and about 16 hours per year, far exceeding the time an average individual spends with his/her primary care physician.'[48] Although the FDA has imposed fines on misleading or dishonest advertising, the inadequacy of the agency's policing is evident from the finding that out of 97 advertisements surveyed '13% promoted off-label use of medications (which is banned by the FDA)'.[49] Off-label prescribing by physicians of medicines not approved for that particular use by the FDA is actually permitted. When supported by strong scientific and medical evidence it is quite normal and has in fact proven quite essential for certain health problems.[50] Nonetheless it is controversial in some respects[51] and the advertising ban makes a lot of sense.

It is hardly an exaggeration to say that US society is addicted to pharmaceuticals. That the industry pays vast sums of money every year on influencing politicians and even patient advocacy groups is surely a large part of the reason for this. The United States market has in fact been a huge success for the industry in terms of finding a huge base of repeat customers:

> Put simply, Americans are on drugs. The average American is prescribed and purchases somewhere between nine and thirteen prescription-only drugs per year, totalling over 4 billion prescriptions in 2011 and growing … Overall healthcare costs were over $2 trillion in 2011, prescription drugs accounting for about 10 percent, or $203 billion, of that amount.[52]

Admittedly, 'on drugs' sounds a little harsh given that medicines generally provide real health benefits, and, aside from the opiates and the benzodiazepines also currently being prescribed at very high levels,[53] most are not addictive. Nonetheless, this level of consumption seems excessive. Despite being probably the world's most innovative country in the biomedical sciences and biological technologies, the US does not rank particularly highly in healthiest nation indices, such as Bloomberg's Global Health Index. All this apparently high-quality and cutting-edge health interventionism, which admittedly is not available to all in that country, and that goes well beyond the prescribing of pills, is not making it the world's most healthy nation. It hardly needs to be said that the industry would love these rates of consumption — or more specifically the revenue thus generated based on well above averagely high prices — to be the global norm. There are US politicians who claim, rather quixotically, that paying the same prices elsewhere is only fair, otherwise the United States is effectively subsidising healthcare innovations for the rest of the world. Obviously, this view carries little weight outside of the Washington Beltway, and virtually none outside of the United States. Meanwhile, as mentioned in the Introduction, overall life expectancy rates there are currently falling.

Despite the wide availability of private health insurance and public insurance schemes to benefit the elderly, the poor, and children (Medicare, Medicaid and the Children's Health Insurance Program), about 30 million people are uninsured, and many others have inadequate cover leaving individuals responsible for high co-payments and deductibles (that is, the amount insured people must pay before the insurer picks up the rest of the tab). The uninsured are left to pay the full list price for the medicines they need. In consequence of the high cost of healthcare generally, including medicines, 'medical bankruptcy' is a known phenomenon and it is widespread. This is so even after the passage of legislation intended to alleviate the problem. Millions of other people struggle with barely affordable medical bills.[54]

On the plus side, the share of the market comprising generics is high by international standards. This is despite the fact market entry of generics can be slow due to regulatory and intellectual property barriers. Moreover, prices can fall as well as rise, and health insurers can negotiate discounts.

But none of this can be relied upon. The decision on whether to cut prices or engage in enhanced access schemes, which undoubtedly benefit many people, rests with individual companies. They are under no legal obligation. Elsewhere, the freedom of countries to set prices is much more constrained. However, there is no country in the world where limitations to full access to medicine is not a concern. We will return to this issue in Chapter 10.

Intellectual Property Rights as Regulation

From patent medicines to patents on medicines

Prior to the 1880s, the so-called 'patent medicines' — 'the first nationally available, branded, goods, sold at a fixed price, apart from books'[55] — were rarely patented. Their purveyors preferred to keep their compositions secret. Why was this? In England from the late eighteenth-century inventors were required to disclose their inventions, and subsequently, written disclosure became the norm elsewhere too. The process of acquiring a patent was difficult but the benefit of doing so was that a patent lent the product the stamp of official approval, or at least the product could be advertised in a way to convey that impression. (The fact that product safety regulations as they came into being also required the contents to be disclosed is of great significance as we will see.) On the other hand, the juridical infrastructure of the day made patent enforcement difficult. In addition, disclosure would reveal part or all of the secrecy, and secrecy was essential to the marketing strategy. Incomplete disclosure of course also makes it hard for judges to find infringement. According to Mackintosh,[56] 'using the approach adopted by the government to decide which medicines should be subject to excise duty, "patent medicines" can be defined as those which had an owner and a secret recipe, and were advertised. By 1830, over 1,300 such owned medicines were listed for excise duty'. Patent medicines, then, were very significant in terms of their abundance and the ways they were marketed but not because they were patented — up to 1830, 'only 117 medicines had ever been patented.'[57] Even during the peak period of medicine patenting, from 1740 to the beginning of the nineteenth century, the number registered per decade only exceeded 20 once.

One interesting pre-pharmaceutical industry patented product is worth mentioning in passing, showing how patenting and branding could, even in those earlier times, operate together — in this case with somewhat dubious intent. As is frequently the case today, as we will see. In 1753, Walter Leake received a patent titled 'Health restoring pill'. Leake was in fact a bookbinder who had cleverly taken advantage of sharing a surname with a certain Doctor John Leake. The latter had published a book concerning a treatment for venereal disease branded as the Lisbon Diet Drink and therefore had acquired a name for himself as an expert on the disease. Walter Leake's own widely-advertised concoction, branded as Leake's Pills, presumably attributed by many to the better known Dr Leake, claimed to have cured 40,000 people over a period of eight years albeit without the evidence that would be necessary today.[58] On the other hand,

Leake could not have obtained a trademark on his branded pills because trademark law did not emerge till the following century. Despite the impossibility of registering a mark such as a product name, litigation by sellers of patent medicines against those using their product names was sometimes successful. We should not be too surprised about this. The trade in remedies and the history of marketing and advertising go hand in hand. Branding has been essential to the medicines trade for centuries, and it still is (see below).

Patents

Patents are property rights that protect inventions typically for a maximum period of 20 years from the date the application was filed with a national or regional granting authority. Despite this attribution to actual persons, patents nowadays function in the modern economy as rather impersonal business assets; like stocks and shares they are a form of intangible capital and are frequently bought, sold, licensed, cross-licensed and pooled. They are typically owned by corporations. Patent licensing is very important for small firms which may be poorly placed to exploit their invention in the marketplace. As for large firms, some of them can amass huge revenues not just from generating new patent-protected products, but also by in-licensing others' potentially valuable inventions and from out-licensing patents to other firms more keenly interested in exploiting the inventions in the marketplace. It is the alienable nature of patents that enables them to function as currency in knowledge transactions. But if patent laws are essentially public policy instruments centred upon inventors and their inventions, how did this modern function and character emerge?

The way patents have been justified in different countries has always depended to some extent at least on the level of industrial development; and also to whom one speaks. Over the years, states have granted patents for a variety of public policy purposes such as to encourage the immigration of craftsmen, to reward importers of foreign technologies, to reward inventors, to create incentives for further inventive activity, to encourage the dissemination of new knowledge, and to allow corporations to recoup their investments in research and development. From a public policy perspective, each of these justifications is as legitimate as the others depending on a country's economic circumstances among other factors.[59] Nonetheless, as with other forms of intellectual property (especially copyright), justice-based arguments for stronger and better enforced rights are also frequently deployed, and such claims can carry strong moral force. After all, many people would consider it just as immoral for somebody to copy an inventor's useful new gadget and claim it as his or her own as to similarly misappropriate somebody's new novel, song or painting.

Patents for inventions have their origins in Renaissance Italy.[60] But the legislative development that shaped patent law for good came in 1624 with the passage of the English Statute of Monopolies.[61] In reality, its primary purpose was to prohibit monopolies rather than to promote invention, and in passing the law the government hoped to encourage continental craftsmen to settle in the country.[62] Monopoly grants were declared illegal except 'the true and first inventor or inventors' of 'any manner of new manufactures within this realm' as long as 'they be not contrary to the law, nor mischievous to the state, by raising prices of commodities at home, or hurt of trade, or generally inconvenient'. Such inventors could acquire a patent or grant allowing up to 14 years' monopoly protection. Strict novelty was not required since courts interpreted the purpose of granting patents as being to introduce new trades to England whether or not they were 'novel' elsewhere in the world.[63] It is unlikely to be entirely coincidental that at this time England was less advanced technologically than both France and the Netherlands.[64] The Statute was amended several times but its legal relevance persisted as late as 1977.

The original role of United States patent (and copyright) law was to implement Article 1 Section 8 of the Constitution, which empowers Congress 'to promote the Progress of Science and useful Arts, by securing for limited Times to Authors and Inventors the exclusive Right to their respective Writings and Discoveries.' US patent law, then, was not founded on a natural rights justification of intellectual property owner-ship. Rather, the granting of exclusive rights *for limited times* was regarded as being beneficial for the country in terms of scientific and cultural pro-gress. It was intended from the start that the patent system should be accessible to all classes of society and not just to the rich and well connected.[65] Soon after independence, two patent laws were enacted. A third law, the 1836 Patent Act,[66] was arguably the first modern patent law. It required all applications to be examined by the government patent office for novelty and usefulness. Although this law did not discriminate between US and foreign inventors with respect to the examination or the extent of rights granted, foreign applicants had to pay much higher fees, especially if they were British. Such discrimination was abolished in 1861 for nationals of countries whose laws were non-discriminatory towards Americans.

The German Patent Act (*Reichspatentgesetz*) of 1877 followed the US example by establishing an examination system. This made these two countries pioneers. Elsewhere, registration systems — which granted patents without the need to convince a specialist that the documentation submitted with the application described a genuine invention — were the norm. The term of protection was 15 years. In common with many countries today, it was possible to except inventions deemed contrary to public order or morality. Inventions regarding luxuries, medicines, articles of food, or chemical products were prohibited.

While national intellectual property regulations (in some countries) have existed for two or more centuries, the history of intellectual property at the international level really begins in the late nineteenth century with the formation in the 1880s of unions of mostly European countries for the protection of industrial property and literary and artistic works. Previously the only instruments for international protection had been based on bilateral commercial agreements involving, again, mostly European countries.[67]

The process of expanded international intellectual property regulation has continued since then to the extent of involving most countries of the world. Previously, countries were held to norms defined in a body of treaties administered by the World Intellectual Property Organization, a United Nations specialised agency established in 1970 to promote intellectual property globally. Countries were free to sign up to these treaties or not. Matters changed quite radically in 1995 when the World Trade Organization open its doors for the first time. Among the collection of agreements to be administered by the WTO and which were binding on all member states — which now includes almost all countries of the world including the EU, the United States, China, India, Brazil and Russia — is the Agreement on Trade-related Aspects of Intellectual Property Rights ('TRIPS' or 'the TRIPS Agreement'). TRIPS, which is administered by the Geneva-based World Trade Organization (WTO), is of special importance in that it establishes global minimum (and high) standards of protection and enforcement for virtually all the most important intellectual property rights such as patents, copyrights and related rights, and trademarks in one single agreement.[68,69] In a sense it compresses what was for today's developed countries about one hundred years of legal and regulatory evolution, into what was for many other countries an approximately ten-year catch-up period.

Whereas non-compliance with the provisions of WIPO treaties carries no legal consequences,[70] the WTO has a dispute settlement structure with teeth that can bite. A violation of the rules of TRIPS challenged by another WTO member can lead to a legally-binding instruction to change or withdraw the national legal provision in dispute. In the worst case, where the violating provision is not changed within a certain time-frame, the winning party may receive authorisation to withdraw trade benefits arising from the WTO legal order that all members are entitled; putting it another way, to discriminate against the losing party to an extent that is proportionate to the scale of the harms[71] to it resulting from the failure of the loser to comply. In reality, this is a weapon that the richer countries are much better placed to deploy than poorer ones.[72]

The relationship between patents and health is complex and constantly changes in response to numerous factors within and outside the law. These factors include legislative reform, court judgements, new business models, advances in science and technology, and new market conditions. The industry is often considered as the one that is most dependent on the patent system. This is due to two main factors.

The first concerns research and development. The costs are very high, and while there is much debate about the average costs, getting new drugs to market is undeniably an expensive and risky business that few companies can afford. To make things worse there is much uncertainty, and lots of money is lost to failures: drugs that turn out after clinical trials not to be effective or safe enough to be approved or that get approved but do not make enough money to recoup the research, development and marketing costs.

The second is that drugs can be copied by those with the requisite technical skill, equipment and resources. Upfront costs may be quite substantial, but the marginal cost of making such copied drugs tends to be very low. This would enable copiers, absent a patent law, to sell their versions at low cost and still make a profit due to their not having to pay any of the research and development costs.

Whether our health would be better or worse without a patent system is a fascinating question that would be difficult to answer. What we can say with a degree of confidence is that the industry would be very different without a patent law, and it would probably be less innovative absent of any alternative system to reward innovation such as funding schemes including those proposed to break the link between research and development costs and price. That said, much of the research is likely to have been paid by taxpayers. Moreover, innovations can come from public institutions that presumably do not require the incentive of, or market power to be gained from, a patent.

Of course, all innovations are not equal in quality or in terms of human welfare. Patent law does not, and never did, discriminate between them. Obviously, industry patents what it thinks it can make money from. Patents offer little in the way of additional incentive to develop an important medicine that would benefit only a small number of very poor people. They will not create a market if the target users have no ability to pay.

What do pharmaceutical companies patent? Nowadays, it is increasingly simplistic if not erroneous to think merely in terms of product and methods of making claims. What types of product and process claims are we talking about? What about uses? Clearly there is much more to patenting than claiming the active ingredient of a drug and the means by which it is produced. We will go into the specifics in Chapter 9, but before doing so one important matter needs to be discussed. Drugs often produce unexpected effects on patients. It might be presumed that all unanticipated side-effects are harmful. However, medical scientists have long known that the opposite can also be the case: side-effects can be good. A treatment for disease x may turn out to be an excellent treatment for similar diseases y and z, or even for more distantly related (or unrelated) diseases d and h. Viagra is an excellent example of this but there are many others. This is why research continues to be done on old drugs, both successful ones and failed ones, that is, natural or synthetic chemicals that were discovered, produced and tested but which failed to work well against drug targets known about at the time. As better knowledge of cell biology, genomics and proteomics increases the number of drug targets, there is a lot of interest in testing known substances against them in the hope of discovering new therapeutic applications. Nowadays this is referred to as drug repurposing.[73] There is much commercial interest in this. Discovering new uses of old drugs is much easier and less risky than discovering and developing new ones, and approval for new indications will be cheaper and most likely much quicker. Patent systems in many jurisdictions encourage such research by allowing claims on newly discovered medical uses of old chemical substances.

Compared to real property, the boundaries between one person's legally enforceable intellectual property and another person's tend to be extremely blurred and are more likely to overlap. Initially, the scope of a patent is determined through an examination by trained specialists. Later on, courts may decide to adjust the boundary line or even remove it by revoking it. Ideally, the 'fence' that is a patent claim 'should be no bigger than the thing you've invented. In particular, the fence shouldn't be extended to existing inventions that are quite close or the same'.[74] This requires patent examiners and the courts to place the fences in the right place so as to keep the invention from intruding, not just on inventions that are someone else's property, but on the public domain of knowledge that is nobody's property. But the intangible nature of intellectual property means this can be an extremely difficult task and a very expensive one. Consequently, users of the patent system must be prepared to spend a great deal of money. Acquiring a patent is expensive enough, but the costs of asserting it in the courts and defending it from competitors may be astronomical. This makes the system much more accessible to larger companies than to small firms and individuals. For this reason, and also because of the fuzzy nature of patent right boundaries, incentives exist for companies, especially the big ones, to perform various kinds of opportunistic behaviour. One can expect, for example, and anecdotal evidence lends credence to this, that large corporations may sometimes seek to free-ride on the intellectual property of smaller firms, independent inventors and other knowledge holders such as traditional healers in indigenous communities that cannot afford to take legal measures to stop them. They may speculatively accuse small businesses of infringing patents of possibly dubious validity, safe in the knowledge that these firms will be so frightened of legal action that they will agree to pay royalties and even withdraw their competing products from the market. Firms may deliberately file excessively broad patent claims in the hope that at least some of these will slip through the examination system and be allowed.

Patent 'systems,' and in fact intellectual property systems generally, can be quite complex and highly contested, comprising not just laws, regulations and the responsible government agencies for granting rights but also the courts, judges, patent attorneys and other legal practitioners, companies and business associations, political lobbyists, academics and public intellectuals, and consumer groups and other civil society organizations that keep the system running or that affect it in some way or another. Pharmaceutical companies and representative associations do not have identical views on patents, or on regulation more generally. Generics associations tend to have somewhat different perspectives to those of 'Big Pharma'. Strong patent rights protection may involve costs as well as benefits for many firms. One can expect generic pharmaceutical manufacturers to oppose extensions to patent terms for pharmaceutical products, and research-based firms, or at least companies that call themselves 'research-based',[75] to advocate against measures allowing generic companies to place their competing drugs on the market as soon as patents expire. Public sector researchers and even pharmaceutical corporations may be opposed to the patenting of basic research tools such as DNA sequences (which is probably why this matter came to be taken seriously by policymakers and patent offices). Even large firms must figure out how to balance their interests as patent owners with their interests in licensing those held by other institutions, and in navigating through what may be a veritable jungle of patents held by competitors, some of which may be extremely broad in scope and even of doubtful validity. Disparate economic power among interest groups may go a long way towards explaining which ones interact most advantageously with politicians and regulators.

National patent offices are the main implementation agencies. However, a number of regulatory spaces are available to be contested. These include patent offices, the government departments in which they are located, the politicians that oversee them, and the courts. But there may be others, such as competition regulators. Clearly, for any one interest group to capture the whole system outright, as opposed to one or more spaces within the system, would be very difficult. Financial clout may not be enough alone. This is where ideological consensus could play its part, often, albeit not necessarily, with positive consequences for industry.

Social scientist Shobita Parthasarathy in her recent comparative study of the United States and European patent systems claims that much of the difference between the two arises from her finding that the United States, uniquely, has what she calls a 'market making' ideology that presumes markets work best when they are left alone, as if free markets by themselves are inherently morally good. It follows that once government frames a system of property rights in inventions, owners should be allowed freely to enjoy them. Patents create markets in information embodied in new and useful things, and society benefits richly from this, so it is assumed. This ideology has not always gone unchallenged. For much of the twentieth century, courts were often suspicious of patents. Once in a while politicians and interest groups called for limitations on the monopoly power of patent owners. Nonetheless, Parthasarathy's claim is true. Perhaps this is due not just to pro-market ideology, but also to a long-standing and deep-seated popular patent culture. As economic historian Zorina Khan has shown us, the US patent system was for a long period quite democratic in the sense of being available to underprivileged individual inventors.[76] At the same time, Britain's patent system — and Charles Dickens's short story *A Poor Man's Tale of a Patent* (1850) amply corroborates this — was largely closed to the general public due to Byzantine bureaucratic obstacles and the high costs involved.

For Europe Parthasarathy coins the term 'market shaping' to capture a very different approach whereby markets, including the grant of property rights, in inventions are seen as requiring more regulatory oversight. Granting a patent is not a morally neutral act, and neither are free markets assumed automatically to produce social welfare-enhancing outcomes. Patents are an element of technology regulation. Thus we find that most European countries fund and support embryonic stem cell research, as does the European Commission, but that patents on related inventions necessarily involving the destruction of embryos are banned. In the United States, such inventions are patentable and this is not controversial even through the research itself *is* controversial. In contrast, the United Kingdom is quite permissive about stem cell research which many be conducted subject to being licensed by the Human Fertilisation and Embryology Authority, a statutory body; yet scientists there must still accept the inherent dignity of human blastocysts as a reason not to file a patent application for practices whose performance requires the destruction of human embryos that may have been done several years previously, and not by those doing the actual research (see Chapter 9).

Suffice it to say that all innovations are not equal in quality or in terms of human welfare and the patent law does not discriminate. Obviously, industry patents what it thinks it can make money from. Patents offer little in the way of additional incentive to develop an important medicine that would benefit only a small number of very poor people. They will not create a market if the target users have no ability to pay. We need to think also about the types of innovation the patent system is, or is not, incentivising and whether the system serves the public interest as well as it should. But the patent system can never be perfect even with a better balance between legal monopoly and public interest safeguards. We also need to come up with additional incentive mechanisms outside the patent system.

For all the reasons given earlier, the pharmaceutical industry has seen a need — and been given the opportunity — to claim a wide diversity of 'subjects', albeit not without limits, in their attempts to protect their investments and secure legal monopoly protection with as much comprehensiveness as the law allows. We will go into the finer points of all this in Chapter 9.

Trademarks and pharmaceutical name regulation

Previously, I coined the name of an imaginary concoction, 'Professor Dutfield's Amazing Anti-Pox Salts'. Had I lived in a time prior to the pharmaceutical industry I could have touted such a product and had I tricked enough people I might have been able to get rich from it. The importance to the public of one not being able to do such a thing or to get it approved as a pharmaceutical product for supply to the public directly or to patients by way of a physician or pharmacist is perhaps obvious. But the regulatory and property rules governing the rights and duties of producers in respect of what their products may be called, and how producers may use these rules to their commercial advantage, are rather specific to this particular industry and have evolved over time. The basic norms and practices were established from quite early in the industry's existence and therefore form one of its essential aspects.

How do pharmaceuticals get their names? Without knowing any better it might seem logical that as brand X denotes active ingredient chemical x, Y should be for y, and Z for z. Accordingly, Aspirin is acetylsalicylic acid, and nothing but ASA. ASA is Aspirin and that is the end of it. However, reality is so often different. To consider some examples, ibuprofen may be sold as Advil by some manufacturers, Nurofen by others, and alternatively as just plain ibuprofen. Losec, Prilosec and Nexium are all used for the same active ingredient. Sildenafil may be marketed as sildenafil, as Viagra or as Revatio. Zantac used to be just a drug but is now also a medical device made of something completely different.

What rules apply to drug-naming? Can companies call their drugs anything they like? Who gets to use which names, and how is this decided? What advantages do companies get from being able to name their products? And how does the naming of products relate to market regulation and the interest of the public and health professionals prescribing or supplying them? This is a key area of interaction between regulation and commercial law that tells us much about the industry. Even from the perspective of business, which of course includes both firms that develop original products and those selling generics, this is not just a commercial issue, but also a regulatory one.

Branding and marketing

In 1888, Bayer's drug Phenacetin first came on the market. It is sometimes claimed that the product, a modified form of a coal tar-based waste product, was the first modern pharmaceutical; not just in the way that science was applied to its discovery and development, but also in the way it was marketed. The basis for this claim is that 'for the first time, a drug had been conceived, developed, tested, and marketed, all by a private company'. As such, and admittedly this is a rather grand statement, 'it marked the creation of the modern drug industry, the marriage of science and business that has transformed this century, making huge profits even as it saves lives'.[77] Phenacetin also represents an early instance of trademark use in the marketing of a pharmaceutical product with known ingredients that was placed on the market to compete against another branded product, one that was not identical but was similar in its chemistry: namely, Kalle's Antifebrin. The latter was a form of aniline whose antipyretic properties were discovered by complete accident.[78] Antifebrin was likewise marketed under its brand name in competition not just with Phenacetin but with chemically identical unbranded products. So, it was from day one an unoriginal product whose sole diffentiating feature was its name. This business strategy was adopted because processes to manufacture the substance were well-known and therefore unpatentable. It succeeded because so many physicians wrote down the brand name on prescriptions rather than the chemical term of acetanilid even though Kalle charged a higher price than its competitors.[79]

We will see in the next chapter how the pharmaceutical industry became research based and that this is one (albeit not the only) defining feature of this industry. Not all pharmaceutical firms invest in research and development to any great extent. Those which exclusively sell generic medicines certainly do not. But the industry as a whole does plough back a pretty substantial amount of sales revenues into research, some of which leads to the development of new medicines. Start-up firms without products obviously have nothing to sell. These businesses must of necessity acquire external funding for research that they hope will lead to products somewhere down the line.

We will also see that the commercial side is every bit as important to firms' success as research, development and manufacturing. Accordingly, while vast amounts of money are spent on research and development (as the industry constantly reminds us), much also goes on the full range of commercialisation activities: advertising, sponsorship, lobbying, hiring and deploying sales representatives, acquiring, using and managing intellectual property rights, and so on. Some at least of the pharmaceutical industry's marketing activities and strategies are specific to the sector. Actions aiming to maximise sales of pharmaceutical products are both similar and different to those employed to enhance the purchase figures for chocolate bars, soap bars, buses and Airbuses.

A few drugs are guaranteed first-in-class life-savers that cure serious disease, keep large numbers of people alive who would otherwise be dead, or otherwise provide substantial relief from suffering, and have no substitutes. But most are not such essential high-stakes products. Whether or not they are essential in any such respects, they are unlikely to be alone in the market even if there is not necessarily a great deal of competition. They may be much better than alternative treatments, just a bit better, or they may be inferior. Some people may get no benefit whatsoever from taking one, whereas others might find the same drug to be highly efficacious. The latter might be due to a genuine pharmacological effect or it could be a placebo response. This matters a lot because marketing strategy can do much to build goodwill in a particular product. Positive views about a branded drug (and perhaps branded drugs generally) seem likely to increase the possibility of placebo effects and there is experimental evidence bearing this out.[80]

For the industry placebo effects have both advantages and disadvantages. Discussion on their implications for public health raises numerous issues. From a *commercial* perspective, placebo effects may be a highly significant factor in how marketing can benefit firms or not. One experiment found that people responded better to a dummy pill said to cost $2.50 than others given the same pill costing, as they were informed, only 10 cents.[81] Similarly, some patients report poorer health when switched from a brand name drug to a generic version.[82] It is important to note here that such is the psychological power of 'the drug' itself that offering a placebo 'packaged' as a tablet has been proven in an experiment involving giving some people no treatment for irritable bowel syndrome and others the placebo to have positive health effects even when patients were informed they were getting 'placebo pills made of an inert substance, like sugar pills, that have been shown in clinical studies to produce significant improvement in IBS symptoms through mind-body self-healing processes'.[83] So perhaps we should not feel too sceptical about reports of people benefiting from apparently ritualistic modes of healthcare in indigenous communities, nor feel too superior about biomedicine to the extent we uncritically treat it as a wholly science- and evidence-based system that has shed all ritualistic aspects.[84]

The fact that a useless pill for something or other can be 'better' than nothing, and that a branded expensive pill with no inherent superiority over the cheaper unbranded alternatives can obtain higher patient satisfaction is of course good for business. It incentivises both brand-based marketing and the pharmaceuticalisation of society exemplified by Ritalin (see above). These placebo effect studies are of course quite recent, but they merely confirm what marketing people have assumed to be true anyway, probably for as long as the industry has existed, hence the priority given to marketing strategy from the start. Marketing is about so much more than just bringing new products to the attention of customers. It is also about persuasion: the art of 'talking up' products, making people believe they *should* buy them, that they should accept no substitutes, and that they are better than they really are. Although pharmaceutical marketing regulations in most countries can be quite restrictive, the pharmaceutical industry is no less dedicated to the art of persuasion than other business sectors if not more so in many cases.

This is not to say the industry always has it easy in this regard. Placebo effects are a two-edged sword. Experimental evidence using clinical trial data from 1990 to 2013 has shown that for painkillers, placebo effects are stronger, and actually getting stronger still, in the United States than in European and Asian countries. At the same time, actual drug responses have not improved during the period surveyed. Other factors, especially changes in the design of clinical trials may be more significant, but a plausible explanation may also lie in the fact that only the US — and New Zealand — allow companies to advertise their prescription drugs directly to consumers.[85] 'So it's possible that hearing the lofty promises pledged by pharmaceutical firms in these ads may have increased consumer expectation of the potential efficacy of any old drug handed to them by a person in a lab coat'.[86] Strong placebo effects have also been identified with antidepressants, though how these effects are manifested is somewhat confusing. One Harvard study on antidepressants found marginal differences in effect between the taking of a placebo and the actual drug.[87] Both helped a significant number of people, but the latter wasn't helping them a great deal more than the former. An Oxford University study, using a different methodology, however, found a big difference in response between the antidepressant and the placebo, in favour of the former.[88]

This situation is of course something of a headache for industry. Perhaps the industry is being hoist by its own petard — over-advertising plus the placebo effect leading ironically to a *reduced* difference in response to the real drug and the fake, making the former effectively ever more redundant. If so, perhaps the solution for the industry is a bigger commitment to innovation and a reduced one to marketing. On the other hand, one public health expert suggests an approach that, if widely acted upon, would be even less convenient for the industry: 'If the major component of a drug in any particular condition is its placebo component, we need to develop non-pharmacological interventions as a first-line response'.[89] Nonetheless, like all addictions, drug-taking alongside the 'epidemics' of mass-scale prescribing and healthcare interventionism have not been contained in the United States.

Given such competitive market conditions, what do companies do to get the purchaser or prescriber to select this drug rather than that one? Or even to prescribe something at all as opposed to advising the patient to take the day off work, exercise more, quit smoking, drink less, deal with the discomfort, or whatever? One product might be markedly superior and be acknowledged as such on the basis of impartial scientific results. Physicians may choose on the basis of treatment guidelines and policies drawn up by experts with no stake in any particular product. But there is much that companies do to influence what the individual person swallows. As we will see trademarks have always been a very important element of companies' marketing strategy.

Although this situation may be starting to change, it remains mostly true that in few cases is there a single treatment that actually works for a specific disease. As long as the drug is under patent protection, the owner is a monopolist in the legal sense. Once it is approved and enters the market, the seller has the benefit of a commercial monopoly, though the strength of the monopoly can vary widely according to whether or not substitutes exist. However, many non-fatal ailments can be treated by other means than by a pharmaceutical product: a good rest perhaps, or simply leaving one's immune system to do its work without chemical aids. The last time I had a headache I decided to go without my usual ibuprofen treatment, opting instead to just ignore the headache till it went away. Had I opted for pills I could have taken generic ibuprofen, the ibuprofen branded medicine Nurofen which is popular despite costing quite a lot more, or else Aspirin or paracetamol or some combination. How about something potentially more serious but not usually life-threatening in itself? I was found recently to have somewhat elevated blood pressure. My doctor prescribed captopril, a so-called ACE inhibitor. I tried them but discontinued pretty quickly, I hope wisely. For more necessary treatments than for headache, the physician may prescribe one branded drug or another using this or that name, or else may write down the generic version using the non-proprietary name. Sometimes there is only one drug for a particular condition. But often there are several. It may be that one is generally acknowledged to be the best and that this has been proven beyond reasonable doubt. However, powerful marketing strategy may lead people to believe drug χ is the best one but it may be that drug χ is *not* better than its competitors (which may include an earlier version of χ). However, the marketing of χ under a new catchy name and publicising its 'superior' qualities may have influenced patient preferences and prescribing and purchasing decisions. As we just saw, it may also affect patients' experiences when taken.

The law and business of sameness, similarity and difference

Central to any marketing strategy is to have a good name for the product, one which directs those purchasing drugs to that product and not to alternative ones. Two closely related but different questions arise. First, are the 'same' products sold under different names precisely interchangeable? And second, are equivalent products with the same active ingredients, but that are differently named, also interchangeable? The first question concerns whether the brand name and the generic name point to the same thing no more nor less. The answer is 'not necessarily'. The generic name is for the active ingredient, not the specific formulation. Tablets contain other chemicals selected, mixed and processed in certain physical forms and proportions with a view to effective admission into the body, transport to its place of dissolution and action, potency, speed and duration of therapeutic effect, and stability. Indeed, the active pharmaceutical ingredient typically comprises less than 10 percent of the drug. So in a sense the generic name and the brand name may not be referring to precisely the same thing: the generic name refers to active ingredient A, whereas the brand name coined (and normally trademarked) actually covers not A alone, but A + B + C etc. in prescribed proportions. This leads to the second question. The generic may well also contain B + C etc. and in the same proportions. But this is by no means certain. For example, it might be that the formulation is under patent after the patent on the active molecule has expired. If so the generic maker cannot offer the drug in the same formulation. Accordingly, it is possible that the patient experience will vary to some extent whether she takes the brand name drug or the generic equivalent as a consequence of the active ingredient being mixed with other chemicals that are not the same.

In this industry names matter hugely, as they always have done. The strategic nature of naming in the pharmaceutical industry tells us much about the pharmaceutical industry and its sustained commercial success as a business sector. The wider regulatory environment on the naming of chemicals and active ingredients of drugs is the context that made strategic naming effective in the marketplace. But business strategy here is in large part dependent on trademark law. However, unlike the patent system, the trademark system has not evolved, or been made to evolve, as the industry has done. Admittedly, the scope of trademark law has expanded to embrace shape, sounds and smells. Such changes have become more important in pharmaceutical branding strategy nowadays (see Chapter 9). In bringing us up to date, using the example of the market in drugs for headaches and mild fevers, the rest of this chapter testifies to this point.

In one sense, there is only one of everything. There are countless numbers of H_2O molecules in the Atlantic Ocean, as there are of hydrogen atoms in the universe. Every one of those is the same if by sameness we mean that they are all identical to each other so that one can stand for another and it makes no difference whatsoever. But in another way, each is different. In what sense is this true? Because every one of those water molecules is an individual. The fact they are indistinguishable is irrelevant. This fact is clear when we think of human twins. They may be genetic copies of each other and very hard to distinguish visually. Nonetheless, they are obviously two separate people.

But often there is a degree of variability among a class of things that many would assume still to be identical to each other. Even twins and cloned animals are slightly different but that is not what I am getting at here. What about single chemicals? This can get tricky. Is a form or variant of a chemical the same thing as that chemical? Or is it something else entirely? What about drugs? We will consider these questions in Chapter 9.

Commercially there is much at stake in the ability of a company to control the borderlines between sameness and difference, and much effort is made to 'impose' differentiation in various ways and through different means:

> Over the past few decades, critics of generic drugs have repeatedly sought new forms of information to differentiate the manufacturing processes of generic drugs from their brand-name counterparts. As controversies over brands and generics have continued, the number of proofs of difference — and protocols for proving similarity — have continued to expand.[90]

Stated plainly, an originator firm seeks as far as the rules allow to achieve a demarcation of the same-different border so that whatever the generic producer would seek to market is either on the wrong side and is therefore significantly different, or else is perceived as being so. The intention is that the generic drug be deemed a poor substitute or not a genuine substitute at all. The originator firm will also try to present its follow-on product, which might in fact chemically be very similar, as being a wholly different thing for marketing and patenting purposes. But it might want to present it as something similar for the benefit of the regulators. For a generic firm's part, it would seek to oppose any move to prevent its equivalent product from being regarded as being different in any substantive sense from the original product (excepting of course the far lower price). However, and here things get even more interesting, a generic seller might see an advantage in marketing its own drugs as being different from identical competing products in order to charge higher prices. Hence we have generic ibuprofen sold as Ibuprofen, and as the pricier Nurofen.

Some over-the-counter branded products muddy the waters of clarity as far as content goes. I tend to think of Alka-Seltzer as a single product, appealingly effervescent, good for hangovers, and containing three active ingredients including Aspirin. But in fact the name Alka-Seltzer is applied to a diverse range of formulations aimed at relieving the various symptoms of colds, headaches, upset stomachs, general body aches and pains, and so on. But at least in every Alka-Seltzer container one will find the same active contents, albeit in different forms and combinations. Anadin (or Anacin in North America), an analgesic launched in Britain in 1932 and currently sold by Pfizer, is far more diverse in terms of what the products contain. Different Anadin products may consist of aspirin[91] and caffeine, paracetamol, aspirin and caffeine, or ibuprofen. At least the contents are clearly labelled and the product range tends to be distinguished by additional words and phrases, often separately trademarked. For example, in recent years Bayer has been selling Alka-Seltzer products specifically for treating hangovers: Alka-Seltzer Morning Relief and Alka-Seltzer Wake-Up Call!

To what extent does pharmaceutical regulation concerning the naming of drugs assist or obstruct the pharmaceutical industry in pursuing its name-based marketing strategy? In fact, beyond trademark law the naming of products has been a subject of both national and international regulation. Such efforts began even before the industry existed, though they only really bore fruit once industrial fine chemistry including in the medical field had emerged.

The nineteenth century advances in chemistry lead to the synthesis of vast numbers of chemical compounds as well as a far more sophisticated appreciation of the complexity of natural chemicals and of their structures, actions and interactions. These rendered obsolete the naming rules formulated by late nineteenth century French chemists, the best-known being Lavoisier.[92] However there was no single logical method by which every substance could be represented textually or graphically in a way that was comprehensible and systematic to all those needing to know what a particular chemical was and how to communicate its features to others. As for names of drugs, there could be immense confusion. Drugs might have many names in a single country, many more across different nations. From the earliest days of the pharmaceutical industry it became necessary to have a shared system of non-proprietary chemical and drug nomenclature.

Regarding chemical nomenclature, the lead really came from chemists themselves rather than companies or governments. The first effort to cooperate internationally on standard setting was headed in 1860 by August Kekulé, who contributed much to understanding of chemical structure, and famously discovered the structure of benzene following a daydream in which he imagined a snake biting its own tail. The *Congrès de Nomenclature Chimique* of the International Commission for the Reform of Chemical Nomenclature took place in Geneva in 1892. One of numerous instances of international cooperation in the late nineteenth century as Europe approached the end of the (arguably mythical) 'long peace'[93] following Waterloo, the meeting adopted 62 resolutions aimed at furthering the standardisation of chemical nomenclature. It was attended by delegates from various European countries: Austria, Belgium, Britain, France, Germany, Italy, Romania and Switzerland.[94] However, it was not until after the First World War that standardisation could be promoted by an effective institutional structure. In 1919 the International Union of Pure and Applied Chemistry (IUPAC) was established, which exists to this day. A federation of national organisations, headquartered in Zurich, its Interdivisional Committee on Nomenclature and Symbols remains the world-recognised authority in the area of naming elements and compounds. All drugs have an IUPAC-compliant name as well as their other names. There never can be just one. To give an example, Zantac, whose generic name is ranitidine, has the IUPAC denomination of N-(2-[[(5-[(dimethylamino) methyl]furan-2-yl)methylthio]ethyl)-N'-methyl-2-nitroethene-1,1-diamine; dimethyl [(5-{[(2-{[1-(methylamino)-2-nitroethenyl]amino} ethyl)sulfanyl]methyl}furan-2-yl)methyl]amine. Obviously this is something of a mouthful signifying nothing to the non-chemist. No pharmacist, doctor or patient is going to prepare, prescribe, request or purchase it under that name. As one might expect, the system is able to accommodate small differences. Thus, omeprazole (Losec) is 6-methoxy-2-[(4-methoxy-3,5-di-methylpyridin-2-yl)methanesulfinyl]-1*H*-1,3-benzodiazole,   whereas AstraZeneca's follow-up drug esomeprazole (Nexium), an enantiomer, is (S)-5-Methoxy-2-[(4-methoxy-3,5-dimethylpyridin-2-yl)methylsulfinyl]-3*H*-benzoimidazole. Unless you are a chemist, you can be forgiven for failing to spot the difference. Needless to say, the system tells us nothing about whether those subtle differences have any therapeutic significance or not. Even less does it give any hints as to whether it is in a company's interests to claim the two as two different things, or as one thing happening to have a level of variation. That is not a matter for science but for business — as well as regulation.

International efforts to standardise the naming of drugs took a much longer time in coming, and only really began from the mid 1940s, another period of international cooperation as was the 1880s, this time following a world war. This period saw the foundation of the United Nations and the Bretton Woods institutions, and the proclamation of the Universal Declaration of Human Rights. The standardisation of pharmaceutical nomenclature was largely initiated by the World Health Organization (WHO), itself founded in 1948, and the American Medical Association. The outcome is the WHO-administered list of non-proprietary names (INNs). These are generic names which are simplified and systematised, and are nobody's property: they cannot be trademarked.

As has been known since the days of Phenacetin and Antifebrin, there are two ways to market a 'new' product. One can advertise it as something new and better than anything we have seen before, which it might even be. Alternatively, one can convey a false impression that it is new and better than what we have now. The industry employs both methods. In order to make such strategies possible, it helps a lot if the legal and regulatory regimes provide an effective, whether or not intended, 'zone of exclusion' to keep out usurpers, that is, rival companies with products that are in competition or that could compete if permitted to approach this zone. Unsurprisingly, from its very start intellectual property rights laws have been essential to how the industry does its business.

The need to name a product with an attractive name in the market-place is fundamental to business strategy, no more so than in the pharmaceutical industry which is one of the biggest users of trademarks. The

German pharmaceutical industry led the way in its sophisticated use of intellectual property including trademarks. There is of course much at stake commercially, but naming products, including natural ones, has wider importance in terms equally of science, business and intellectual property protection. Attribution, credit, priority and property claims are strengthened when individuals or a company establish an association between themselves and a 'thing' they have discovered or brought into existence in a sufficiently 'real' manner to be claimed. One of the best ways to construct that association is to devise a name. Not any old name but one that sticks. Zantac, for example, has been hugely effective enabling it to be used quite creatively. It used to be *solely* the brand name for the medicine whose generic name is ranitidine — no more nor less. The name has been acquired by another company and the use of the name has undergone a shift (see above and Chapter 9).

Clearly we cannot rely on a trademark to inform us of what something is as if it signifies a single thing, is the only way to signify that thing, and as if it means only the thing and not something else too. This point serves to remind us that the 'name' is of crucial importance, and that the industry has always understood this. From the start, drug companies had a commercial incentive to encourage the generic adoption of complicated chemical names and nomenclature for drugs, leaving their products with much simpler more memorable ones. Why? For one thing, physicians would be more inclined to write down a brief and easy to spell brand name on the prescription if the chemical name were especially complicated. Second, in some cases it allowed for a certain product differentiation that could be advantageous once the patent had expired. Thus Bayer came up with the generic name 'monoacetic acide ester of salicylic acid' in the United States, 'the theory being that few American physicians would ever remember such a complicated term or know that it was the same thing as acetylsalicylic acid. Most would continue to put "Aspirin" down on their prescription pads just as they always had.'[95]

Notes

1   Braithwaite and Drahos (2000).
2   Arikha *op, cit.*, 252.
3   Lee (2012).
4   Ravetz (1971), 64.

5 Arikha *op. cit.*, 302.
6 Intriguingly this applies also to European rules concerning traditional agricultural products and foods. The *European Council Regulation (EC) No 1151/2012 of 21 November 2012 on quality schemes for agricultural products and foodstuffs* provides that such a good can be labelled as a Traditional Speciality Guaranteed. 'Traditional' means having 'proven usage on the domestic market for a period that allows transmission between generations; this period is to be at least 30 years.'
7 Caulfield (2016).
8 Goldacre *op. cit.*
9 WTO, (2000).
10 Engelberg (1999), 390.
11 *Ibid.*, 392.
12 *Ibid.*
13 Bouchard *et al.* (2011).
14 *FTC v. Actavis, Inc.*, 570 U.S. (2013).
15 Miller (2015).
16 For a critical commentary on the European Commission's more assertive approach, see Straus (2016).
17 T-472/13 — Lundbeck v. European Commission.
18 For discussion, see Unni (2015).
19 *Bayer* MANU/DE/0316/2010.
20 For a discussion on the relationship between intellectual property and competition law in the health context, see Yu (2016).
21 The relative lowness of the barrier is implied in a 1968 US government estimate that for every sale dollar earned, only 2.5 cents was devoted to 'quality control', as compared to 9 cents on research and as much as 20 cents on promotion. United States Department of Health, Education and Welfare (1968), 13, quoted in Silverman and Lee (1974), 29.
22 Bouchard *op cit.*, 408–9.
23 Buick (2019).
24 DeGrandpre (2006).
25 Its official chemical name is a great deal longer than this.
26 And yet nothing is impossible in this regard. Lithium carbonate which is now the standard treatment for bipolar disorder and on the World Health Organization's list of essential medicines, actually *was* developed in a kitchen by one John Cade, an Australia psychiatrist. The urine samples with added lithium that he used for experiments were stored in his home fridge. Brown (2019).

27   Marley (2000).
28   Haynes (1999); Cochrane (1972).
29   Some types of patient may not have been studied in a clinical trial, e.g. children, the elderly, or those suffering other sicknesses.
30   Select Committee on Patent Medicines (1914).
31   *Ibid.*
32   Abraham (2002), 224–9.
33   Harrison (1986), 6.
34   Quirke (2013) *op cit.*, 154; Marks *op cit.*, 230.
35   Dumit (2012), 23.
36   *See* Sneader (1985), 87. Carl Djerassi, the renowned steroid chemist, went further, suggesting aspirin might not have even been developed in the first place. He pointed out that aspirin causes birth defects in various animals but only rarely in humans. Since new drugs must now be tested on animals, most companies would likely have dropped aspirin as a potential drug candidate. Djerassi (2001), 282–3.
37   Quirke (2013), *op cit.*, 154.
38   On the other hand, in the US at least, there was a plunge in the number of fixed-ratio combination products. These had formed the majority of new products. The decline started in the late 1950s, and then dropped quite dramatically. Whether regulation caused this is arguable. Silverman and Lee (1974), 39.
39   The EMA was founded in January 1995. Initially known as the European Agency for the Evaluation of Medicinal Products, or alternatively the European Medicines Evaluation Agency, its name was changed in 2004 to European Medicines Agency. Previously, the EU Committee on Proprietary Medicinal Products served to assess new medicines and recommend their approval. Now known as the Committee for Medicinal Products for Human Use (CHMP), it continues to operate, but within the EMA.
40   Greene (2019).
41   Marquand *et al.* (2016).
42   Allison (2008), 517.
43   Richter (2014) 291–3.
44   It means 'black bile'.
45   Kirsch (2014).
46   Shorter (2009), 10. There is continued debate about the effectiveness (or otherwise) of SSRIs. However, there does appear to be an emerging consensus that while they can reduce severe depression in some people and on balance may be beneficial, physicians should be cautious about prescribing

them for milder cases. Wilson (2018). However, DeGrandpre is highly critical, arguing that their positive impacts are mostly placebo in nature, and that for some people they are highly dangerous, being linked to self-harm including suicide and murder. See also Healy (2004, 2012). If so, the approval of SSRIs represents a gross failure of the regulatory system.

47 'The attribution of tuberculosis and Koch's bacillus to Ramses II should strike us as an anachronism of the same calibre as if we had diagnosed his death as having been caused by a Marxist upheaval, or a machine gun, or a Wall Street crash. Is it not an extreme case of "whiggish" history, transplanting into the past the hidden or potential existence of the future?'. Latour (2000), 248.

48 Parekh and Shrank (2018).

49 *Ibid.*

50 Dresser and Frader (2009).

51 Hamzelou (2019), 36–7.

52 Dumit, *op cit.*, 2.

53 Hamzelou (2020).

54 Himmelstein *et al.* (2019). For a rigorous examination of the problem of health inequality in the United States, its underlying causes, and its tragic consequences, see Case and Deaton (2020).

55 Mackintosh *op. cit.*, 542.

56 *Ibid.*, 542.

57 *Ibid.*

58 Macgregor (1955) Eighteenth-century V.D. publicity. *British Journal of Venereal Diseases* 31: 117–18.

59 For an interesting discussion of how the justifications of patents have evolved over time, see Lai (2017).

60 Kaufer (1980), 5–6.

61 Officially, '*An act concerning monopolies and dispensions with penal laws and the forfeitures thereof*'.

62 MacLeod (1991), 891.

63 A 1602 court case (Darcy v. Allin) determined that 'the introducer of a new trade into the realm, or of any engine tending to the furtherance of a trade, is the inventor' (in Webster 1844:756). A 1691 patent dispute (Edgeberry v. Stephens) clarified that

> if the invention be new in England, a patent may be granted though the thing was practised beyond the sea before; for the statute speaks of new manufactures within this realm; so that if they be

new here, it is within the statute; for the Act intended to encourage new devices useful to the kingdom, and where learned by travel or study, it is the same thing. (in Hayward (1987), 118).

64   Cornish (1999), 111.

65   Khan (2005).

66   Officially titled 'An act to promote the progress of useful arts, and to repeal all acts and parts of acts heretofore made for that purpose'.

67   A total of 69 bilateral industrial property-related conventions to protect the rights of foreigners were signed between 1859 and 1883. *See* Ladas (1930), 54–57. All parties to these conventions were either European, North American or Latin American, but the vast majority were European countries.

68   These also include geographical indications, industrial designs, layout-designs of integrated circuits, and protection of undisclosed information (trade secrets). Among the few IP rights excluded from TRIPS are utility models and plant breeders' rights (although plant varieties must be protected whether through patents or by an alternative system such as UPOV-style PBRs, or a combination thereof).

69   Prior to the TRIPS Agreement, the main IP conventions played the biggest role in the world wide adoption of national IP systems sharing common standards. However, the conventions still allowed these systems to vary widely. So when 33 developing countries joined the Paris Convention for the Protection of Industrial Property and 25 joined the Berne Convention for the Protection of Literary and Artistic Works during the 1960s and 70s, this did not mean that national IP systems would begin to look like each other. In fact, because these new members were allowed to have a say in the further development of the conventions, harmonization was unlikely to go too far if it meant they would have to adopt high standards of protection before they thought they were ready.

70   Although diplomatic consequences are certainly possible.

71   Or in legal terminology, the 'nullification or impairment'.

72   For more on TRIPS, see Braithwaite and Drahos (2000); Correa (2007, 2010); Deere (2008); Dutfield and Suthersanen (2020); Kennedy (2016); Sell (2003); UNCTAD-ICTSD (2003, 2005). On the particular challenges for developing countries with respect to the dispute settlement system: Shaffer and Meléndez-Ortiz (2010).

73   Cragg *et al.* (2014); Mullard (2012).

74   Aharonian, quoted in Stix (2001).

75 As Marcia Angell, former editor of the *New England Journal of Medicine* rather cynically puts it: 'Big pharma likes to refer to itself as a "research-based industry," but it is hardly that. It could best be described as an idea-licensing, pharmaceutical formulating and manufacturing, clinical testing, patenting and marketing industry.' *See* Angell (2004), quoted in Mirowski (2007).

76 Khan *op cit.*

77 Mann and Plummer (1991), 23.

78 Armstrong (1935), 1023.

79 Mann and Plummer *op. cit.*, 22–3.

80 Faase *et al.* (2013). Placebo responses have been observed in a range of product types, not just pharmaceuticals, suggesting in many cases that pricing and branding can influence consumers' expectations which in turn affects their consumption experience. So there is nothing remarkable about finding that placebo responses do occur among users of pharmaceutical products. Borsook and Becerra (2005); Shiv, Carmon and Ariely (2005).

81 Waber, Shiv, Carmon and Ariely (2008).

82 Winslow (2008).

83 Kaptchuk *et al.* (2010).

84 Ehrenreich (2018).

85 Tuttle *et al.* (2015).

86 Dahl (2015).

87 Kirsch *op cit.*

88 Cipriani *et al.* (2018).

89 Marchant (2015).

90 Greene (2014) *op. cit.*, 15.

91 In this context, aspirin is an ingredient not a branded product, hence the lower-case initial letter.

92 Guyton de Morveau, Lavoisier, Berthollet and de Fourcroy (1787). For a critical discussion on the *Méthode* in its contemporary context, see Simon (2002).

93 Anderson (2007).

94 The resolutions were published in an issue of the *Bulletin de la Société Chimique* (1892) vol. 8, series 3.

95 Jeffreys (2004), 96.

Part 2

Antecedents, Origins, and the Emergence of a New Industry

Chapter 4

Cells, Germs, Receptors, and Magic Bullets: From Ancient to Modern Theories of the Body, Disease, Drugs, and Drug Action

Introduction

In Part 1, I looked into how this new industry broke with the past enabling us, albeit with some difficulty, to view the industry as something different to what was there before, and what currently exists in health product provision, namely traditional, alternative and complementary medicine – as we call them today. The first two chapters cast doubt that the science of pharmaceuticals captures all of what the pharmaceutical industry is, does, and stands for. It might well be the 'science-based industry' it claims to be, one that comes up with products that improves lives like no other, but that does not sum up what it is that makes it special, distinctive or otherwise interesting. This is not meant to deny the role and importance of science and scientists and their life-enhancing products. Without question, the industry did — and of course still does — tap into scientific advances and new theories coming out of university and hospital laboratories that were and remain essential to science-based pharmaceutical discovery and commercial production and sale. And as we will see, the industry has contributed scientific advances of its own albeit often in collaboration with scientists working elsewhere. But we need a much more rounded and detailed approach which this part of the book aims to provide. Here we start with the science; the coming chapters will fill in the remaining gaps.

This chapter first maps out the state of the relevant arts of the time just preceding the industry's beginning. In so doing it seeks to address this question: how far, and in what ways, had the medical sciences progressed to that point in time? It then goes on to identify specific fields of scientific advance which made it possible for the industry to exist, to get started, and to grow into something like what we have today. This part of the chapter is organised around seven individuals. The purpose is not to single out these particular people as 'founding fathers' of the industry, nor am I seeking to construct, or to justify, a 'great man' version of pharmaceutical history which places excessive weight on the acts of a small number of males to the exclusion of everybody else. I appreciate my selectivity might make it seem that way, but I hope the reader can accept my disclaimer. I focus on these people as a way to organise the narrative around times, places, institutions and people in a way that makes sense in the present context whilst applying a human touch to the narrative. In my view, most great innovations stem from the wisdom of small crowds, building on the ideas of other and earlier small crowds. Often the first one to discover, invent, or think something turns out not to be first but the second or third, or else to be one of a group not necessarily more brilliant than other members but who, by dint of good fortune, self-promotion, friends in high places, patent acquisition, litigation, or by other means, happen to be accorded the credit.[1] Nothing in this chapter including praise accorded to certain people should be used to undermine what I believe to be the essential validity of this point.

The Evolving State of the Arts — From Early Modern Era to the Nineteenth Century

For pharmaceutical science to even start to become a true science with industrial application, reliable insights, effective approaches and insightful theories needed to be developed. Such scientific advances shed much necessary light on the functioning of living systems, and on how to discover and manufacture substances affecting these systems in controlled ways generating therapeutic effects on the human body. Let us start with a brief survey of what European science had achieved by the mid-nineteenth century before turning to those achievements most relevant to what became the pharmaceutical industry.

A number of discoveries in the new and in some ways overlapping sciences of biology and chemistry, starting from the late eighteenth century, finally refuted some very long-held misconceptions that were holding back these sciences from emulating the amazingly steep learning curve achieved in sixteenth and seventeenth century astronomy, mathematics and physics. Alchemy, which Newton himself practiced, was discredited and became mostly a matter for ridicule.[2] Though not particularly relevant to this book, the great chain of being concept, whose essential tenets dated back to ancient Greece,[3] was replaced eventually by modern taxonomy and evolution through natural selection thanks to Carl Linnaeus (1707–1778), Charles Darwin (1809–1882), and the underrated Alfred Russel Wallace (1823–1913).[4]

Experimental evidence virtually disproving spontaneous generation in macroscopic life was published by Francesco Redi in 1668 in his book *Experienze intorno alla generzione degl'insetti*. (Disproof of spontaneous generation of microbes took two more centuries). It is astonishing now to think that highly intelligent people really did believe mice emerged fully formed from dirty clothes and wheat, and flies from smelly socks.[5] Jan Baptista van Helmont (1579–1644), an important figure in the history of science who coined the word 'gas' was a believer and even devised a recipe for the production of mice: 'If a dirty shirt is stuffed into the mouth of a vessel containing wheat, within a few days, say 21, the ferment produced by the shirt, modified by the smell of the grain, transforms the wheat itself, encased in its husk, into mice.'[6] William Harvey was another prominent adherent.[7] But perhaps it was not quite so silly. Not only was it taken for granted by most people, and was supported by no less an authority than Aristotle, but as philosopher Joachim Schummer points out, 'Everybody had ample evidence from ordinary experience: under favourable conditions, faeces, dung, meat, straw, and so on are all perfect materials to generate different kinds of organism'.[8]

Admittedly disbelief in spontaneous generation was nothing new either: to the ancient Roman poet and philosopher Lucretius (ca. 94 BC — ca. 49 BC), 'nothing from nothing ever yet was born' was one of the laws of nature,[9] a notion updated in the 1850s by Rudolf Virchow who popularised the phrase

Omnis cellula e cellula ('every cell originates from another existing cell like it'), an idea that apparently came from Robert Remak (whose lack of fame and professional success may be connected to his being Jewish).[10] But it was fatally discredited at last in the nineteenth century by Louis Pasteur who came up with a pretty irrefutable experimental disproof.

Vitalism in its chemical form, according to which only living things could produce organic chemicals,[11] which is to say those containing mixes of carbon, hydrogen, oxygen and nitrogen, was disproved when scientists began to make them in the lab. In 1828, Friedrich Wöhler (1800–1882) accidentally synthesised, albeit partially, a naturally-occurring biochemical, urea (CH_4N_2O), boasting incontinently that 'I can no longer, so to speak, hold my chemical water and must tell you that I can make urea without needing a kidney, whether of man or dog; the ammonium salt of cyanic acid is urea.'[12] Antoine Lavoisier (1743–1794) showed that living processes are chemical processes. From that time, the chemical basis of living things and biological processes became ever more apparent. The importance of this cannot be overstated. Gradually, what could be explained by a materialism founded on the laws of chemistry and physics was so comprehensive as to leave less and less room in science for forms of vitalism holding that life had some special immaterial essence or attribute not shared with the animate dead and the inanimate. Vitalism had to change in order to survive, which it did quite successfully. The emergence of cell theory in the mid eighteenth century undermined spontaneous generation but gave vitalism a new relevance. Indeed, Rudolf Virchow who did more than anyone to substantiate cell theory talked of *lebenkraft* (life force) and sought to reconcile his 'new' vitalism with mechanistic and reductionist views on life.[13] But what could no longer be disputed was that life is made of the same stuff that non-life is, nothing more nothing less. In other words, living organisms were made of bits of non-life. Justus Liebig may have been the first to realise, following his friend Wöhler's breakthrough, that these bits could be made artificially in a laboratory.[14]

Generally old theories and belief systems do not get substituted overnight by new ones at the moment when people begin to consider them obsolete. Likewise, vitalism was not replaced by materialism just like that. Wöhler's urea 'synthesis' was not considered at the time to have been of great import and it was only decades later that the achievement was elevated to the status of a 'crucial, significant, epoch-making event.'[15] The great French chemist Pierre Eugène Marcellin Berthelot (1827–1907) was perhaps the first to use chemistry to attack vitalism. Meanwhile, great pioneering scientists like Virchow and Bernard appeared to see merit on both sides of the debate. Liebig was unable to abandon vitalism while contemporaries such as Berzelius were rejecting it. Indeed, the special qualities of stem cells might seem to offer a way to reconcile vitalism in a modernised form whilst reinforcing the centrality of the cell as the basic unit of life. Enduring theories about life and sickness going back to the ancients proved to be highly persistent, perhaps more than we might think. The humoral theory of ancient Greece, associated with Hippocrates and later with Galen, retained some relevance to medical treatment until the beginning of the twentieth century even in the face of sixteenth and seventeenth century challenges from the likes of Paracelsus and Van Helmont, and the blood circulation discoveries of William Harvey (1578–1657). Even now people take ginger to relieve nausea (and ginger beer for hangovers): 'In humoural terms, ginger is 'warming'.'[16] Over the preceding two centuries, 'in practice, the theory continued … to sustain medicine and to offer a general scheme within which anatomy, physiology, and psychology could be made to fit'. The humours, originally black bile, yellow bile, phlegm, and blood, have still not gone away. They are embedded in modern English and are used metaphorically. Indeed, one could say that rather than disappear from medical usage, they have been subjected to a kind of transformative expansion. No person or movement did deliver humoral theory a fatal blow. Indeed, arguably rather than die out one could say it was updated in light of modern biomedicine. The theory behind it has mostly been replaced, yet humours remain albeit by other more reliable names and descriptions.

According to Noga Arikha in her history of the humours: 'By now, the original four humours imagined by the ancients have been multiplied by the hundreds into hormones, enzymes, neurotransmitters, particles, and the like, constituting the hydraulic system that is our body, providing us with a partial picture of what is going on inside our organism.'[17] If we are prepared to accept this, what we have is a refusal of an apparently falsified theory to die overnight but rather a lingering on, not in the shadows but more openly, embedding itself in modern biomedicine, rather like biological relics such as pelvic bones in whales and pseudogenes in humans or our appendix that are presumed obsolete but may continue to serve some residual function or other. Given the huge apparent differences between humoral theory and biomedicine, this suggests that a conservative, gradualist view of theory change may be more valid than one that sees paradigms shift overnight: evolution rather than revolution. According to Max Planck: 'a new scientific truth does not in general prevail because its opponents are convinced by it and declare themselves to be so, but rather because these opponents gradually pass away and the coming generation is intimately familiar with the truth from the beginning'.[18] So old and deeply-rooted ideas only die when their believers do. But he is talking here still about revolution, albeit in slow motion. Instead, it may be the case often that the 'new' theory is actually another version of the 'old' one that makes better sense in light of the scientific state of the art. Regarding humoral theory, if Arikha's view is correct, it was less a case of a wholesale abandonment than a transformation of sorts.

Harvey, for his part, managed to reconcile his circulation system with humoral theory (and as mentioned spontaneous generation);[19] indeed he continued to perform traditional Galenic practices like bleeding, though the difficulty in doing so plus his dislike of the Paracelsans who he colourfully referred to as 'shitt-breeches' failed to immunise him from the attacks of conservative Galenists.[20] Apart from a difficult to shake off deference to the wise ancients, one possible reason might be that the nature of humours as fluids was quite compatible with early articulations of mechanical philosophy. Just as nowadays we tend to imagine and talk about science in relation to the most advanced technologies of the day,[21] Harvey in the pre-steam power era thought in terms of hydraulics when treating the heart as a pump, a metaphor that continues to hold water (or should that be blood!).[22] Similarly, as Stephen Gaukroger observes in the cardiovascular context, 'Descartes' mechanistic model is not that of a clock, but one of hydraulic systems, such as those that worked the fountains and moving statues in the gardens of Saint-Germain'.[23] Perhaps, at least for a time, it mattered less what the fluids were and what they comprised than that the human body functioned according to hydraulic principles.[24] After Descartes and Harvey, a prominent Dutch physician of the time, Herman Boerhaave (1668–1738) of Leiden University, continued to combine mechanical philosophy with hydraulic notions of body function, thereby synthesising 'into a satisfactory whole the various strands derived from the new mechanical philosophy, the new chemistry, and the remnants of classical Galenism'.[25] His chief critics came from then important hotbeds of medical training, the Universities of Göttingen, Edinburgh and Montpellier where vitalism now held sway.[26]

Moving into the eighteenth century, medical theory was at least becoming more heterogeneous — even if much of it still wasn't very good. As with humoral theory talk, the mechanistic language which was supposed to be replacing it was not convincing to everybody either. As early as the mid eighteenth century it had become apparent already to some that 'there was more to life than the mechanical philosophy had dreamt of'.[27] But organism-as-machine language and thinking are still with us too, especially in the study of brains and consciousness but also in science generally,[28] and are deeply embedded also in currently the most advanced areas of applied life science like biotechnology and synthetic biology. Indeed, as an analogical device, organism-as-machine continues to perform effective theoretical, heuristic, and rhetorical roles to the extent that it is probably not even considered by its users as metaphorical at all but as an authentic and literally correct perspective.[29] According to historian of science John Hedley Brooke, 'the assimilation of natural processes to machinery continues to be a conspicuous feature of scientific investigation. The legacy of the seventeenth century mechanical philosophy is apparent in such terms as genetic engineering'.[30] Thus he identifies some of the most recent, and apparently revolutionary, scientific terminology as an extension of a scientific worldview that emerged centuries earlier.

Eighteenth century medical science was not without its triumphs as experimentalism and observation began to bear fruit, at least towards the century's end. According to one historical account, 'While the 18th century might have seemed like a long arid period in medicine actually it was the gestation period, from which was eventually delivered the flourishing progress of the mid-19th century.'[31] In the 1750s naval surgeon James Lind identified a link between citrus fruits and the reduction of scurvy, and proved it with the first ever clinical trial on the HMS Salisbury. In 1796,

Edward Jenner inoculated an eight-year old boy called James Phipps successfully immunising him from smallpox. He is not due all of the credit. In the early part of the century, Turkish peasant women were reported to be able to immunise people through inoculation, and from there the practice spread to England and then to other countries. The period also marked a high point in the art of quackery and in no country does this seem to have been a bigger curse than in England where the principle of *caveat emptor* applied.[32]

As regards scientific medicine specifically, France paved the way initially. The idea that achieving advanced healthcare was a matter of translating the successful results of laboratory experiments to the bedside emerged in that country and came into its own in the nineteenth century, persisting to this day.[33] The French experience demonstrates the importance not just of great individuals, groups and professional networks, but also of *institutional factors*. A new national system of medical institutions was established during the Revolution by legislation passed in 1794, ironically the year of Lavoisier's judicial murder by guillotine.[34] It sought to integrate the medical education system, but it also united medicine with surgery, emphasised the centrality of the hospital in medical education and research, and encouraged empiricism. It was not perfect. Moreover, the emergence of experimental physiology out of the much older discipline of anatomy did not happen without a struggle against the existing (post-revolutionary) order. Reliance on hospital medicine had its shortcomings, emphasising, as Claude Bernard alleged, passive observation over the elucidation of causation.[35] The fact remains that from this country and out of this system came crucial advances in the emerging science of animal and human physiology, as well as biochemical attainments from the isolation of natural substances, notably alkaloids from exotic medicinal plants, to the preparation of such chemicals in purified forms.[36] This progress was through experimentation rather than reliance on long-established theories, and can be attributed to François Magendie, his successor Claude Bernard, and their numerous contemporaries who contributed to the state of the art during the times these individuals flourished.[37]

Germany, or at least the states that were later merged into what we now call Germany, was hardly a laggard for long. As the nineteenth century progressed its university system became pre-eminent in Europe if not the world, 'the centre of organized research', where 'the system of academic science may be said to have achieved its greatest moments'. By the end of this century, 'the systematic institutionalized connection of an important science with industry was established. This was chemistry, which had always had a very close relation with practice, but which in late nineteenth century Germany became a sophisticated, capital-intensive industry on the pattern which is now dominant.'[38] Specialist institutes attached to universities became powerful, autonomous and entrepreneurial. Justus von Liebig (1803–1873) at the University of Giessen, who had gained a chemical education in France which initially was in the lead, did much to enhance the reputation of German chemistry and related sciences and the university system there.[39] Students from the rest of Europe and the United States began to flock there.

One of the major achievements from Germany in addition to chemistry was an enhancement in our understanding of the basic units of life: cells, and their central structural, functional and organisational contributions to life as we know it. This achievement is commonly associated with Schleiden, Schwann and Virchow. As far as medicine is concerned, Virchow stands out here (see below).

A better understanding, albeit still far from complete, was also required concerning the causes of disease, and of how one should find or make substances to treat them. Such theories were devised during the 60-year period from about the mid-1830s. Louis Pasteur and Robert Koch demonstrated beyond reasonable doubt that incidences of infectious disease could best be explained by germ theory. Later, Paul Ehrlich heralded the age of chemical therapy ('chemotherapy') as opposed to the biological therapies of Koch and others. He also advanced and inspired drug discovery with his selective affinity, magic bullet and receptor ('side-chain') concepts that inspired pharmaceutical chemists as they seemed to provide a rational underpinning for their work that was not there before.

There are reasons why the industry emerged when it did. But scientific advances cannot possibly be the only reason, besides which much of the science discussed in this chapter took time to be absorbed by industry. Nonetheless, they had a catalysing effect even if one must be careful not to exaggerate it. Consequently, we also look at a very important figure who helped take science from the laboratory to the market and was very successful and influential in doing so. This was Carl Duisberg. But we must start with two Frenchmen, both of whom were not just great scientists but un-squeamish vivisectors that in their lifetimes provoked both acclaim for their medical science achievements and condemnation for their unfeeling mistreatment of animals.

François Magendie (1783–1855)

Magendie was a versatile scientist who made numerous contributions, as befitted his being considered by many as 'the father of experimental physiology'.[40] Only a few need to be mentioned here. Although educated in medicine he also worked as a clinician. Accordingly he was at home both in the laboratory and at the bedside. He owed much to being in a post-Revolution France that had 'abolished distinctions between surgery and medicine, which produced surgical procedures helpful to the advancement of scientific physiology', and for a time was, as we saw, the most advanced nation in scientific medicine.[41] Empiricism was no longer in thrall to theory. The institutional environment of the time was conducive to radical progress, though not necessarily supportive of the individual scientist.[42]

Magendie, who after a period struggling to get established became chair of medicine at the elite Collège de France in 1826, was a devoted experimentalist, dedicated to translating findings in the laboratory to bedside care.[43] He had no time for theory as had previously dominated physiology, or for outdated notions like vitalism ('childish nonsense')[44] and Cartesian dualism.[45] Among his numerous achievements, he was among the first to advocate drug purity and to study toxins to gain insights into human physiology and the possibility of the knowledge acquired being useful in finding effective treatments for disease. For him, as stated in his Preface to the sixth edition of the Formulary published in 1827, 'the impossibility of isolating by chemical analysis the elements of medicines, has much retarded the progress towards perfection of the Materia Medica'. With such analysis becoming possible, the remaining obstacle to 'the ultimate principles of remedies from being investigated' was the lingering belief 'that medicinals act altogether differently on man to what they do on animals.'[46] The latter was far from being something that he believed in.[47]

Magendie was in the right time and place to experiment on and test out newly identified, isolated and purified single plant-based active ingredients, such as alkaloids, often of exotic origin; indeed, that he was one of the first scientists to promote this approach makes him such an important early actor in facilitating the later emergence of the pharmaceutical industry.[48] In this sense he was fortunate that his career coincided with a series of remarkable achievements in chemistry, mostly taking place in France. From around 1805 to the early 1830s, numerous therapeutically significant alkaloids were isolated from plants (see Table 4.1 below). Among the most important were morphine from opium (by Sertürner), emetine from ipecacuanha (by Pelletier with Magendie himself), quinine from *Cinchona cordifolia* (by Pelletier and Caventou), and codeine also from opium (by Robiquet). Magendie worked with Pierre-Joseph Pelletier (1788–1842),[49] the son of an apothecary personally acquainted with Lavoisier,[50] to whom has also been attributed the notion that purity has therapeutic value. They tested emetine on animals and recommended it as a treatment for amoebic dysentery.[51] Magendie was also one of the first to experiment with quinine whose effects impressed him greatly.

Table 4.1. Discoveries about some alkaloids[52]

Source	Alkaloid	Isolated	Uses
Opium	Narcotine	Derosne 1804 (a)	Relief of cough
Opium	Morphine	Sertürner 1806	Relief of pain; addictive
Ipecacuanha	Emetine	Pelletier & Magendie 1817	Treatment of amoebic dysentery
St. Ignatius's beans	Strychnine	Pelletier & Caventou 1818	Tonic (obsolete): (b)
Autumn crocus	Colchicine	Pelletier & Caventou 1819	Relief of gout
Jesuit's bark	Quinine	Pelletier & Caventou 1820	Treatment of malaria: (c)

(Continued)

Table 4.1.   (*Continued*)

Source	Alkaloid	Isolated	Uses
Coffee beans	Caffeine	Robiquet; Runge 1821	Mental stimulant
Hemlock	Coniine	Geiger 1831	(d)
Opium	Codeine	Robiquet 1832	Relief of cough
Nightshade	Atropine	Geiger & Hess 1833	Reduction of secretions etc.
Opium	Papaverine	Merck, 1850	Relief of spasm of involuntary muscles
Coca beans	Cocaine	Niemann 1860	Local anaesthetic
Calabar beans	Physostigmine	Jobst & Hess 1873	Treatment of glaucoma

(a) Derosne's, a minor constituent of opium, was identified some years later. (b) Strychnine has important uses in the physiological analysis of spinal reflexes. (c) Quinine was synthesized for the first time in 1944. (d) Coniine was the first alkaloid to be synthesized, in 1886. Its use as a relaxant of muscles is limited and obsolete.

Pharmacist turned historian Walter Sneader explains the wider significance of the 1820 paper that Pelletier published with Caventou on their isolation of quinine.[53] As he put it, the article 'marked a new departure, for previously the active principles of plants had been isolated for analytical rather than therapeutic purposes. By urging their medical colleagues to study pure plant principles, Pelletier and Caventou set the course of drug discovery in a new direction.'[54]

Magendie's work displays a clear understanding of the importance of obtaining a consistent formulation and producing the right dosage. With respect to the fever-reducing cinchona alkaloids which of course include quinine, he remarked as follows:

If it always be of importance to the physician to know the exact quantity of the active ingredient in the medicine he employs, it is especially so with reference to the cinchonas, whose activities vary greatly according to the nature and quality of the barks. It is also of great advantage to be able to administer this medicine in a sufficiently small volume and in a form that is not disagreeable. Patients have perished in remittent fevers merely for want of resolution to swallow the necessary quantity of cinchona in powder, or from its exciting vomiting or diarrhoea; even in more favourable cases the stomach is obliged, as it were, to analyse the bark and extract its febrifuge principle; this, however, is a difficult and toilsome process even for the healthiest stomach, and chemistry has therefore rendered a real service to medicine by discovering a method of effecting this separation before hand.[55]

It should be noted here that isolation and purification are not the same thing. Isolation means extricating particular chemicals in a laboratory from the confines of their natural source. It does not mean separating them from other chemicals liberated at the same time. That is the task of purification techniques. Few if any of these therapeutic substances of the period were devoid of such unwanted impurities. But processes were discovered over the course of the century, largely in Germany, France and Britain, which much improved purity levels.

Pelletier and Caventou's work also had immense and far-reaching practical significance. In short time, their published work on isolating quinine was to lead to mass production with factories opening in Paris, Barcelona and in Germany. It helped that they took out no patents on their work so others could freely apply their published methods, not that they were left unrewarded: 'The Paris Institute of Science awarded these French chemists a sum of ten thousand francs for their valuable work'.[56] Pelletier became a producer himself, his factory 'processing more than 15,000 kg of cinchona bark yearly, yielding around 3,600 kg of quinine sulphate.'[57] From this time onwards, 'Isolation of the active principles from any therapeutically-active material became an established procedure. It required collaboration between chemist and physiologist in order to show that the substances had the same actions as the parent material. This required trials in man … or, less hazardously, experiments on animals, in which some analysis of the mode and site of action was also possible.'[58]

It is worth mentioning also that alkaloid production was an entry point for some firms that later became important pharmaceutical corporations. A good example is Merck, a German company set up in Darmstadt that much later on became two companies with the same name, one remaining in Germany, the other being based in the United

States (see Chapter 5). As Sneader claims, these early alkaloid makers and traders 'quickly recognised the economies obtained through large-scale production of quinine and morphine, and also acquired specialised knowledge that enabled adulterated or inferior plant material to be rejected. *In this way, the modern pharmaceutical industry gradually became established.*'[59]

Claude Bernard (1813–1878)

Claude Bernard, apprentice and successor to Magendie, struggled for much of his career with poor working conditions and scarce funding, but eventually was feted and showered with honours. Unlike Magendie, he was a pure researcher and not a clinician. In fact, he never practiced medicine except as an intern, discovered no drugs, did not heal a single person, and none of his great discoveries — 'the role of the liver in synthesizing glycogen and in keeping blood glucose levels within a defined range; the digestive function of the pancreas; the vasodilator nerves; the site of action of poisons such as carbon monoxide and curare'[60] — *individually* transformed the world of medicine.

He was, though, the most important experimental physiologist of the nineteenth century and a giant of medical science, who dramatically enhanced our understanding of how the whole human body works by providing numerous ground-breaking insights into the *internal environment* of humans and other higher animals. The idea that human and other mammalian bodies are able to maintain a stable temperature-controlled inner world through numerous feedback and other mechanisms that assured stability despite the vagaries of the external environment was perhaps his most original contribution to science. Admittedly, this was not particularly useful at the time in part because understanding of the endocrine system was still fairly rudimentary.

It is interesting to note, given our discussion earlier on humoral theory, that the term 'internal environment' may have been borrowed from a contemporary of his 'who used *milieu de l'intérier* as a synonym for "the humors"'.[61] Balance, equilibrium, constancy and self-regulation are concepts that seem so integral to Bernard's *milieu de l'intérier* whose essential characteristic was later named homeostasis. Interestingly, others extended the general notion of homeostasis through self-regulation 'from the realm of bodily fluids to the wider social environment',[62] whilst Norbert Wiener much later on absorbed it into a field he named cybernetics which embraced self-regulation and its dynamics in both animal and machine.[63] It is noteworthy also that Arikha describes *milieu de l'intérier* in a chapter of her book titled 'Contemporary humours'.[64] Hence the relationship between the 'obsolete' theory and the cutting edge idea can be more creative, more intricate, and less mutually antagonistic than one might suppose.

According to two mid-last century biographers:

> His earlier discoveries were concerned with the functions of particular bodily organs, the pancreas and the liver; but as his work progressed, it gave greater prominence to the unified activity of the whole body. His conception of the blood as furnishing an internal environment which mediates between living tissues and the external environment is a striking illustration of this tendency.[65]

His physiological focus on the internal environment might sound rather abstract. However, there was nothing of the ivory tower in him. As with Magendie, theoretical obscurantism had no appeal. His work did much to enhance understanding of how foreign substances introduced into the body interact with it. This was crucial to both toxicology and pharmacology, which were opposite sides of the same coin. Medical historian William Bynum summarised his approach to medical research, according to which the triad of physiology, pathology and pharmacology 'constituted for him the pillars of experimental medicine'[66]:

> Bernard used his own work to illustrate the complex interaction but essential integrity of their three pillars: how, for instance, diabetes could be more comprehensively grasped as a disease after his elucidation of the glycogenetic functions of the liver; or how the pharmacological action of curare (admittedly, a poison rather than a common mainstay of the pharmacopoeia) could be pinpointed to the neuromuscular junction. He was under no illusions that a medical millennium was at hand: the laboratory was just beginning to make its presence felt in medicine.[67]

His discoveries relating to curare and the workings of the pancreas formed major early staging posts along long learning trails leading to the use of curare products in surgery from the 1940s, and the 1920s discovery and production of insulin. With regard to the former, first, curare eventually inspired the discovery and development of better surgical muscle relaxants. Secondly, and more importantly, follow-on scientific investigation of curare from the 1930s was incredibly fruitful. Using curare as a research tool proved the essential role of chemicals in channelling messages within the brain and from the brain to the rest of our body, thereby radically enhancing our understanding of physiology and brain function. This led directly to the subsequent development of numerous spin-off drugs including the beta-blockers, anti-depressants like Prozac, and treatments for afflictions ranging from Parkinson's disease to asthma and diarrhoea.[68] All this subsequent work was of course done by others, but somebody had to come first and channel research in the right direction.

As mentioned, Bernard did not come up with any medicines himself. Yet his investigations into exactly how it is that poisons kill revealed much that would inspire future drug discovery. His studies on curare and carbon monoxide uncovered the specific ways they cause death by reference to particular modes and sites of action.[69] *If poisons work in such specific ways that laboratory experimentation can demonstrate, the same should apply to drugs. It is a well-known truism that understanding how existing drugs work aids the discovery of new and better ones.*

Rudolf Carl Virchow (1821–1902)

Rudolf Virchow was trained as a pathologist and served as professor at the University of Würzburg. He is one of the more interesting and rounded characters among this illustrious group. He was not just a laboratory scientist but a political activist during turbulent times, and one whose politics informed his views on the social aspects of medicine. Indeed, to him doing medicine and doing politics were indistinguishable. But what mainly interests us here is his formulation of a cell theory of human biology which seems to be irrefutable, and its application to a better understanding of disease.

Robert Hooke coined the word 'cell'. The first mention in print is this passage in the famous *Micrographica*, published in 1665, in which he describes looking at the bark of the cork tree though his microscope:

> '... I could exceedingly plainly perceive it to be all perforated and porous, much like a Honey-comb, but that the pores of it were not regular. ... these pores, or cells, ... were indeed the first *microscopical* pores I ever saw, and perhaps, that were ever seen, for I had not met with any Writer or Person, that had made any mention of them before this.

However, not until the mid-nineteenth century did microscopes attain the quality to reveal the far less distinct cell walls of animals, thereby demonstrating that cells are the fundamental units of both plant and animal life, that is, all visible life. This insight is commonly attributed to two Germans whose discoveries preceded those of Virchow by just a few years: Matthias Schleiden and Theodor Schwann. It is to them that 'cell theory' is normally attributed. Soon after, Karl von Siebold extended the theory to include protozoa which he showed to be unicellular. It was Virchow, though, who made this basic fact of life medically interesting. According to Siddhartha Mukherjee, author of the modern classic on cancer, *The Emperor of All Maladies*, Virchow 'launched a project that would occupy him for his life: describing human diseases in simple cellular terms.' What led him to this? Again, according to Mukherjee:

> It was a project born of frustration. Virchow entered medicine in the early 1840s, when nearly every disease was attributed to the workings of some invisible force: miasmas, neuroses, bad humors, and hysterias. Perplexed by what he couldn't see, Virchow turned with revolutionary zeal to what he could: cells under the microscope.[70]

Virchow's views on normal cell reproduction and growth framed his observations of disease arising from pathological growth, whereby for certain reasons yet to be determined, cancerous cells fall out of the control of the body system, escaping from any 'switch off' mechanisms there might be, leading to disease and eventual death. Virchow's name for this phenomenon was neoplasia: the disease itself is of course cancer, a name that goes back to the time of Hippocrates and which Galen had associated with excess black bile, a body imbalance also responsible for melancholia.[71]

Virchow provided vital insights, mainly into non-communicable diseases of the body itself, including cardio-vascular ailments, as well as such phenomena as inflammation. A harmful proliferation of white blood cells was coined 'leukaemia' by Virchow. That he disclaimed any full understanding of its causes does not detract from the value of what he contributed here. Paradoxically, such an admission of incomplete knowledge was an advance when one thinks of the false and misleading causation theories of the day.[72] It fell to others later to see leukaemia for what it was: 'cancer in a molten, liquid form', in Mukherjee's eloquent almost humoral words.[73] Virchow recognised two forms of leukaemia. Currently, about 40 have been identified.

Virchow did not ignore infectious disease. He discovered the link between human infection by a parasitic nematode (*Trichinella spiralis*) and consumption of contaminated pork, and identified a heating method to make meat safe, thereby leading to public inspection of meat products. He was a courageous individual with a social conscience and was prepared to stand up for his views on the essential social and political aspects of public health and on militarism. According to one colourful account:

> He was opposed to Bismarck's excessive military budget, which angered Bismarck sufficiently to challenge Virchow to a duel. Virchow, being entitled to choose the weapons, chose two pork sausages: a cooked sausage for himself and an uncooked one, loaded with *Trichinella* larvae, for Bismarck. Bismarck, the Iron Chancellor, declined the proposition as too risky.[74]

Virchow was not a supporter of the germ theory of disease, holding that sickness was either caused by problems internal to the human body at the cellular level, or else infectious disease outbreaks were a consequence of poverty and injustice thus requiring more a political than a medical response. Whilst correct to see that reduced poverty and better education is bound to improve public health overall, and one must admire his devotion to improving sanitation and public health, the germ theory is certainly proven. But there is no necessary conflict here. He and the germ theorists, Pasteur and Koch, were each correct: as we all now know, some diseases are caused by infective agents such as bacteria and viruses whereas others are non-communicable and linked to malfunctions at the cellular level that may or may not be attributable to external factors.

Louis Pasteur (1822–1895)

Louis Pasteur is of course one of the most famous scientists of all time, and not just because of his undoubted brilliance: he was also an excellent self-publicist.[75] He achieved great esteem in his lifetime in France, and for good reason. As the late science historian John Pickstone put it, while intriguingly suggesting an odd instance of scientific progress seeming to reinforce belief in charms and evil spirits:

> The agricultural and industrial technologies supported by his work — on wines and beer, and on plant, animal and human diseases — were central to the 'modernisation' of France and its empire. His experiments promised action against disease; the success of immunisation confirmed the potential and made him a national hero. In the cottages of rural France, charms against spirits could now keep germs away.[76, 77]

Pasteur came to scientific medicine by a circuitous route. He began as a chemist but in studying fermentation, putrefaction and infectious disease he came to see that these chemical reactions were in fact biological and related to each other. He realised that different types of microbe do different things including causing specific diseases, and the distribution of microbial life is truly ubiquitous: they are on land, in the air, in the water, and inside the human body. So some microbes ferment wine and beer,[78] others cause milk to go sour, and then there are germs that cause anthrax and rabies.

By no means an ivory tower chemist,[79] and with industry becoming aware of the industrial applications of his expertise, he frequently acted as a consultant. The commercial food, beverage, silk and livestock sectors all benefited from his work, and he filed numerous patents protecting food and beverage production methods (but not on his vaccine work due probably to certain exclusions in the patent laws of the time).[80]

Though trained as a chemist, and not as a doctor or physiologist, public health definitively enhanced as a result of his work. We all have him to thank for pasteurised milk and other perishable products rendered safe by a process he may not have invented but that he did give a rational and convincing scientific basis to. His work made possible its standardisation and efficiency thereby enabling its widespread adoption. Like Koch and unlike Virchow, his key scientific contribution to medicine was in the ambit of infectious disease, whereby sickness is caused by foreign agents entering the body. Whereas Virchow founded cellular pathology, Pasteur was at the right place and time to be recognised as the founding father of bacteriology. This embraced industrial biotechnology (as we now call it) including food hygiene, but also the study on relationships between human disease and bacterial infection, and the production of vaccines. The germ theory of disease is of course consequent on a bacteriological mode of thinking.

So what *was* the general state of knowledge in the mid-nineteenth century that Pasteur was driving into obsolescence? According to René Dubos, himself an esteemed scientists who did ground-breaking work on the antibiotics, in his biography of Pasteur written a century later, 'the man of science as well as the layman of 1850 regarded fermentations and putrefactions as caused by chemical agents', that is, involving nothing that was living.[81] Admittedly, a number of people were challenging this just prior to Pasteur. Jacob Henle, a friend of Schwann and teacher of Koch had hypothesised in 1840 that 'the material of contagion is not only organic but living, endowed with individual life and standing to the diseased body in the relation of a parasitic organism'.[82] Yeast as a product having life-like properties had been known about for a long time:

> All ancient folklores have associated the activity of yeast with the phenomena of life; indeed, bread and wine became the symbol of Life Eternal in the Mediterranean religions. In addition to the magic of their results, the nature of the processes initiated by yeast caught the fancy of philosophers and chemists. The bubbling that takes place

spontaneously in the mass of vintage, or in the flour paste, appeared to them as the manifestation of some living spirit.[83]

Great scientists like Lavoisier and Berzelius had sought to understand fermentation. But their failing was not to realise both that yeasts were living — in fact they had been unconsciously domesticated by humankind over thousands of years — and that fermentation was a living process. How fitting that wines, spirits and the staff of life were all made by life itself! Pasteur was not the first to hold that yeasts were alive but 'the vitalistic theory of fermentation'[84] was rejected by the scientific establishment: 'As a reaction against the romantic and confused airings of the German *Natur philosophie*, the new prophets had pronounced anathema on anyone who preached the doctrine of vitalism.'[85]

From then onward, Pasteur did much to turn biology into a human technology: bio-technology before biotechnology, if you like. He accurately hypothesised that 'the purity of a ferment, its homogeneity, its free unrestrained development by the aid of food substances well adapted to its individual nature, these are some of the conditions which are essential to good fermentation'.[86] This approach led not only to the improvement of industrial production but also to the germ theories of hygiene and disease.

Pasteur's first projects applying the germ theory to understanding of infectious disease and identifying ways to treat or prevent it were on silkworms, chicken cholera and anthrax. Economic importance rather than human therapeutic potential took priority. The interests of government and industry were initially first in line rather than the needs of the sick which came later. This later pathological turn in his work became very comprehensive indeed, covering studies on anthrax, gangrene, septicaemia, childhood fever, chicken cholera, rabies, cattle erysipelas, and human cholera. In 1879, using anthrax bacillus produced by Koch, he discovered immunisation using attenuated cultures. He proved it worked in a public demonstration two years later. This marked the beginning of the age of vaccines. In 1884, he produced rabies vaccine, a much bigger challenge given that rabies is caused by a virus not a bacterium or protist. Therefore, it is invisible with a microscope. A year later, a nine year-old boy, Joseph Meister who had been bitten by a rabid dog, was given a course of injections and stayed well. In the coming years thousands of people were treated and by 1915 the death rate in the number of people killed after being bitten by rabid animals had declined markedly.[87]

Robert Koch (1843–1910)

Robert Koch has something in common with Charles Darwin: for much of his career his home was his laboratory, which in his case was well stocked with the latest technology. He had a state-of-the-art microscope, microphotographic devices, and even a darkroom.[88] But he was in no way a gentlemen scientist of independent means as was Darwin; rather, like Pasteur and others, he was a practitioner. Koch's career illustrates the importance of technological innovation in medical instrumentation for medical and pharmaceutical research. For much of his life Koch worked as physician and district medical officer in a region now in Poland though later in his career he worked for five years each at the Imperial Health Bureau and the University of Berlin where he obviously enjoyed the institutional support he lacked earlier. He also travelled widely doing medical research in Egypt, India, New Guinea, South Africa and the German African colonies.

Koch's achievements are interesting in various ways. He gave disease-related and therapeutic bacteriology a stronger scientific basis. He and his students were responsible for a number of innovative experimental procedures and techniques including the so-called Koch postulates, and the use of agar and Petri dishes (named after one of his students) for growing bacteria. He isolated the causative agents of several diseases, including cholera, anthrax and most notably tuberculosis for which he was awarded a Nobel Prize. He also did much to enhance hygiene and public health in Germany.

Pasteur, Koch and their colleagues, students and successors had an excellent run from 1879 to 1900 when 'the micro-organisms responsible for major diseases were being discovered at the phenomenal rate of one a year.'[89] This did not mean effective therapies though, except in a few cases such as diphtheria, cholera and tetanus antitoxins which were curative. But identifying the sources of infective microbes and their channels of transmission to humans did enable avoidance measures to be taken that must have saved many lives. Vaccines for cholera and tetanus, not attenuated live vaccines, but blood sera antitoxins first developed by two workers in Koch's laboratory, Emil von Behring and Shibasaburo Kitasato, were marketed by Hoechst in the 1890s. These were among the first undeniably novel and modern pharmaceutical products marketed by this new industry.[90]

The anti-diphtheria serum therapy first developed by Behring with Wernicke and Ehrlich was ground-breaking in several ways, in terms of what it stood for, the procedures employed to turn it from a laboratory discovery to an approved therapeutic substance, and of its commercial potential. By attacking and eliminating the disease agent rather than the symptoms it 'was seen as a major therapeutic innovation, and celebrated as a milestone in bacteriology and a revolution in pharmacology'.[91] Moreover, its development 'covered all the aspects of "modern" pharmaceutical research, that is, the sequence of numerous *in vitro* and *in vivo* experiments were followed by clinical trials that were critically supervised.'[92] As for its industrial attractiveness, it 'promised high profits for manufacturers who would be able to stabilize the production process and produce serum in large quantities in so-called industrial production plants.'[93] Another precedent set by this new product is the engagement of the regulatory state, in this case the new Germany of Bismarck, which brought in institutional reforms and oversight procedures both to protect patients from harm and to guarantee the integrity of the product which was recognised as being novel and as very much an item of trade and profit.

The idea that drugs could be made from bacterial and other microbial products that are toxic to other microorganisms but harmless to humans was not something Pasteur or Koch had contemplated. Nonetheless, to the extent that antibiotics are an extension of bacteriology — a move from prevention to cure — there is a clear learning trail from Pasteur's and Koch's work to the later discovery of penicillin and the other antibiotics that saved many lives and generated huge profits for industry. The route of the trail goes via the finding by two of Pasteur's students, Roux and Yersin that, at least with diphtheria, it was not necessarily the bacterium itself that causes disease but a particular toxin it produces, and the discovery by others in Germany that immunity and even cure could be achieved using serum from an immunised animal targeted at such a toxin. As we will see, success in antibiotics decades later led to huge profits and increased research funds that did much to justify the industry's claims to being 'research-based'.

Vaccines remain important products, but they have never been the most lucrative type of pharmaceutical product, and are difficult to develop. (As I finish off this book, the world eagerly awaits a vaccine for Covid-19, but we are warned that despite the genetic code being publicly available we will still have to wait 12 months at a bare minimum). Generally speaking, commercial gains will tend to be higher for cures than they will for preventive treatments to be taken once; and higher still for the pill one needs to keep taking for the rest of one's life to stay alive. As legal scholar Ana Santos Rutschman explains in relation to Covid-19 while discussing vaccines more generally:

> Large pharmaceutical companies with the infrastructure necessary to produce massive amounts of vaccines tend to allocate resources elsewhere, as vaccine manufacturing is widely deemed unprofitable. Second, outbreak-spiked funding for vaccine development is likely to decline precipitously as soon as the pandemic begins to wane, cutting short many of the development projects now underway, as was the case in the recent outbreaks of Ebola and Zika. And third, for the vaccines that are fully developed, there is no guarantee that they will be made available at affordable prices to all populations in need.[94]

That said, the size of the vaccines market has increased dramatically in recent years for several reasons including the shorter development timespans as compared to drugs, and it will quite likely continue to expand.[95] Moreover, funding mechanisms and Gavi, an international agency promoting public-private partnerships, are helping to get vaccines to those who need them around the world.

Paul Ehrlich (1854–1915)

The work of Koch and his immediate successors forms a bridge between biological and chemical therapeutics. The turn from biology to chemistry, or perhaps better said the addition of chemistry to the pharmaceutical arsenal, including the making of molecules not found in nature, is of tremendous importance as we will see. Chemotherapy is a word nowadays confined to cancer drug treatment regimens, but in the late nineteenth century it referred to the use of new laboratory-made chemicals targeting a variety of infectious diseases. Paul Ehrlich, who worked with Koch at the University of Berlin and later moved to Frankfurt to head the Royal Prussian Institute of Experimental Therapy, took things further. Much could be said about Ehrlich in the present context. He won a Nobel Prize for his work on immunology, and he is credited with the invention of the anti-syphilis drug Salvarsan. But it will suffice to focus on just a few of his contributions to the medical arts in addition to chemotherapy and his use of dyes: his theory of selective affinity and the allied concept of the 'magic bullet', a term he is supposed to have coined.[96]

Ehrlich was certainly not the first scientist to use dyes to aid the visibility of human blood and tissue samples through microscopes. One essential feature of such staining was its selectivity: different kinds of dye highlighted different types of cell. This selective affinity has, at least in itself, no obvious health implications. However, if certain dyes are shown not only to stain but also to affect the behaviour of certain cells *and* unicellular organisms, therapeutic possibilities become more apparent, at least to the insightful scientist. Ehrlich began to realise that there must be something about the specific structure of chemicals that causes them to 'fix' to particular cells leading, in some cases, to physiological or pharmacological effects. He had the idea that dyes and drugs work in the same ways and that dyes can be used to deliver attached chemicals that are toxic to the infective agents the dyes are fixed to. As historian John Lesch expressed his reasoning here, 'just as with dye compounds, where part of the molecule attaches to the substance to be dyed while another part is responsible for the colour, so too with therapeutic compounds: one part will attach to a specific tissue while another part is responsible for the therapeutic effect.'[97] As we will see in Chapter 8, this, in essence, is exactly what today's antibody-drug conjugates (ADCs) do: the antibody does the targeting, and the toxin covalently linked to it does the rest.

Such potential specificity led Ehrlich to adopt the word *Zauberkugel* ('magic bullet'), which he borrowed from an operatic work by Carl Maria von Weber called *Der Freischütz* (The Marksman).[98] The concept was first applied to the highly specific antibodies which he believed cells released in response to attack by foreign substances called 'antigens', although what antibodies actually were was unclear to Ehrlich. A few decades after it became evident that they were proteins. Ehrlich subsequently widened application of the term to include artificial counterparts to natural antibodies. The current term in vogue which most closely embodies the magic bullet concept is precision medicine.

For Ehrlich, chemotherapy was one of three modes of experimental therapeutics. The other two were 'organotherapy (the use of organ extracts, or what we would call hormones)' and 'bacteriotherapy (the use of immunological agents such as antitoxins)'.[99] The fact that Ehrlich did not get his theory entirely correct is not to belittle the scale of his influence. He held out the possibility of rational and finely targeted drug discovery which proved to be inspirational and enduring.

From the 1880s, the German synthetic dyestuff firms, who as we will see, later became big pharmaceutical concerns, were producing vast numbers of dye products, and Ehrlich was able to experiment with them. One dye he did try out was methylene blue for which the malaria parasite had an affinity (as did some human cells). He also tested large numbers of dyes for activity against sleeping sickness, a highly dangerous tropical disease. In this endeavour he competed with the Pasteur Institute which availed itself of dyes provided by the world's biggest dye-maker Bayer. Many of Ehrlich's came from Casella, a Frankfurt-based company.[100] Both teams came up with Trypan Red as the most promising candidate but it was ineffective in mammals.[101] I note in passing that such sharing with industry is an excellent example of 'open innovation', a supposedly novel industrial knowledge management paradigm much in vogue today. Indeed, Ehrlich had a number of collaborations with industry involving exchanges of knowledge and resources, including with Hoechst.

Thanks to Ehrlich and others working in collaboration with industry, the application of synthetic chemistry to drug discovery began to bear fruit from the late nineteenth century, and the dyestuff firms were at the forefront, along with a small number of longer established pharmacy firms. The first ever pharmaceutical products were developed in-house or by chemists based in German universities and licensed to companies, most of which were primarily dyestuff firms.

Ehrlich's endeavours led him to the development of dyes as selective toxins for pathogenic microbes. The publication of a report by Guttman and Ehrlich in 1891 dealing with the cure of two malarious patients using the phenothiazinium dye Methylene Blue represents the first record of successful antimicrobial chemotherapy using a synthetic chemical... The work of Ehrlich was carried on by his students, such as Browning and Roehl. The former was responsible for the introduction of acridine dyes as topical antimicrobials during the exigencies of base hospital treatment in World War I, while the latter carried on Ehrlich's tropical research and was responsible for the development of the trypanocidal drug Suramin (also known as Germanin) from azo dyes such as Trypan Red.[102]

Despite this, there were limits to what was possible. The therapeutic potential of dyes' light absorbing properties was — and is[103] — genuine, but these same properties could also be harmful:

However, despite their undoubted efficacy in treatment, dyes were (and remain) unpopular due to associated tissue coloration. Thus workers at I G Farben in Germany in the 1920s used Methylene Blue as a principle compound for their antimalarial research, but rejected improved compounds on the basis of blue coloration in animal testing.[104]

To sum up so far, advances in bacteriology and immunology associated with Louis Pasteur, Robert Koch and Paul Ehrlich catalysed the emergence of the modern pharmaceutical industry. As we saw, Pasteur and Koch showed that many illnesses were caused by invasive bacteria, identified the microbes causing several of the major diseases, and a certain number of highly effective vaccines were produced by them or as a direct consequence of their work. Discovering the role of white blood cells in destroying disease-causing bacteria not only gave scientists a much better idea of how the body defends itself from hostile microbial invaders and the toxins they produce but inspired the idea of using biological agents to fight disease. This, and the realization mentioned above that toxins made by bacterial cells can cause disease, led eventually to the discovery and industrial production of penicillin and the antibiotics.[105] These are substances produced by fungi or bacteria which inhibit or destroy other bacteria yet cause no harm to humans. This huge advance for pharmaceutical science and, as it turned out, for the pharmaceutical industry, was nonetheless somewhat slow in coming, not taking place until the 1940s. Typically, the industry could not have achieved any of this all by itself.

The insight that blood serum also contained anti-bacterial agents inspired another scientific approach to pharmaceutical research and development. Ehrlich, impressed by the specificity of coal tar dye staining applied to human and animal tissue, and the way that dyes attach to fabric, investigated the chemical structures of various dyes. As we saw, his aim was to discover synthetic versions of natural antibodies. Eventually this strategy led to the first chemotherapeutic revolution — the sulphonamide drugs, discovered in 1932 by a scientist working for a German company (see Chapter 7).

Carl Duisberg (1861–1935)

It is impossible to overlook a major figure to whom we shall return in the coming chapter. Carl Duisberg differs from all the scientists whose achievements we covered above in that he spent his whole career in industry. Hired by Bayer as an ambitious young scientist when it was not a pharmaceutical company but a synthetic dyemaker, Duisberg during his long career, much of it spent in corporate management, did much to establish the modern science-based corporation, one generating *incremental* inventions on an unprecedented scale, filing large numbers of patents and trademarks, and marketing products with skill, aggression and clever strategy. One could even go so far to suggest that Duisberg created the modern pharmaceutical company as we know it today. One might well consider him a European Thomas Edison.

Duisberg's influence started at quite a young age. As a young company scientist employed by Bayer, he provided evidence in an absolutely seminal court case in Germany that set a very important precedent: that incremental differences from the state of the art could be patentable inventions as long as what was done had a 'new technical effect'. We will see why this is so important in Chapter 5.

He was instrumental in Bayer's building of the most advanced company research laboratory in the world, and setting up a large manufacturing facility alongside it. He did much to turn Bayer into a pharmaceutical company, perhaps the first one anywhere when in 1888 at his initiative it placed on the market an anti-pyretic drug that it sold as Phenacetin.[106] At the very least, it is due to him that the industry became recognisable not just by its harnessing of medical science and industrial fine chemistry, but by its use and management of intellectual property and sophisticated marketing. This to my mind is a definining feature of the industry.

This is not to suggest that use of intellectual property rights, especially patents, has ever been uncontroversial. Scientists over the years have considered patents in the field of health to be unethically questionable or even downright wrong. There are those who still do. Many countries were reluctant to allow full patent protection over medical substances so as not to enable companies to wield undue power over national health policy. Hostility to patents on medicines, and more generally in the biomedical field, endures to this day. Noenetheless, there has never been a time when the industry's mode of doing business did not involve the acquisition and market deployment of intellectual property rights. Arguably, Duisberg started this off.

It would perhaps be remiss not to mention that Duisberg, judging by today's standards, was a war criminal who enthusiastically contributed to the production of poison gases including mustard gas to be used against enemy troops in the First World War.[107] The ease by which industrial chemistry could switch from the production of dyes and drugs to toxins designed to kill is of course obvious given the discussion above. I will have more to say about Carl Duisberg in the next chapter but not on this specific matter. The fact he was not a nice person was tragically relevant of course to the Allied troops who were gassed (one of whom was a great uncle of mine), but it is immaterial in the context of this book.

Notes

1 For the role of the patent system and litigation in assigning individual credit during the late nineteenth century, albeit in a different industry, see Arapostathis and Gooday (2013).

2 Intriguingly, Joseph Wright of Derby's well-known painting 'The alchymist in search of the philosopher's stone', completed towards the end of the

eighteenth century, possibly depicting Henning Brand's discovery of phosphorus a century earlier, suggests a more ambiguous view. The position of the man rather implies he is about to find what he was seeking. This was an age when it was quite common to depict men in moments of inspiration.

3   'The Chain of Being is the idea of the organic constitution of the universe as a series of links or gradations ordered in a hierarchy of creatures, from the lowest and most insignificant to the highest, indeed to the *ens perfectissimum* which, uncreated, is yet its culmination and the end to which all creation tends.' Formigari (1973–74). For a detailed history and commentary, see AO Lovejoy (1936) Arguably, the persistence of words like 'higher' and 'lower' to divide complex and relatively less complex forms of life suggest that the great chain of being has not been abandoned in its entirety. This has had legal implications. In 2003, the higher/lower distinction was drawn by the Canadian Supreme Court in a 2002 decision concerning the patentability of a genetically engineered mice used in cancer research (Harvard College v Canada (Commissioner of Patents) 2002 SCC 76).

4   Historian of biology Staffan Müller-Wille sees the decline of the chain of being concept in the context of a replacement of natural history with history of nature around 1800 following Carl Linnaeus's formulation of his hierarchical taxonomic classification system. Müller-Wille (2015).

5   Davies (2003), 60.

6   Harris (2002), as quoted by Louis Pasteur in an 1864 lecture. Pasteur (1922–39).

7   Harris, *op. cit.*, 5.

8   Schummer (2007).

9   From *De Rerum Natura*. Downloaded (gratefully) from Project Gutenberg website.

10   Porter (1997) *op. cit.*, 331; Wikipedia entries on Rudolf Virchow and Robert Remak (visited: 20 September 2020). Allegedly Virchow plagiarised Remak's work on this.

11   Hence the artificial distinction we still draw between inorganic and organic chemistry.

12   In Hunter (2000), 56–9. For discussion on the sometimes overstated significance of Wöhler's achievement, see also Bensaude-Vincent and Stengers (1996), 145–6; Brooke (1968); Goodfield (1960); McKie (1944).

13   Channell (1991), 93–4.

14   Hunter *op. cit.*, 57–8.

15   Goodfield, 126.

16   Arikha (2007), 301.

17   Arikha *op cit.*, xix.

18   Planck (1958), quoted in Harris *op cit.*, 155.

19 Arikha *op cit.*, 187–91.
20 Porter (1997), 216.
21 Rose (2003), 79.
22 *Ibid.*
23 Gaukroger (1998), xxiv.
24 Intriguingly Mukherjee identifies a correlation between the emergence of humoral theory in ancient Greece and 'a revolution in hydraulic science originating with irrigation and canal-digging and culminating with Archimedes discovering his eponymous laws in his bathtub.'
25 King (1970), 3; Porter *op. cit.*, 246–7.
26 Porter *op. cit.*, 247.
27 *Ibid.*, 248.
28 Ruse (2010), 142.
29 Dutfield (2012); Nicholson (2013, 2014).
30 Brooke (1991), 117.
31 King *op. cit.*, 3.
32 Porter *op. cit.*, 284.
33 Marks (1997), 1.
34 Bynum (1994), 25–30.
35 *Ibid.*, 103–5.
36 Burgen (1996).
37 Lesch (1984).
38 Ravetz, *op. cit.*, 38.
39 Bynum (1994) *op. cit.*, 96–7.
40 Stahnisch (2009).
41 Bloch (1989).
42 Bynum (1994) *op. cit.*, 103–4.
43 *Ibid.*, 104.
44 Bloch *op. cit.*, 1260.
45 Cunningham (2002).
46 Magendie (1828).
47 Though dedicated to animal experimentation Magendie was not averse to trying things out on himself at some personal risk: 'Having been rendered sleepless by drinking green tea, I was induced to take black drop, in which citrate of morphia predominates; the consequences were most alarming to myself and those around me, and it required large and frequently repeated doses of brandy to prevent the utter annihilation of the pulse, and the sinking of the powers of life.' Magendie (1835), 28–9.
48 Magendie (1821), 165–172.
49 Pelletier and Magendie (1817); Rossignol (1989).

50   Buckingham (2005), 44.

51   Pelletier came up with the name emetine. Sneader (2005), 92.

52   Weatherall, *op. cit.*, 20.

53   Pelletier and Caventou (1820).

54   Sneader (2005) *op. cit.*, 93.

55   Magendie (1835) *op. cit.*, 57.

56   Le Couteur and Burreson (2004), 336.

57   Sneader (2005) *op. cit.*, 94.

58   Weatherall (1990), 17–18.

59   Sneader (2005) *op. cit.*, 94 (emphasis added).

60   Bynum (1994) *op. cit.*, 104.

61   Gross (1998), 383.

62   Gross *op. cit.*, 384.

63   *Ibid.*, 384.

64   Arikha *op. cit.*, 285.

65   Olmsted and Olmsted (1952), 5.

66   Bynum (1994) *op. cit.*, 105.

67   *Ibid.*, 105-6.

68   Feldman (2009), 227.

69   Porter *op. cit.*, 338.

70   Mukherjee *op. cit.*, 14–5.

71   Mukherjee *op. cit.*, 48.

72   Mukherjee *op. cit.*, 14. See Virchow (1860), 167–72.

73   Mukherjee *op. cit.*, 16.

74   Schultz (2008), 1481.

75   Bucchi (1997).

76   Pickstone (2000), 51–2.

77   'Such achievements prompted even an Englishman, Thomas Huxley, to assert that Pasteur's discoveries alone had reaped sufficient wealth for France to repay her enormous reparations to Germany after the 1870 war.' Bud (1993), 14.

78   Pasteur was not the only outstanding chemist with industry experience, specifically beer brewing. During the nineteenth century, the English brewing industry came to regard chemistry as a necessary area of expertise, requiring the setting up of laboratories and the hiring of top chemists including Germans. One of these, Peter Griess, was a pioneer in the development of synthetic dyes and was consulting to BASF while simultaneously employed by Allsopp, a brewery based in Burton upon Trent, the English beer town. Sumner (2013), 182; Yeates and Yeates (2016). It is worth adding in passing that neither Pasteur nor Griess had ideological or moral objections to the patent system.

79 As he famously stated, 'There are no such things as pure and applied science — there are only science, and the applications of science.' Quoted in Dubos (1951), 152.
80 Cassier (2005).
81 Dubos (1951), 117.
82 Quoted in Dubos *op. cit.*, 240.
83 Dubos *op. cit.*, 117–8.
84 Dubos *op. cit.*, 121.
85 Dubos *op. cit.*,123.
86 Quoted in Dubos *op. cit.*, 128.
87 Porter *op. cit.*, 435.
88 Watson (2010), 386.
89 Porter *op. cit.*, 442.
90 Chandler (1992), 94.
91 Hüntelmann (2013), 45.
92 *Ibid.*, 45.
93 *Ibid.*, 45.
94 Rutschman (2020).
95 'Between 2000 and 2013, the market value for vaccines soared from US$5 billion to almost $24 billion; by 2025, that value is expected to quadruple. Groups around the world are trying to devise effective vaccines for dozens of diseases, especially the "big three" — HIV/AIDS, malaria and tuberculosis.' Nelson (2015).
96 Parascandola (1981).
97 Lesch (2007), 18–9.
98 Marks (2015), 5.
99 Parascandola *op. cit.*, 21.
100 Parascandola *op. cit.*, 30.
101 Lesch (2007) *op. cit.*,19; Parascandola, *op. cit.*, 30.
102 Wainwright (2004), 95.
103 Following the introduction of penicillin, the use of dyes in photodynamic therapy was neglected by industry. However, the effectiveness of some dyes and dye derivatives against microbes and even cancer tumours has recently led to a revival in commercial interest in dyes as drugs. *See* Wainwright (2004) *op. cit.*
104 Wainwright (2004) *op. cit.*, 95.
105 Bynum *op. cit.*, 160.
106 Morris (2015).
107 Harris and Paxman (2002).

Chapter 5

From the Dyeing Arts to Drugs: *Or* Dye-making, Pharmacy, and the New Research Corporation

The last chapter provided the scientific background to the industry's beginnings. It showed how scientific achievements made elsewhere began to interact with the world of commerce in which the appliance of science was of course targeted at the discovery and manufacture of commercial products. This chapter picks up where the last one ended, shifting focus onto the emerging industry itself. It traces the evolution of the pharmaceutical industry from its origins up to the First World War by which time it was clearly recognisable as a distinct industrial sector sufficiently important to be strategically valuable to national governments.

As I mentioned in Chapter 2, the pharmaceutical industry evolved as part of the second industrial revolution from pharmacy shops, branded retailers of medicines and related products such as food additives, and plant and mineral-based drug wholesalers, some of which were already quite old. However, the importance and influence of the quite new synthetic dyestuff-making firms, mostly German, who began to move into pharmaceuticals from the 1880s, was enormous in representing the most radical break with the past, and in shaping the sector for at least another hundred years. Bayer, Hoechst and BASF are the most notable of these. Several companies producing processed foods and food and nutritional supplements became successful drug companies too, sometimes continuing to sell such products alongside pharmaceuticals. Glaxo, or GlaxoSmithKline as it is now called, for example, started life in New Zealand as a shop selling its own powdered milk for babies, and then shifted to medicines via food supplements.[1] Of course there was a thin and indistinct line between supposedly health-giving food substances and medicines, at least insofar as marketing is concerned. A visit to a retail chemist or health food store suggests that there still is, though regulated pharmaceutical products are of course something different, as we saw in Chapter 3. Of course, in some respects the lines continue to be somewhat blurred. What is a vitamin tablet? It is a nutritional supplement if one is healthy, but a medicine if you have a deficiency-related disease. And if given in purified form to prevent or treat such a disease, it is a modern pharmaceutical product no more or less than is, say, paracetamol, ibuprofen or ranitidine.

If we look separately at Germany, Switzerland, the United States and Britain we find that the industry has somewhat different roots in each country. Germany presents the most interesting and important case of the four and will get much of the attention in this chapter. Before the industry properly emerged, drugs were sold by pharmacies but all of the research including the discovery and testing was done by academic institutions and hospitals, as may be inferred from the previous chapter.[2] What changed everything was the synthetic dyestuff industry which came up with the research-based approaches to discovery and the intellectual property management strategy that made them leading pharmaceutical companies once they moved into drugs as they started to do in the 1880s. Behind this rapid evolution were advances, trends and new research priorities in pure chemistry, fashion, and the need to dispose of coal tar, a waste product of gas lighting that was produced in high volumes during this age.[3] While the scientific advances of the time made this new industry possible, its initial attractiveness as a potentially profitable business was due to the high demand for new colours, especially in the fashion-conscious French high society. But as we will see its beginnings were to some extent serendipitous. Switzerland largely followed Germany albeit some years behind, benefiting from German leadership *and* the absence of domestic patent protection, meaning anything could be copied.

Britain, like France got into synthetic dyestuff discovery and production rather early. However, these products did not lead to medicines. Instead, the transition to research-based pharmaceutical manufacturing took much longer and came about largely through natural products, rather than those synthesised in the laboratory, and mostly made by old firms. For example, Allen & Hanburys, which was acquired by Glaxo in 1958, started as an apothecary shop in 1715. Initially, the company made and sold what were then known as 'drugges', and 'chemical and galenical medicines'.[4] Beecham's was a trader in branded medicines and food supplements. Indeed, during my childhood its most famous product was the cold treatment Beechams Powders, which is still sold despite the company having been taken over. That the brand has outlived the company that first made it testifies not only to the importance and value of trademarks but specifically to the commercial value of a branded product whose ingredients may be quite commonplace: in this case aspirin and caffeine. As business historian Jonathan Liebenau put it:

> The major British manufacturers of medicines were usually first and foremost importers and wholesalers of materia medica. With a well-integrated and hierarchically organised medical profession there was not a great pull for novelty in therapeutics, and new drugs were rarely introduced through hospitals. The leading firms of the 1890s were long-established, most dated from the early part of the century.[5]

The United States was somewhat similar. Again, according to Liebenau:

> In the United States the outstanding characteristic of manufacturing pharmacy was its recent development out of the practice of pharmacy. Ethical pharmaceuticals production was boosted because of the particular interest in the new medicines of the 1890s. Production was stimulated by a public health system which was on the lookout to incorporate esoteric medical science. Transportation and advertising were transforming the production and sale of drugs nationwide.[6]

In his historical account of the origin of the US pharmaceutical industry, Joseph Gabriel highlights the importance of a change in attitudes towards intellectual property rights. Previously, medical patenting and trademark use were deemed to be unethical in creating monopolies over health products.[7] For various reasons this stance changed from the late nineteenth century, albeit not exactly overnight. Given intellectual property's role as a defining aspect of the industry, this change in perspective and practice was a necessary, albeit not sufficient, condition. As he puts it, 'this transformation in values was an essential component of the corporate reconstruction of the American pharmaceutical industry and its subsequent growth in the decades following.' This might also be largely true for Britain but with the difference that compared to the United States, which was not more advanced than Britain in medical science, it was largely a follower with respect to intellectual property and marketing strategy. Indeed, Burroughs Wellcome, which was established in London by two American immigrants, did much to import US-style business practices into Britain including the heavy use of trademarks, perhaps most famously the word mark 'Tabloid' for their compressed tablets. Arguably firms in the United States were influenced by those in Germany. According to one view, Sir Henry Wellcome's 'introduction of a research and development laboratory was a direct effort to adopt methods which his American colleagues had originally brought across the Atlantic from Germany'.[8] However, Church and Tansey's detailed biography of Burroughs Wellcome reveals Silas Burroughs as the real innovator, not Henry Wellcome: 'While Burroughs may have been a year or possibly two years later than Allen & Hanburys in introducing American compressed medicines into Britain, he was the first to introduce American methods of marketing drugs to the trade by 'detailing' physicians. He promoted his vision of a company possessing extensive overseas markets through energetic travelling'.[9]

Targeting doctors rather than the general public was extremely important in terms of establishing respectability — something obviously good for business. It carved out so-called 'ethical' drugs from the masses of quack remedies and other dubious substances being purveyed elsewhere; that is, patent*ed* drugs made from recipes provided to the authorities (written disclosure being required under patent law from the late eighteenth century) from patent medicines made from secret ones, advertised directly to the public and sold over the counter with no questions asked. Ethical drugs were thus defined substances patented and marketed under a distinct and newly coined name (e.g. Phenacetin, Aspirin). The patent medicines typically comprised an extract or mixture sold in one form or another under the name of the inventor, producer, trader or perhaps even an unknown or imaginary person (e.g. Dr Johnson's Yellow

Ointment,[10] Stevens's Consumption Cure,[11] Beecham's Pills) that as patent law evolved became ineligible for protection. In due course the stigma attached to the patenting of medicines lessened as the pursuit of profit from medicines was frowned upon less and patenting came to be seen as a legitimate means to this end. As investment in research and development increased in the twentieth century, patenting came to seem more justifiable morally. Nonetheless, many European countries did not allow drugs to be patented until the late twentieth century, and the stigma has certainly not disappeared. Indeed, it seems to be enjoying a revival for reasons we will look into later.

As we will see, the industry which emerged largely in late nineteenth century Germany was unique in the way it effectively integrated science, especially synthetic chemistry, with impressive commercial acumen including sophisticated intellectual property strategy. Other new companies, often British and American, emerged largely from pharmacy shops and sought to glean treatments from natural products. American firms proved especially adept at marketing and in doing so helped to make the industry what it is today.[12] During the industry's history vast amounts of money have been spent on marketing as well as research. For critics a result of this devotion to marketing and to research is that the industry now has a kind of identity crisis. Is it a research-based industry or a marketing-based one? Or is it both? We will return to this question later in the book.

Whilst initially less scientific than the German 'big three', British and American companies came to rival them. This was by no means immediate, though. They achieved this in large part both organically and, especially, by acquiring knowledge from outside, often from universities. The synthetic chemistry practiced by the dye-makers and the isolation and purification achievements in natural product chemistry attained by the other firms both shaped patent law and intellectual property management strategy in Europe and North America in ways that have proved enduring and defining characteristics of the industry. *In terms of what the industry is and represents, these legal and business aspects are just as significant as the underlying science and the products themselves arising from the application of ever-evolving scientific effort and achievement.*

An Accidental New Industry

According to most accounts,[13] the synthetic dyestuff industry dates back to 1856, when William Henry Perkin created one of the first coal tar dyes, aniline purple ('Mauve'). In that year Perkin, based at the recently established Royal College of Chemistry in London, was set the task of making quinine using coal tar, an industrial waste product of gas lighting that was being produced in high volumes at the time. This was in fact a futile task since the state of the chemical arts had not then reached a level that would have made it possible, feasible as it appeared to Perkin and his professor, August Wilhelm Hofmann.

Coal tar happens to be a rich source of interesting organic compounds like benzene and phenol. Starting with aniline, a coal tar derivative discovered several years earlier, Perkin produced what appeared initially to be a worthless black gunk. Many other scientists would just have thrown it away and tried again or done something else. But curiosity was clearly part of Perkin's nature. He added methylated spirits and water and found that the substance stained his test-tubes bright purple. After that, he lost any interest he had in cures for malaria and turned to the possibilities of dyeing. He tested it on cloth, and realising the commercial potential, filed a patent and set up a company to manufacture and sell it. Perkin's dye was not the first aniline dye to enter the market, but it was one of the first to be commercially successful, and its implications were far-reaching.

Although it was Hofmann who told Perkin to conduct such an experiment, the credit for discovering the properties of mauve and in effect establishing a completely new science-based industry rightly goes to Perkin. In any case, the task of making quinine was way beyond the means of anybody at the time. It was one thing to know the chemical formula of a molecule like quinine, which chemists at the time did; it was quite another to know its three-dimensional configuration. Indeed, so challenging was the task of synthesis that it was not to be achieved for almost another century. But ignorance and error can lead to unforeseen achievement if the timing is right. 'If Perkin had been born twenty years later, he would have known how fruitless his search would have been, and thus would not have blundered into mauve.'[14] Perkin conducted the experiments leading to the discovery of mauve in his own home and without Hofmann's oversight. Besides, Hoffman was rather under-whelmed by Perkin's discovery and felt that he should stick to doing scientific research rather than enter the risky world of commerce.[15]

Soon after, Perkin patented his discovery in Britain and formed a company to commercialize it. Perkin's discovery paved the way for new coal tar-based industries to emerge rapidly and become incredibly productive in terms of the variety of products discovered and entering the market and in the extent of the wealth created. One of these industries was pharmaceuticals, but there were several others. As an eminent British scientist writing at the beginning of the twentieth century put it rather presciently:

> The manufacture of synthetic medicinal agents, artificial perfumes, sweetening materials, antitoxines, nutritives, and photographic developers are all outgrowths of the coal-tar industry, and in great part still remain attached to the colour works where they originated. Of these subsidiary industries the most important is the manufacture of synthetic medicinal preparations, which has already attained to large proportions, and bids fair to revolutionise medical science.[16]

The aniline dyes, which were derived from benzene, were the first generation of the coal tar dyes. The most commercially important aniline dye was aniline red, otherwise known as fuchsine or magenta, invented by Françoise Verguin. The French firm Renard Frères patented fuchsine in 1859 in both France and Britain. Apart from being a lucrative product in itself — it is still on the market — fuchsine is an intermediate for making many other dyes. During the 1850s and early 1860s, other companies in Britain and France developed a growing number of new products and processes. At the same time, significant breakthroughs in elucidating the chemical structures of the coal tar derivatives were being made in industry and academia, not just in these two countries, but also in Germany.

The second generation of synthetic dyes were the azos. Peter Griess, a German chemist and soon to become a long-time employee of an English beer brewery, came up with the principle behind azo manufacture. Once August Kekulé, another German chemist, had figured out the ring structure of benzene in 1865, it became possible to generate countless numbers of synthetic dyes through molecular manipulation and recombination and to determine their chemical structures. The azo era took a while to take off, but within 40 years more than 50 per cent of the commercial dye products were azos.[17]

The third generation of synthetic dyes appeared in 1869 with the synthesis of the natural dye, alizarin. A year previously, two German academic scientists, Carl Graebe and Carl Liebermann, developed a formula to synthesize alizarin from anthracene. After they patented their discovery a race began to find a way to produce it on a commercial scale. Heinrich Caro at BASF developed a promising process and filed a patent jointly with Graebe and Liebermann in Britain just one day before Perkin, who had come up with a very similar process also using anthracene. Unlike the anilines and azos, the commercialization of synthetic alizarin actually substituted for a natural product, madder — a fact that had legal repercussions in the United States as we will see below. Indeed, the need for legislatures, patent offices and courts in different countries to consider the correctness or otherwise of treating artificial copies of natural substances as new inventions, as raised by this early example, has continued to this very day to be a pressing matter. The same may be said for natural phenomena revealed to have practical applications. Again, where does the invention lie — and even if there is inventiveness, should the result still be patentable?

The fourth stage in the evolution of the synthetic dyestuff industry arrived with the manufacture and successful commercialization of synthetic indigo. This achievement was especially important. It required an unprecedented commitment to in-house research and development, which turned out to be one of the defining features of the second industrial revolution. More specifically, it stimulated the development of the twentieth-century fine chemical and pharmaceutical industries. It also ensured the dominance of German firms in various chemical product markets.

The French dyestuff industry dominated the aniline phase, while the early part of the azo phase marked the leadership of the British firms.[18] So by the mid-1860s Britain was pre-eminent with France in second place. There did not appear to be any serious rivals at the time, but from the beginning of the alizarin phase, the synthetic dyestuff industry came to be dominated by new German chemical firms like Bayer, Hoechst,[19] BASF,[20] and AGFA.[21] The first of these soon became more famous for drugs than dyes. *Indeed, the modern pharmaceutical industry can be said, in part, to be an offshoot of the dyestuff industry.*

As for patenting, Perkin's invention heralded a major change. With the patenting of fine chemicals and processes to make them, new science-based industries appeared almost from nothing and these generated huge revenues. The patent stakes for such firms, whether they were innovators or imitators, were immense. Consequently, success depended often on clever use of the patent systems of their own countries *and* of their overseas markets. Their ability to be strategic about patenting (and, increasingly, trademarks) depended on what patent laws allowed them to protect, or to get away with. As a result, the chemical industries became active lobbyists influencing as far as they could the drafting of patent laws. Where they found under-protection (as they saw it), companies would join with rivals to persuade the government to strengthen protection. Where they found overprotection, they would lobby either for less protection, or alternatively collaborate with other firms to mitigate market distortions arising from either too many patents or from the monopolies created by small numbers of overly broad patents. They would do this, for example, by pooling their patents or shifting their operations to neighbouring countries. When patents were insufficient to keep prices high for lengthy periods, companies sometimes formed price-fixing cartels. When one looks at the business practices of today's pharmaceutical and biotechnology companies, it becomes obvious that these lessons were learned from the dye-makers 140 years earlier when they were starting also to make drugs. Furthermore, governments became aware of the economic stakes involved and consequently became very interested not only in their own patent laws but in those of their perceived economic competitors. Again, this is very much the case today.

There are several reasons why the rapid emergence of west European firms set up around that time to develop synthetic dyestuffs derived from coal tar is of historical *and* current significance. First, this period is associated with the appearance of the corporate research laboratory. German companies such as the ones just mentioned above, were pioneers in in-house research and development in which teams of scientists collaborated to solve technical problems in the development of collective innovations. Among other things, this marked a decline in the economic importance of independent amateurs, inventor-entrepreneurs, small firms, and countries that had tended to rely on 'practical tinkering' and were thus rather slow in moving into organized industrial research and development.[22] As it turned out, the first mover advantages of the first research-based companies were tremendous and enduring. Most of today's pharmaceutical giants were founded in the nineteenth century or, despite having quite new names, are direct descendants of old companies established over a century ago. The former group includes Pfizer, Merck, Roche, Eli Lilly and Bayer, whilst the latter counts Novartis, GlaxoSmithKline, Sanofi and AstraZeneca among their number.

Second, a fruitful marriage between the synthetic dyestuff industry and the new fields of bacteriology, biochemistry and human biology provided a huge impetus for the modern pharmaceutical industry. Third, some of the largest life science corporations that dominate the chemical, pharmaceutical and seed and agrochemical sectors of the modern global economy are direct descendants of the original late nineteenth century European synthetic dyestuff companies like the German ones just mentioned and also Swiss firms like Ciba and Geigy that are now Novartis. Fourth, the synthetic dyestuff industry provides an interesting example of how countries appeared to benefit from adopting a strategic approach to designing and using their patent systems, and how others were harmed by not doing so. The fact that companies themselves were involved in the process of drawing up the law is of course highly important. However, nothing in this book should be construed to imply a belief that there is a natural alignment of interests between a prominent industrial sector and the citizens of that country. What is good for General Motors is not necessarily good for the USA, and the same goes for Bayer and Germany.

The Rise of Germany and Switzerland

In 1862 August Hofmann, the London-based German scientist who had trained Perkin, expressed firm confidence that Britain would be the leading synthetic dyestuff producer for many years to come because of its coal reserves, its huge production of coal tar, and its enormous market for textiles.[23] He was wrong. By 1913 German companies had captured 85 per cent of the global market for dyestuffs. Switzerland, the only other major exporter was in second place albeit with a mere 10 per cent. Germany was equally dominant in the pharmaceutical sector.

The rise of Germany from the 1870s as a major industrial power with its dominant chemical and pharmaceutical industries can be attributed to at least three main factors. These are government investment in education and training, in-house research and development and company/ academic collaborations, and government industrial and trade policy.

The Prussian government provided a great deal of support for scientific and technical education and training throughout the nineteenth century.[24] As well as introducing mass primary education from the late eighteenth century, Germany established the world's foremost technical higher education system. Its research universities educated large numbers of organic chemistry students. During the middle of the century some highly talented graduates moved to Britain and carried out research that was of enormous benefit to the British chemical industry. When chemists like Hofmann, Caro, Martius and Witt returned to Germany during the 1860s[25] they helped to turn the new firms from imitators into the most innovative chemical companies in the world in less than two decades.

Concerning the second factor, new German firms like Bayer, Hoechst (both founded in 1863), BASF (1865) and AGFA (1867) were established to copy French and British dyes, and were able to do so because there was no single patent law covering all the pre-unification German states and of course the German system of technical education was producing large numbers of competent chemists able to do the copying. This is similar to India today, which is not an innovator in the fine chemicals/ pharmaceuticals context, but is able to copy pretty much anything. (That said, the German switch to consistent innovativeness has not yet been matched by India.) For foreign firms, the only alternative was to file patents in each of the different states that had patent laws at the time. Since this was troublesome, often they did not bother to file in any state.

Nonetheless, the main German dyestuff firms decided early on both to invest in research and development and to collaborate with university researchers. Thus Germany missed the inventor-entrepreneur era exemplified in Britain by Richard Arkwright and by James Watt and Matthew

Boulton, moving straight to research and development departments[26] comprising teams of scientists collaborating to solve technical problems. 'It was the German dyestuff industry which first realized that it could be profitable to put the business of research for new products and development of new chemical processes on a more regular, systematic and professional basis'.[27]

The huge profits from products like alizarin based on highly advanced new processes helped companies to expand and to invest in even more expensive research and development such as the successful synthesis of indigo and the early twentieth century development of a process for producing ammonia from atmospheric nitrogen (the Haber-Bosch process).[28] Academic researchers were often invited to collaborate with company chemists or hired as consultants and this was very good for industry.[29]

Turning to government industrial and trade policy, despite the political dominance of the Prussian Junkers (the land-owning elite) during the early years, the new German state identified the national interest with the success of its emerging industrial sector and decided actively to support it. Consequently, while 'the British industrial revolution was more or less carried out by the hands of private individuals, ... Germany's entry into the industrial era was orchestrated by government bureaucracies'.[30] Not only did the government actively seek to facilitate a business climate that was conducive for its companies to flourish, such as by protecting them from foreign competition, but it took a permissive if not supportive stance towards cooperative inter-firm alliances to fix prices and rationalise sales networks.[31] Such industrial cooperation also spurred the formation of trade associations by companies to further their common interests. For example, the chemical industry set up such an association to promote the intellectual property interests of its members.[32] Alfred Chandler, the eminent business historian, appropriately referred to this system as 'cooperative managerial capitalism'.[33] Quite a contrast with British *laissez faire* capitalism that prevailed for much of the nineteenth century.

Switzerland, like Germany, experienced rapid growth in its chemicals sector during this period. Many of the first synthetic dye chemists in Switzerland were actually French chemists and entrepreneurs who had relocated to Basle, a city with long established textile and dye-making industries.[34] Like Germany, academy-industry collaborations encouraged by government were crucial to the enhancement of scientific and technological capabilities,[35] while close relationships between companies and financial institutions allowed businesses to secure credit necessary to expand their research and development capabilities. The Swiss firms began by manufacturing such bulk dye products as fuchsine and alizarin but soon found themselves unable to compete with the German firms, which were the main suppliers of their intermediates and base products.[36] In response, firms like Ciba, Geigy and Sandoz shifted their production to high quality dyes and pharmaceuticals mostly for export. This strategy was so successful that, by the 1890s, Switzerland, *with no help from a national patent system*, was already the world's second biggest dyestuff producer.

Patents, Dyestuffs and the European Chemical Industries

If we accept that the advance of globally competitive domestic high technology firms is likely to be beneficial for a country in terms, for example, of foreign exchange receipts, increased income per capita, job creation, technological spillovers, and the availability of useful new products,[37] and the relative decline in competitive position of such firms is probably disadvantageous, it seems fair to conclude that Germany and Switzerland gained from the success of their chemical firms at the expense of France and Britain. If it is true that their respective patent systems helped determine whether countries' national industries were 'winners' or 'losers', they clearly had implications — positive or negative — for the public interest. In fact, it is highly likely that the patent systems of each country, including the fact that they were so different, played a major role in determining the outcome of the race for supremacy in the global dyestuffs market and later in the early years of the pharmaceuticals sectors as well — albeit not in the ways that supports any clear correlation between enhanced availability, scope and enforceability of rights, and more innovation.

Germany

The development of German patent legislation, jurisprudence and practice in the late nineteenth century was very much driven by newly-organized stakeholder groups and an emergent wider patent community. 'This patent community gathered the employees of the *Reichspatentamt* [Patent Office], those of the legal departments of big companies or private lawyers specialized in intellectual property rights, and scientists working in academic institutions, such as the *Kaiser-Wilhelm-Gesellschaft* research centres.'[38] Although German industrialists had limited involvement in party politics, they 'were represented in politics through extraparliamentary lobbying channels. An elaborate system of well-organized and well-financed employers' associations acted as very effective mouthpieces for their interests'.[39]

The *Deutsche Chemische Gessellschaft* (German Chemical Association) was founded in 1867 under the presidency of Hofmann, and consisted of academic scientists and private sector chemists and businessmen. Its aim was to stimulate academic-industrial collaboration.[40] The Association strongly favoured a patent law and sought to convince Bismarck of the need for such legislation. Without a country-wide patent system barriers to entry were low, enabling many new chemical firms to spring up in the early 1870s. This was obviously a very good thing at such an early stage of the industry's development.

However, the industry was changing. With the economic recession that began in 1873, many small firms went bankrupt and the chemical industry consolidated so that the market became dominated by a few large firms. Many of these surviving businesses understood that to become research and development intensive and truly innovative, some kind of a patent system was needed.[41]

In 1874 a group of high-technology firms jointly set up a pressure group called the *Deutsche Patentschutz-Verein* (German Society for Patent Protection) to lobby for a patent law that would protect German industry during a time of economic difficulty. The prime movers were in fact the engineers not the dye-makers. Nonetheless, the latter were still involved. Carl Alexander Martius and Hofmann represented the interests of the chemists in the Society.[42]

Within German industry as a whole there were a number of conflicting views. While the Society of German Engineers lobbied in favour of a patent law, there were still differences about the kind of patent law needed. Werner Siemens, who was one of the most powerful industrialists of the time, was gravely concerned that rival British and American firms would take out many patents for inventions that they would not work in Germany, and which would severely restrict the research and commercial opportunities of German companies.[43]

The chemical industry was also divided. Some firms (for example, BASF) favoured a patent law which protected processes but not products, and were thus unhappy that the first draft of the patent law would have provided protection of chemical products as such. They argued that this created no incentive to improve production processes.[44] On the other hand, the co-founder of Hoechst,[45] Adolf Brüning, wanted the chemical industry to be completely excluded from the patent system.[46] His view was that the French and British chemical industries had been harmed because the laws there had allowed excessively strong monopoly protection for intermediate products, whereas — as he saw it — the lack of a German patent law had allowed the chemical industry to expand. Although the synthetic dyestuff firms had not completely reached a consensus, the board of the Chemical Association submitted a petition to the Reichstag which argued in favour of patents for methods of manufacturing chemical products but not the products themselves. The stated grounds were that 'a chemical product can be obtained by various methods and from different starting materials; the grant of a patent for the product itself would prevent better processes discovered subsequently from being brought into effect in the interest of the public and of the inventors'.[47] In the event, the Chemical Association's position was heeded and adopted by virtue of Section 1 of the 1877 Patent Law, according to which

> Patents are granted for new inventions which permit of an industrial realization. The exceptions are: ... 2. Inventions of articles of food, drinks and medicine as well as of substances manufactured by a chemical process in so far as the inventions do not relate to a certain process for manufacturing such articles.

The language is somewhat vague, but implies that while processes alone could be patented, chemical products could only be protected if manufactured by a specific process and by no other. Since the interpretation of the courts (until 1888) was that sale of a chemical made through a patented process did not constitute infringement,[48] chemical products were effectively excluded. While this provision encouraged chemists to be creative and devise original processes, it also encouraged anti-competitive 'blocking patents' intended to close off broad areas of research from competitors.[49] Another noteworthy provision, which also appears to have reflected the interests of many German firms, was Section 11, according to which a patent could be withdrawn after three years, either

> if the patentee neglects to work his invention in the Country to an adequate extent or to do all that was requisite for securing the said working; [or] when it appears conducive to the public interest that permission to use the invention be granted to others and the patentee refuses to grant such permission for a suitable compensation and on good security.

A third provision of great importance to the chemical industry was the publication of patent applications and awarded patents, ensuring the rapid dissemination of state-of-the-art knowledge. It had already become evident that keeping chemical processes secret did not necessarily provide more than a few months' lead-time,[50] so the industry as a whole probably saw publication as being advantageous. In fact, dissemination of technical information has from as far back as the late eighteenth century been considered to be one of its most important functions,[51] and for Germany it was a key objective. Similarly, the Japanese patent system has over the years treated dissemination as being at least as important as rewarding invention, on the basis that the circulation of knowledge accelerates the rate of further invention.

A fourth feature of the law that served the interests of the larger research-based companies (for reasons we will soon come to) was the exclusion of all mention of 'inventors'. The right holders were 'applicants'. This was justified by the argument propounded by these firms that modern inventions were collectively achieved and depended primarily on capital investment in laboratories, equipment and skilled employees.[52]

Most historians of the European synthetic dyestuff industries with a view on the matter[53] agree that the 1877 patent law had a positive effect overall, encouraging the establishment of research and development departments in all the major firms. Not only did it contain the right provisions for the industry, but its timing was just right. According to Johann Peter Murmann, this was the case

> because it came after the industry had already developed strong firms and science was providing the tools to do systematic R&D on new dyes… Had the German patent law arrived in 1858, it is doubtful that as many German firms would have developed into such strong competitors. Fewer firms would have entered the industry, and inefficient firms would have been more likely to survive, as was the case in Britain. The most important institution in the early success of the German dye industry was the university system, but patent laws were a second key factor that allowed the German firms to capture a dominant position.[54]

The availability of protection for chemical processes but not products reflected the prevalent commercial and research strategies of the German firms at that time. They soon realized that chemical dyes were not only products but were also likely to be intermediates for other products. Therefore, patenting dyes directly could have inhibited the kinds of innovation that allowed German firms to compete with their British counterparts. Process innovation was all-important for them because the concern of German firms was to develop processes enabling them to improve efficiency and cut costs while also meeting the requirements of the dyers for the widest possible range of colours for all fabrics. But they soon found they could achieve cost efficiencies best by putting on the market a massive range of colours for all fabrics, using the same production equipment to create them. Emphasizing process innovation as a research strategy and product diversity as a marketing strategy resulted in the cost-effective generation of an extraordinarily large range of new and relatively inexpensive products. On the eve of the First World War, Bayer had 2000 different dyestuffs[55] while Hoechst made as many as 10,000.[56] The development of such huge product portfolios was not demand driven, but with them the big three German firms 'had a firm grip on every conceivable composition of hydrocarbons, *firmly shielded by a wall of patents and tacit knowledge*'.[57]

Allegedly, this grip was strengthened by submitting patent specifications that not only failed to disclose sufficient information to repeat the invention, but also included deliberate mistakes.[58] It is very possible that such accusations are more a reflection of hostility towards their nation than a true account of German companies' patent filing behaviour.[59] Nonetheless, copying German inventions by reading patent specifications could clearly be a frustrating task whether that was due to the lower competence of British chemists or for other reasons.

On the other hand, the development of the azo dyes brought to the fore some of the difficulties in applying patent law to chemistry, the patent doctrines of the period having been formulated with mechanical inventions in mind and not chemical processes.[60] It is useful to look at this situation and see how the aforementioned German patent community responded to it in the context of three reasons why innovation in the field of industrial chemistry, particularly during its early stages, challenged the patent system in hitherto unforeseen ways.

The first reason has to do with the danger that broad patent protection can stifle innovation in new industries where the learning curve is particularly steep. The dyestuff industry was a case in point. During its infancy, some of the most innovative activity centred on *existing* chemical substances. This was, first, because compounds may have many uses that would have been inconceivable to the original discoverer or manufacturer of the compound. For example, research on some of the dyestuffs revealed that they also had pharmaceutical properties. Second, it was likely that ways would soon be found to manufacture the substance in a more efficient and cost-effective way than its original inventor had managed to do. Third, the substance might have turned out to be an intermediate for the manufacture of a host of other useful substances which individually could have required minimal additional effort, expense or inventiveness to discover. For these three reasons, allowing chemical substances to be patented may have fatally discouraged innovation by allowing excessively strong monopolies. This explains why the German chemical industry lobbied against product patents on chemicals in the 1870s. That this situation has changed in more recent times explains why the trend in Europe since the Second World War has been to allow patents for chemical products.

The second major difficulty is that a whole family of compounds may share the same useful characteristic. Thus, the application of a chemical process may generate large numbers of related substances producing the same effect. How broadly should patent applicants be allowed to extend their claims? Should it be allowable only to patent a process for one and only one substance? Or should it be possible to go to the other extreme, casting the net as widely as possible to claim as many classes of related substances as is theoretically conceivable 'besides the substances actually used in the "invented" process'?[61] The dilemma is that protection could be so inadequate as to be worthless, or so strong as to inhibit innovation. Striking the right balance between rewarding inventors adequately without hindering follow-on innovators is never easy. But patent offices, courts and legislators had no prior experience and had to wait until problems arose and then figure out how to deal with them. Industry sought to deal with the situation by filing large numbers of patents so as to shield products from almost identical competing ones. In 1887, the German Patent Office decided it had to respond to the proliferation of chemical patent applications indirectly claiming not just the actual substances used in the process that was the subject of the application, but also various classes of analogue, homologue and isomer.[62] It did so by introducing a new regulation requiring chemical patent applicants to provide samples of all substances claimed in the application.[63]

The third problem, which azo dyes in particular raised, is that stringent standards of novelty and inventive step could have made most such products unpatentable. It was in fact rather easy to generate vast quantities of dyes without doing anything particularly original. So what should the law do concerning the patentability of known processes when applied to the manufacture of 'new' dyes that were really hardly different to those that already existed? This latter problem was not settled — as it happened to the advantage of patent holding corporations — until an 1889 Supreme Court case relating to the Congo Red dye.

Congo Red and the new technical effect

Congo Red was an azo dye, the process for making of which was patented by Paul Böttiger, a former Bayer chemist. Sold to AGFA, it became a very profitable product, the first that could dye cotton directly. Carl Duisberg at Bayer came up with a chemically very similar dye albeit more brilliant in

(*Continued*)

colour and less sensitive to acid than Congo Red called Benzopurpurin 4B and filed a patent. This was also commercially successful. AGFA and Bayer agreed not to challenge each other's patents and made an arrangement by which AGFA held both patents but both companies would be able to commercialize the two dyes.[64]

Subsequently, a small firm called Ewer & Pick began selling both products made by a slightly different process. AGFA sued for infringement and Ewer & Pick counter-sued to have the patents nullified. Some very eminent chemists provided written or oral testimony that the patents should be made void, including Heinrich Caro of BASF who argued that so lacking in inventiveness was Congo Red that one of his young lab assistants would be able to make it just by reading the title of the patent. Duisberg, representing Bayer, cleverly responded that his assistants could also make BASF's dyes merely by reading the titles of the patents. This was to make the point that if Congo Red were unpatentable then so would the azo dyes generally be too. Such an outcome would obviously have been highly undesirable for both firms.

Duisberg's defence of the patent won the day. But much the most important outcome was the expansion of 'the new technical effect' doctrine which henceforward made it possible for the requirement of true inventiveness to be softened where the result of the disclosed method was a product with 'unexpected and valuable technical qualities'. According to one account:

The court argued that the process for making Congo red, lacking any inventiveness of its own, would as such not have been patentable. In this case, however, the application of the general method resulted in a dyestuff of undoubted technical and commercial value. Its unexpected and valuable technical qualities more than compensated for the lack of inventiveness of the process. In other words, the court said that, if the requirement of utility is particularly emphasized, it is no longer necessary to look at whether the requirement of inventiveness is also satisfied.[65]

The doctrine was a solution to a problem at a particular time but remains an element of European patent law to this day. It has, however, led to much uncertainty since an agreed definition of 'technical' in concepts like technical effect and technical character continues to elude inventors, practitioners and jurists.

(*Continued*)

(*Continued*)

For industry there were two advantages arising from the downgrading of true inventiveness — apart from the obvious one that confirmation that azo dye-making processes were patentable was highly desirable. First, companies were in a better position to accumulate massive patent holdings. Having to demonstrate a genuine flash of genius — that is to say, a significant inventive step — would have made this strategy more difficult.

Moreover, companies preferred to hire inventors and make them assign their inventions to their employers rather than to have to compete with them or at least to have to pay to acquire their patents.[66] Treating inventorship as a collective activity placed each scientist in a more subordinate position than would have been the case otherwise. Therefore, it was not necessarily advantageous for corporations in Germany or elsewhere to extol the genius of the 'inventor-heroes' when promoting their intellectual property interests. Collectivising the inventive process had the effect not only of marginalising the individual inventor but also of defending the patent system from its detractors. As historian Andrea Maestrejuan expressed it: 'When the drafters of the German patent law sought a compromise to silence anti-patent resistance to a unified patent law, they codified this notion of invention as a collaborative process between an inventor with the technically creative skills and a businessman with commercial and marketing skills. Claims to inventive priority included 'juridical' as well as 'physical' persons, acknowledging that inventive activity was just one part of a larger set of human and physical capital brought to bear on advancements in technology.'[67] Moreover, in adopting the first-to-file principle, whereby there is no need to identify a true and first inventor in order to establish who has priority and thus entitlement to a patent, the first German Patent Act favoured well-resourced firms especially with the very high patent renewal fees.

Similar challenges to patenting came up in the United States but took longer to resolve. In 1941, Charles Kettering of General Motors commented — it must be said erroneously and perhaps dishonestly — that 'a one-man invention isn't very possible these days', and argued that it would be unfair to reward individuals for what were basically collective endeavours.[68] Kettering's comment may well have been inspired by a controversial US Supreme Court judgment that same year[69] which denied the patentability of a mechanical device on the grounds that the inventor's skill had not 'reached the level of inventive genius which the Constitution authorizes Congress to award'.[70] But it had no effect on statutory law and the United States did not abandon first to invent until the second decade of the twenty-first century. Having said all this, the naming of inventors in patent documents was made compulsory for all parties to the Paris Convention on the Protection of Industrial Property in 1934 following a revision to that effect, and one can argue that the requirement can in fact serve the interests of companies as long as ownership is retained by the employer.[71]

In 1877, another chemical industry lobby group, the *Verein zur Wahrung der Interessen der chemischen Industrie Deutschlands* (Society for Safeguarding the Interests of the German Chemical Industry) was founded to influence the government, including its trade policy and patent regulation.[72] In the event, German law was reformed in 1891 to incorporate the new technical effect doctrine, which is now part of modern European patent law, and statutorily recognise another Supreme Court decision in 1888, the Methylene Blue case, which placed the burden of proof on alleged infringers to demonstrate that their product was made using a different and unpatented process and clarified that whole families of chemicals could be claimed in the same patent.[73] Recognizing the 1888 decision benefited the German chemical industry since it became easier to prevent Swiss firms from exporting such chemicals to Germany.

The prohibition on the patenting of chemical substances as such remained. This was in accordance with the demands of the Society, which held that 'such comprehensive protection has ... always been considered by the German chemical industry as an obstacle prejudicial to the discovery of new and improved processes'.[74] All of this makes evident, to borrow the words of two recent commentators, that 'the interface between the German chemical industry and the government was well-developed in the last quarter of the nineteenth century, allowing such important collective policy initiatives as the passage of a patent law to be especially tailored to the needs of the chemical industry'.[75]

Finally, it is worth mentioning here that the German companies' attempts to use patents to exclude competitors in foreign markets were assisted greatly if they could acquire protection of chemical substances, and not just of processes. So their control was particularly strong in Britain and the USA, where both kinds of protection were available, and where they were able to sue infringers in the courts. A 1912 US Tariff Board study found that as many as '98 per cent of applications for patents in the chemical field had been assigned to German firms and were never worked in the United States'.[76] Complaints about this situation prompted the drafting of several patent reform bills in the early twentieth century to abolish product protection, and to require the working of patents. These were opposed by other interest groups representing more successful — and influential — American industries, patent lawyers, and prominent entrepreneurs like Thomas Edison and Leo Baekeland, the inventor of Bakelite.[77] Unsurprisingly none was passed, though one important measure was adopted around this time.

In 1894, the US Supreme Court held that patent infringement was a tort for which the federal government had sovereign immunity. In 1910, Congress introduced a balancing measure giving patent owners the right to sue the government for compensation in the Court of Claims, including, as confirmed by the same court in a 1918 case, when the use or manufacture was by a person or entity contracted or subcontracted by the government. This absence of immunity for contractors, in this case the constructors of warships for the navy to be used for the conflict the United States had joined the year before, caused some concern, and the acting navy secretary (Franklin D. Roosevelt no less), intervened to have this part of the law changed so that any liability would fall on the government. Section 1498, Title 28 of the United States Code (as it later become codified), was the result.[78] Accordingly, the patent owner had the right to sue the government for compensation in the Court of Claims, including when the use or manufacture was by a person or entity contracted or subcontracted by the government. Of course, in wartime governments have to take decisive action for the national interest and the industry will not always get its way. Nonethless, the provision remains in the US legal code. For medicines, it came into use in the 1950s when the Military Medical Supply Agency, which bought medicines for the US military, unable to secure a satisfactory price from American companies, placed an order with an Italian company for a consignment of tetracycline powder.[79] In recent years, though, there has been resistance to resorting to Section 1498. Probably, this is not unrelated to the industry's lobbying and election-related funding activities.[80]

Switzerland

The Swiss chemical industry has been seen as an unplanned and ungrateful child of the French patent law, which is said to have driven French dyemakers to Basel due the excessively strong monopolies that it enabled.[81] While such claims can be overstated,[82] the combination of the French patent law and the absence of a domestic one undoubtedly provided a huge impetus to the incipient Swiss dyestuff industry from which the country's chemical and pharmaceutical sectors have benefited to this day.

The Swiss chemical industry first opposed the patent system, but when it became inevitable that there would be one[83] it demanded to be kept outside the system.[84] The companies justified this position with the argument that patent law cannot accommodate the complexities of innovation in the field of chemistry and is therefore inappropriate. But they were mainly concerned that they would be left vulnerable to their German competitors. While the second concern was understandable, the first was somewhat hypocritical given that some Swiss chemical firms were becoming very active users of other countries' patent systems. In consequence of such opposition, the 1888 patent law required inventions to be demonstrated by a model, thus effectively excluding chemical substances and processes from patentability. It also provided compulsory working and licensing.[85] This prohibition on chemical process patents continued until 1907. One important factor was that Switzerland was pressured by Germany to do so. Such pressure was effective owing to the dependence of natural resource-poor Switzerland's chemical industry on the German market (which was its biggest) and on German chemical firms for supplies of coal tar distillates and other chemicals needed to produce the dyes.[86] However, it is also true that the Swiss chemical firms were already building independent capacity, were filing patents in other countries, and felt themselves ready for the change.[87] The ban on product protection continued for seven more decades, though.

Britain

Unlike the cases of Germany and Switzerland, the British dyestuff industry inherited an ancient patent system which, in spite of some reforms during the nineteenth century, failed to meet its requirements. The 1852 *Patent Law Amendment Act* had been passed four years prior to Perkin's great discovery, but apparently without any consideration of chemical inventions. It took several years for the courts to establish rules for interpreting claims in chemicals and in the meantime litigation was a frequent and very serious distraction for many companies, as well as a disincentive for investors.[88] The early patents, including Perkin's, and a series of expensive court cases served as a barrier to entry so the number of new firms was quickly exceeded by new German companies with no patents or litigation threats at all to worry about.[89] Furthermore, compared to their German counterparts, the dyestuff firms were slow to form an industry-wide interest group to pursue their interests,[90] and it took a long time for the government to take account of their needs. With its huge textile industry, Britain was the world's biggest market for dyes, and German companies had filed many patents there even before their country had its own unified patent law.

In later years, the British firms had to contend with ever increasing numbers of patents by German companies that were adept at strategic patenting. In doing so, they effectively blocked many potentially lucrative research and development possibilities,[91] thereby using the law to stifle innovation in Britain at the same time as they were helping to develop, and then benefit from, an innovation-friendly patent law in their own country. Concerns about this situation were raised in the House of Commons in April 1883[92] and again at various times in the early part of the following century. The Act passed that same year sought to allay them by providing for compulsory licensing in certain cases including failure to work the patent in the UK. Unfortunately, this provision was difficult to put into practice and failed to make the British firms more competitive.

At the turn of the century, the government established a committee chaired by Sir Edward Fry to investigate the working of the patent system. Patent agents, inventors and businessmen were among those giving evidence. The dyestuff industry was represented by Ivan Levinstein, a

German-born industrialist from Manchester, and a passionate and dedicated activist for patent reform. Invited to be as radical as he wished by the Master of the Rolls, Lord Alverstone, he proposed that, 'if the department [that is, the Board of Trade] is anxious to bring back an important industry which we have almost lost in this country, principally through our patent laws, then we ought to follow the example of France and Germany and say that a patentee must manufacture the patented article in the country within a certain time, otherwise the patent may be revoked'.[93] In response to the Committee's Report, the patent law was amended in 1902 in a way which allowed for the possibility of revocation in the case of non-working.

In part it was the threat to the Indian indigo trade posed by imports of BASF and Hoechst's patent-protected synthetic indigo, a matter that Levinstein had been wise enough to stress, that convinced the government to reform the patent system. This is hardly surprising given that 'the indigo trade was important to the Empire, unlike azo dyes that had little or no impact on natives, planters, traders, the stock market and other vested interests'.[94] The other big issue, mentioned above, was the way that German chemical firms were said to be flooding the country with unworked blocking patents. Their British rivals complained about this situation, as did their parliamentary allies. Undoubtedly, the German firms were patenting on a huge scale compared to their British counterparts and a large proportion of these patents were never worked (see Table 5.1).

Table 5.1. Comparison of the number of completed English patents for coal tar products taken during 1886–1900, by six largest English and six largest German firms[95]

German Firms	English Firms
Badische Aniline Works (BASF) 179	Brooke, Simpson & Spiller 7
Meister, Lucius & Brüning (Hoechst) 231	Clayton Aniline Co. 21
Farbfabriken Bayer & Co. 306	Levinstein 19
Berlin Aniline Co. 119	Read Holliday & Co. 28
L. Cassella & Co. 75	Claus & Rèe 9
Farbwerk Mühlheim, Leonhardt & Co. 38	W. G. Thompson 2
Total of six German firms 948	Total of six English firms 86

But the amendment act was a very watered-down version of what Levinstein had proposed, and it made little if any difference. By this time the German dyestuff producers had achieved such economies of scale that they could reduce prices to undercut their domestic competitors and still make a profit. However, Levinstein was persistent and managed to impress David Lloyd George, President of the Board of Trade (and future Prime Minister) with his views.[96] In 1907, Lloyd George introduced new legislation with strengthened revocation provisions intended to put stronger pressure on the German synthetic dyestuff makers to work their patents in Britain. The *Act to consolidate the enactments relating to Patents for Inventions and the Registration of Designs and certain enactments relating to Trade Marks* which was partly modelled on its counterpart German legislation, successfully induced the main German dyestuff companies to set up factories in Britain to manufacture their patented dyes as well as drugs like Salvarsan and Novocain, though its full effects were nullified by a court judgement which effectively made 'it virtually impossible to bring a successful patent revocation suit' for non-working.[97] It was not until after the First World War that the government took a strategic approach towards the development and regulation of its key high technology industries such as organic chemicals and pharmaceuticals.

France

As mentioned before, the French patent system allowed patent scope to be stretched very broadly so that process patents included the resulting product and a patented product would embrace all possible methods of manufacturing it. In addition, the law required patented inventions to be worked. Both features turned out to have perverse consequences.

Soon after Renard Frères patented fuchsine in 1859, the company asserted its monopoly position by taking alleged infringers to court. In 1863, Renard Frères successfully sued a rival firm, Monnet et Dury, which was making fuchsine by a different process.[98] With such a strong monopoly position over what was not only a product but a key intermediate for other dyes, the firm grew into a much larger company, the Société la Fuchsine. Instead of diversifying its product range and improving its manufacturing processes it devoted its efforts to asserting its monopoly position by charging high prices and aggressively suing infringers.[99] The result was that many dye chemists and even some dyestuff firms relocated abroad, some of those that remained reverted to production of natural dyes, and smuggling of dyes from Germany and Switzerland increased.[100] The Société, which evidently had no incentive to be innovative, declined and went bankrupt in 1868. As one historian put it rather dramatically:

> The first men to bring their expertise in the manufacture of synthetic dyes to Basel were French. They carried their knowledge into neighbouring countries. They soon arrived in large numbers, fleeing the unusual situation in France. Their contemporaries compared this to the Revocation of the Edict of Nantes as if they were fleeing religious persecution, escaping the orthodox religion ordered by the government. The knowledge those Huguenots imported proved to be of economic advantage to the adjacent countries; this time, however, the refugees were fleeing the dictates of the French patent law.[101]

The French patent law cannot really be blamed for the demise of the French dyestuff industry, which did not completely disappear anyway. But the patent law did not reflect the fact that rapid innovation during these early stages in the development of the industry meant that enabling strong monopoly protection did not only discourage innovation, at least within the country; such monopolies could never be secure for any length of time anyway if neighbouring countries did not have patent laws.[102] 'Verguin and Renard's patent on magenta ... did not prevent the Gerbers of Mulhouse from developing a cheaper process... they simply emigrated to Basel in order to be able to exploit it freely'.[103] Moreover, the rule that merely importing a patented product would lead to revocation of the patent did not necessarily serve the interests of the domestic firms. Indeed, the French chemical firms were apparently well aware that compulsory working rendered them even more vulnerable to the capture of domestic markets by German and Swiss firms setting up branch factories in France.[104] Most likely the domestic chemical industry had never achieved sufficient economic importance for its concerns to be taken seriously enough by policymakers or the politicians.

The United States

Like Britain, the United States was a follower, not an innovator. The sense of dependence on Germany was very much felt. However, as in Britain the textile industry was hardly hostile to the availability of high quality foreign dyes that could not have been made in that country by domestic firms. Chemicals were patentable but a court decision created some limits to patentability in synthetic chemistry. The 1884 *Cochrane v Badische* case of the Supreme Court ruled that a synthetic copy of alizarin, the dye hitherto extracted from madder was not patentable for being identical to the plant-based chemical that it sought to replace in manufacture; that is to say, it lacked novelty because it was already available to the public from another source.[105] Notwithstanding the fact that this product had been separately patented twice in Britain, by Perkin, and one day earlier by Caro, Graebe and Liebermann, the latter of which was for the same invention at issue in this case, it was held in consequence to lack novelty. This is what the Court had to say:

> the article produced by the process described was the alizarine of madder, having the chemical formula $C_{14}H_8O_4$. It was an old article. *While a new process for producing it was patentable, the product itself could not be patented, even though it was a product made artificially for the first time,* in contradistinction to being eliminated from the madder root. *Calling it artificial alizarine did not make it a new composition of matter,* and patentable as such, by reason of its having been prepared artificially, for the first time, from anthracine, if it was set forth as alizarine, a well known substance.[106]

Patents and Industrial Development — Lessons from the Dyestuff Industry

Evidently, patents were not a prerequisite for economic and technological advancement in all countries, and may not have been in any. But, since we cannot turn the clock back and re-run past centuries without a patent system, there is much that we will never be sure of. On the other hand, it is very likely that patents did in at least some cases stimulate the development and diffusion of new technologies that were the foundation for rapid industrial development.[107] It is also probably true that inappropriate systems hindered such progress. Unlike the French and British governments, Germany had a patent strategy in the nineteenth century. The 1877 law was intended to benefit German industry and the economic well-being of the new nation. The involvement of industry in drawing up the legislation was therefore only to be expected. Indeed, it was a sensible course of action. The patent law appears to have been successful given Germany's subsequent rapid industrial development, and its emergence as an economic rival to Britain. However, it could not have succeeded on its own, that is, without public investment in technical education which at the time had become the best in the world. In Switzerland, the delay in introducing a patent system was largely due to the country's unique constitutional complexities. Nonetheless, as with Germany, the Swiss chemical industry from its earliest days strongly influenced the development of national patent law.

If we accept that the development of world class industrial sectors is likely to benefit the national economy, we can conclude that allowing such a policymaking role for industry was probably a good thing in Germany's and Switzerland's cases. But the lesson is not that private industry should dictate to governments how national patent systems ought to be designed because we all benefit by allowing them to do so; even less that firms and industrial associations should be able to dictate to foreign governments in countries where they have — or intend to have — commercial interests. Rather, countries should have the freedom to design patent systems for strategic purposes. As major stakeholders, companies and others who benefit economically from patent systems, such as patent agents and attorneys, may reasonably advise governments on patent policy, but they should certainly not monopolise this role. They represent the interests of their profession and their clients, and these may be different from those of the consuming public.

The Modern Pharmaceutical Industry — Early Decades

As we saw in Chapter 4, the nineteenth century experienced some major medical science breakthroughs, especially in the extraction and purification of the active principles of plant-based drugs. Pharmacists and doctors were able to sell and administer powerful alkaloid substances such as morphine, codeine, quinine and cocaine whose purity, strength and dosage could at last be regulated.[108] There is little doubt that such advances made the use of traditional natural product remedies, which tended to be mixtures, appear unscientific (unless they were exploited as sources of single active compounds rather than as drugs themselves). Purified lab-made standard-dose products developed by teams of salaried scientists became something the new companies could consistently deliver and make good profits from. Such new products must surely have looked like progress to many people. Consequently, '*since the late 1800s, when specific agents were isolated and characterized, the need for standardization and synthesis of natural substances favoured the development of the drug industry*'.[109] Favoured is of course not the same as 'determined'. Other factors were at play, and nothing about the industry's emergence and growth was inevitable.

As the century drew to a close, though, the ability to synthesise chemicals in the laboratory, both new ones and artificially produced natural products, really came to the fore. Patent law may originally have had something to do with this orientation towards synthetic chemistry. In Germany, among the court decisions from 1888 to 1890 which expanded the scope of patentability in chemistry was one which to some extent circumvented the pharmaceutical exception in applying these changes to medicines as long as they were chemically synthesised substances.[110] These changes probably encouraged German and Swiss dyestuff firms (which were dependent on the German market) to move into pharmaceuticals and to manufacture synthetic rather than natural products. As for the United States and Britain, those countries' patent systems did not incentivise one of the approaches over the other. In both those jurisdictions, synthetic chemicals were patentable as long as they were deemed to be novel, as were isolated natural products.

Modern pharmaceutical science is inherently multidisciplinary. Apart from synthetic organic chemistry, it is based on pharmacology, physiology, immunology, biochemistry and fermentation science, among other life science disciplines. While scientists and institutions from various countries contributed to the development of these new fields of enquiry, the modern pharmaceutical industry was invented in late nineteenth-century Germany. Bayer and Hoechst were the most prominent pioneering firms. In hindsight, there are very good reasons why the industry can be said to have emerged first in Germany and is, to some extent at least, an offshoot of dyestuff research, development and production.

The application of synthetic chemistry to drug discovery began to bear fruit from the late nineteenth century, and the dyestuff firms were at the forefront, along with a small number of longer established pharmacy firms. The first ever pharmaceutical products were developed in-house or by chemists based in German universities and licensed to companies, most of which were primarily dyestuff firms. Several reasons may be given to explain why these companies decided to move into drug development and were successful in doing so. First, there was good reason to believe that the research strategies they had adopted and the mass production capabilities they had acquired could be harnessed to drug discovery. Second, the same equipment they used for dyestuff production could also be used for drug production. Third, they soon realized that pharmaceutical compounds could be developed from analogous or even identical raw materials.[111] Investigating Paul Ehrlich's hypothesis that some dyestuffs have properties allowing them to treat infective agents but without harming human tissue, it seemed feasible to carry out research aimed at discovering dual-use substances to dye clothes and heal the sick.[112] Fourth, as their dyes became increasingly profitable, large funds became available to plough back into research and development. In short, since pharmaceutical research and development could be carried out with the same research strategies and technologies,[113] drug development was a commercially attractive and feasible proposition. Even the same substances could be used.

By the turn of the twentieth century, Bayer, Hoechst, AGFA and the main Swiss dyestuff firms were all producing pharmaceuticals as well as dyes. But that was about all the companies that were. Until well into the century virtually all the important new chemotherapeutic drugs were developed by German firms. This was despite the fact that most were still primarily dyestuff producers that treated drugs as no more than a promising sideline. Apart from Phenacetin (1888),[114] these included Hoechst's Antipyrin (1883) Pyramidon (1896) Novocain (1905) and

Salvarsan (1909), Bayer's Sulfonal (1888) and Aspirin (1899), and Kalle's Antifebrin (1886).

Most of the early chemotherapeutic drugs came out of the laboratories of the German dyestuff companies or of chemists at universities or state research institutes, as was Ehrlich, who had connections with these firms. Perhaps the most important of these early drugs were Salvarsan and Aspirin. Salvarsan is an arsenical compound that was synthesised by Paul Ehrlich, and discovered by him and his colleagues to be effective against syphilis. It was patented in 1909 by Hoechst. However, Aspirin is of course by far the most famous and the one that has commercially been the most enduring. There is much that is very old about Aspirin and much that is also quite new. Patented and trademarked in the late nineteenth century, Aspirin's natural precursor was known about for thousands of years, yet nobody knew how it worked until the 1970s. New discoveries about Aspirin continue to be made. The history of Aspirin is an intriguing one, and is worth looking into at some length.

Aspirin occasioned a great deal of learning in terms of marketing and intellectual property management based on levels of innovation that were quite modest. One might even go so far as to suggest that it was in the marketing and intellectual property management that the real innovation could often be found, and not so much in the science. This is true for more drugs than the industry would like us to know. Indeed, Aspirin is a prime example of how much money can be made from some fairly mundane tinkering in the lab as long as the marketing is done well. The lesson was well learned by the pharmaceutical industry. As with mauve, there is a malaria connection.

The long, long history of Aspirin

Bayer, an early manufacturer of synthetic dyestuffs, is the company that patented and trade marked Aspirin. As we will see, the company's patents on Aspirin proved to be quite controversial, as did the identity of the true inventor. But what is even more fascinating about (small 'a') aspirin — as opposed to Bayer's branded Aspirin — is its surprisingly long history.

(*Continued*)

The notion that willow bark has therapeutic qualities dates at least as far back as 5000 years BC in ancient Ur. It was also known to the ancient Egyptians. Later on, it was recommended by Hippocrates in fifth century BC Greece as an analgesic, the Roman Celsus as an anti-inflammatory agent, and the famous Claudius Galen, physician to Roman emperor Marcus Aurelius, also as an analgesic.[115]

In the modern era, scientific attention was turned towards willow bark following a discovery made in 1757 by one Rev. Edward Stone, a vicar in Chipping Norton, Oxfordshire. He sucked on a piece of willow in a marshy area near the town and noting its bitter taste, which made him think of quinine ('the Peruvian bark'), he wondered if this might be useful in treating the ague. His reasons for trying willow are not difficult to surmise given the similar source of quinine, and being guided by the long-established notion that the places where diseases are considered to originate, in this case marshy ground, tend also to be those where their cures reside. There is no evidence, though, that he was inspired by the writings of those ancient Greeks or Romans. He dried some of the bark, reduced it to a powder, and tested it on 50 fever sufferers over five years. It was particularly effective on mild fevers but offered some relief to more severe ones. He reported this to the Royal Society's journal, the *Philosophical Transactions*, which published his findings six years later, mistakenly under the name of Edmund Stone.[116] Stone's discovery soon piqued the interest of scientists both in England and on the continent.

In 1828, a German scientist, Johann Buchner, isolated a crystalline form of the active compound from willow bark, naming it salicyn after *Salix*, the Latin name for willow. Others improved the method, including the Italian Raffaele Piria, who named the crystal salicylic acid.[117]

Willow is not the only source of the raw active principle. A Swiss pharmacist, Johann Pagenstecher, found that an extract of the meadowsweet flower, *Spirea ulmaria*, relieved toothache and rheumatism. The article he published was read by a German chemist called Karl Jacob Löwig, who conducted experiments and discovered that the extract he made from this plant was salicylic acid.

Salicyn and salicylic acid share the drawback that swallowing them in the doses necessary to be effective causes an irritating burning sensation in

(*Continued*)

(*Continued*)

the stomach. In 1853, Charles Frederic Gerhardt, a chemistry professor at Montpellier University modified salicylic acid to produce a crude form of acetylsalicylic acid (ASA) that was less irritating. In 1859, Herman Kolbe of Marburg University came up with a very efficient process for making ASA from coal tar, and this formed the basis in 1874 for the first industrial scale production of the chemical, by the Heyden Chemical Company which was founded by a former student of Kolbe's, Friedrich von Heyden. Heyden's product was not a great success because it was insufficiently pure to eliminate stomach irritation, but the company came to play its part in the Aspirin story 30 years later. Another form was produced by Karl Johann Kraut in 1869.

While drug extraction, purification, synthesis and production were becoming scientific activities, the sale of medicines continued to lack respectability. One reason is that in the absence of trade and production regulation, there was a plethora of so-called 'patent' remedies on the market, often with unknown ingredients, that simply did not work, while others that may have worked were not subjected to tests which might have differentiated them better from the useless ones and given them scientific validation.

Thomas Maclagan was a Scottish doctor who worked for several years in a Dundee hospital and then moved to London. Acquiring quantities of salicin, he conducted a controlled clinical trial and reported his positive findings concerning treatment of acute rheumatism patients in an 1876 edition of *The Lancet*.[118] This article attracted the attention of doctors in France and Germany who wrote to the journal that they had obtained similarly good results from salicin and also salicylic acid. As Dormandy put it, 'if in modern times the Reverend Edward Stone was the 'discoverer' of salicin as a potential drug, it was Maclagan who gave it medical standing.'[119] Nonetheless, the unpleasant side-effects had not been eliminated.

The story now shifts to the laboratories of Bayer. Like its competitors, Bayer had become aware from an early time that drugs that were no more than modest improvements on competing ones could sell well with an aggressive marketing and intellectual property strategy. Accordingly, whether a new drug was 'new' enough to be patentable in overseas markets (only process patents were available in Germany at the time) was not

(*Continued*)

necessarily as important as a commercially attractive name that could be trademarked. German law became quite friendly to firms seeking to use trademarks in marketing. Along with the 1877 patent legislation, 'the German Trademark Law of 1894 had a powerful influence on German pharmaceutical companies. The latter's protection of trade names, packaging, and even the way companies wrote their names justified heavy investment in advertising to associate companies with health, quality, and serious research in the public mind.'[120] A major marketing innovation was Bayer's decision to stop selling powdered ASA to wholesalers and instead make its own Aspirin pills, stamping the Bayer cross logo on each one — and with it the association between Aspirin and the company in the minds of each consumer.[121] For Bayer, it was important to keep 'Aspirin' the Bayer-owned brand from becoming 'aspirin' the generic product associated with no particular company. As it turned out, war was the biggest threat to the success of this strategy. But Bayer was not just about clever marketing and intellectual property policy. The company was well aware of the value of recruiting good scientists and doing its own research and development.

In fact, around this time, Bayer was following up on two competing possibilities. One was diacetylmorphine, discovered originally by a scientist at St Mary's Hospital in London, where Alexander Fleming worked some decades later.[122] Bayer had hoped to market this unpatentable product (due it its lack of novelty) under the name 'Heroin'. The other was acetylsalicylic acid. While Carl Duisberg and his head of pharmacology, Heinrich Dreser favoured heroin, two Bayer chemists, Arthur Eichengrün, who was head of pharmaceuticals, and Felix Hoffman, took matters into their own hands and arranged for a trial of their modified form of ASA. The trial was a great success with none of the usual side-effects. Duisberg and Dreser were far from happy that the two of them had gone behind their backs. Nonetheless, the commercial possibilities were undeniable. Before marketing, a name had to be chosen for the product. It was apparently Eichengrün's suggestion that it be named Aspirin after acetyl, the Latin name for meadowsweet (*Spirea*) and the added suffix '-in', which had become common at the time in drug names.

Hoffman, Eichengrün and Dreser are all associated with the 1897 'discovery' of Aspirin, though there is some controversy as to who played the

(*Continued*)

(*Continued*)

most important role. Recent research suggests that Eichengrün's contribution was deliberately understated in the 1930s, presumably because he was Jewish, and is still not properly acknowledged even by the company.[123] Whatever the case, while these three came up with the specific form of ASA that became Aspirin, several other people played their parts. Indeed, Aspirin evidences how the last piece in the innovation 'jigsaw' puzzle is often a rather tiny one compared to the size of some of the pieces put in earlier. What the three scientists most closely involved achieved was rather modest, important as it nonetheless was. Piria, Maclagan and Gerhardt are obviously key people, but there were other contributors going all the way back to Edward Stone, who arguably was the one indispensable actor in the whole story. But as far as Aspirin the product is concerned, credit must really go to Carl Duisberg and Bayer.

But was there an invention at all? ASA was of course a known substance and Heyden had been selling it for some years. Patents were filed in Germany, the United States and Great Britain. The German application was accepted at first but was then rejected because only processes were patentable at the time and not chemicals themselves, and also because it was not new anyway. The British patent was filed in 1898 but was invalidated in a 1905 infringement case. The court accepted the defence of Chemische Fabrik Von Heyden, which had been marketing a very close equivalent to Aspirin since 1901, that it lacked novelty. If the rather sarcastic allegation made by a British obituary writer of Duisberg published in 1935, the year of his death, is true this was correct: 'Some genius in the firm, if not Duisberg, lifted into a patent specification a paper in *Liebig's Annalen* describing the preparation and properties of acetylsalicylic acid. Of course, the patent was lost when attacked in the Courts'.[124] The US patent, on the other hand, which was filed in 1900 and named Hoffman as the inventor managed to survive a 1909 infringement case.

The aspirin story is still not over. It is as long as the pharmaceutical industry itself — one reason why it is such a fascinating and illuminating one, and worth covering here (despite its possible chronological disruption to our account). Due to the First World War, Bayer lost control of its Aspirin trademark in various countries, including the USA and the UK.

During the inter-war years, an increasing number of rival products became available. These included Aspro, another ASA product developed in Australia and sold by Nicholas Proprietary, and others that contained mixtures of Aspirin with other ingredients.[125] Nicholas is now owned by the Indian firm Piramal. Interestingly, Bayer currently owns the Australian Aspro trademark — perhaps a revenge of sorts.

Just after the Second World War, Reckitt and Colman's soluble aspirin called Disprin came on the market. There was also Anacin (or Anadin), Bufferin and Excedrin. All of these were marketed aggressively and at times successfully. Interestingly, three old compounds gave rise many decades later to a revolution of sorts in the market filled by these products. The first of these was acetaminophen, synthesised by Bayer in 1878 but rejected on toxicity grounds. Like Antifebrin it also turned some people blue. The second and third were Antifebrin (acetanilide) and Phenacetin (acetophenetidine). In the late 1940s, scientists at Yale and New York Universities discovered, first, that acetanilide was converted in the body into acetaminophen, and second, that acetophenetidine was similarly transformed into acetaminophen. The substance seemed to be safe, suggesting that Bayer might have been testing contaminated samples all those decades earlier. In the 1950s it was marketed in the UK (but not the US) as Panadol, and like Aspro and Disprin, was a great success. When it became an over-the-counter product, it was given the generic name paracetamol instead of acetaminophen. Sterling, which had acquired Bayer Aspirin in the United States, chose not to market Panadol in the US as it would have competed with its Aspirin branded product. But a branded acetaminophen came on the market anyway in the late 1950s. This was McNeil Laboratories' Tylenol, which fell into the hands of Johnson & Johnson when it took over the company soon after.

During all this time, aspirin's mode of action was unknown. It remained that way until 1971, when it was discovered by John Vane, a pharmacologist at the Royal College of Surgeons who won a Nobel Prize for this achievement. Vane had become interested in a class of fatty acids called prostaglandins which perform a variety of functions and are produced in the body from another chemical found in cell tissue, arachidonic acid. One weekend in April 1971, it struck him that aspirin and related drugs known nowadays as the non-steroidal anti-inflammatory drugs (NSAIDs), a category that includes ibuprofen and naproxen but not acetaminophen, worked by inhibiting the biosynthesis of prostaglandins from arachidonic acid. This would account for the therapeutic effects of aspirin, which are to reduce fever, pain and inflammation, as well as for the two main side-effects: stomach pain caused by weakening of the stomach lining, and thinning of the blood due to interference with anti-platelet activity. Both result from absence of the right prostaglandin caused by aspirin.[126]

Subsequent research showed that the prostaglandin manufacture process requires the intervention of an enzyme called cyclo-oxygenase (COX), which is especially important as it is also involved in converting one type of prostaglandin to another. COX comes in two forms and the way that different NSAIDs work depends on the dose and on whether the drug in question is more or less active against COX-1 as compared to COX-2. The COX-1 enzyme is involved in the making of prostaglandins concerned with the gastro-intestinal tract, while COX-2 assists in the synthesis of prostaglandins relating to inflammation and pain.

Vane suggested that understanding aspirin's mode of action could well lead to further medical applications. Since then, it has turned out to have other therapeutic applications, especially in preventing heart attacks and strokes, though several other uses seem to be feasible too. Indeed, aspirin also instances how new uses of a drug may continue to be discovered as scientists learn more about the chemical, the ways the chemical interacts with the cellular machinery of humans (or infective agents of humans such as bacteria) and about human biology and the diseases that afflict us. As we will see later on, the fact that revisiting old drugs in this way can lead to commercially interesting new discoveries explains the increased availability nowadays of patents for new uses of old things. Indeed, patents relating to aspirin continue to be filed.

It should not be assumed that just because these products have been on the market for so long and are available over the counter, they are perfectly safe in all circumstances especially when used over a long time. Initially paracetamol became popular due to concerns about the side effects of other NSAIDS. In recent years paracetamol itself has come under scrutiny for harmful side-effects on people suffering chronic pain such as arthritis and some medical experts have questioned whether the drug should be so widely available for self-medication given its fairly modest painkilling abilities.[127]

Let us now get back to the turn of the last century. Another important early drug, E. Merck's Veronal (1903), the first of the barbiturates, was an exception to the other early synthetic pharmaceutical substances that became products listed earlier. This is because its producer was not a dyestuff firm but had begun as a pharmacist shop and subsequently became a bulk producer of alkaloids. In common with another former pharmacy business, Schering, E. Merck's US branch separated and eventually became a major research-based pharmaceutical corporation that outgrew its parent by some considerable measure. In Merck's case the separation took place after the First World War. The Schering split took place during the Second World War when the US branch was confiscated by the government. It was privatized in 1952. The main German chemical companies merged in 1925 to form I.G. Farbenindustrie, which immediately became a dominant player in various types of chemical product, including pharmaceuticals.[128]

The Swiss pharmaceutical industry,[129] like its German counterpart, benefited from early advances in synthetic chemistry. Three of the four most successful companies during the twentieth century — Sandoz, Ciba and Geigy — began as dyestuff manufacturers. In 1895, Sandoz was the first of these companies to graduate to pharmaceuticals when it began producing Antipyrin, originally developed by Hoechst. In 1917, the company established a pharmaceutical research laboratory. Five years after Sandoz, Ciba moved into pharmaceuticals, developing two products, Vioform (an antiseptic) and Salen (for rheumatism).

This might all suggest that very little happened in Britain and the United States before the First World War changed everything — for reasons I will go into soon. It is certainly true that these two countries were far behind Germany in their chemical prowess and their firms were not at all competitive. While the German and Swiss drug discovery approaches were based on synthetic organic chemistry, the North American and British strategy was initially geared towards extraction and purification of natural products.[130] The German and Swiss firms were the most successful and their dominance continued at least up to the mid-1930s.

The impetus for early growth of the US pharmaceutical industry came from such factors as the growing population, the availability of chemists and medical scientists trained in American and German universities, and the close links between university scientists and companies.[131] In addition, drug regulation introduced in 1902 requiring a government laboratory to monitor the production of new drugs for safety increased competition and encourage innovation and growth. 'The Act made possible a new means of competition: competition based upon the quality of laboratory facilities that the company could provide and the stringency of the standards which they could meet. It also implied that the leading producers could benefit by extremely tough standards which would be difficult for smaller companies to equal'.[132] Company laboratories no longer 'used simply to standardise basic products or to fiddle with new combinations of drugs, but rather they were now in the business of setting standards, meeting the requirements of the regulators, and producing as many novel products as they were capable of doing which would distinguish their product lines from those of their competitors'.[133]

Even before the antibiotics and corticosteroids eras, American companies began to achieve some good results from their research. A few pioneering firms such as Abbott Laboratories, Parke Davis & Co., and E.R. Squibb began from the 1920s to invest profitably in research in such areas as vitamins and hormones.[134] Eli Lilly, as we will see, became the first commercial producer of insulin, which had been discovered by University of Toronto scientists.

In the main, the British pharmaceutical industry in the pre-First World War era consisted of rather conservative small and medium-sized family firms. Most of these companies extracted drug ingredients from imported plants and minerals for wholesalers, pharmacists and physicians.[135] Some of them also prepared their own proprietary remedies from these ingredients. Often, these companies were originally retailers that had later on moved into manufacturing. Examples include Boots and Allen & Hanburys.[136] Other firms, like May & Baker, began as manufacturing chemists before becoming retailers.

Burroughs Wellcome, formed in 1880 by two American pharmacists who had immigrated to Britain, was an exception to the rule that the industry had little interest in research and development but other firms followed in their footsteps. The Wellcome Chemical Research Laboratories, set up in 1896, played an important role 'as providers of qualified and experienced research scientists to other companies, including Boots, Glaxo, and May & Baker'.[137] This firm also introduced the tablet form of drug manufacture and delivery from Germany and the USA.[138]

In spite of its relative backwardness in pharmaceuticals, Britain enjoyed a trade surplus on the eve of the First World War. In 1913 drug imports were worth £2 million, whereas exports were valued as £2.4 million.[139] This made Britain second in world pharmaceutical exports, 21.3 percent as compared to 30 percent for Germany and figures of 13 percent for the United States and 11.9 percent for France.[140] Even so, the outbreak of the war made plain to the government how dependent the country had become on German dyestuffs and drugs, and how the patent system seemed to reinforce such dependence.

International Competition and the Impacts of the First World War

After the USA joined the First World War in 1917, the government realized how dependent it was on Germany for chemicals and felt a need to do something about it. That same year, the Office of the Alien Property Custodian was established under the *Trading with the Enemy Act*, and in 1918 started to confiscate German owned business assets. After the War, in 1919, Francis Garvan, who as Alien Property Custodian 'had become aware of the strategic importance of the synthetic dye industry and of previous US dependence on German industry for its products',[141] set up a semi-public institution called the Chemical Foundation to act as trustee for American industries which had been affected by the German chemical patents. He arranged for the transfer of 4,767 German-owned chemical patents as well as trademarks, which included drugs such as Novocain and Salvarsan, to the Chemical Foundation for around US$270,000. These were then licensed to companies.[142] Even though many of these patents apparently turned out not to sufficiently disclose the inventions claimed, the Chemical Foundation provided a huge shot in the arm for the US chemical industry.[143] At least as important as the transfer of these patents and trademarks, the war resulted in the loss by some German companies of their US branches. US Merck became an independent company. Bayer's US assets were auctioned off and acquired by Sterling Drug. These included a factory, Bayer's dyestuffs business and rights relating to 64 medicines including the Aspirin trademark.[144] Perhaps the most transformative outcome of the crisis created by the War was that the US government (as did the British government) finally decided to follow Germany in adopting industry policies specifically geared to promoting the development of their domestic chemical (including pharmaceutical) industries.[145] For example, 'American manufacturers, concerned that the Germans might regain their former dominance in the field of synthetic dyes and drugs, pressed successfully for tariff protection.'[146]

For Britain, the drug whose unavailability caused most concern was Salvarsan. Unfortunately, it was extremely difficult to manufacture in a form safe enough to administer to patients. The Board of Trade authorised Burroughs Wellcome, Poulenc Frères and May & Baker to manufacture the drug, which, once produced needed to be tested for impurities. This was carried out by the recently-founded Medical Research Committee (later renamed the Medical Research Council).

The lessons of the war were not lost on the government or industry. For one thing, the government took a more mercantilist approach to strategic industries. The 1921 *Safeguarding of Industries Act* imposed import tariffs on certain goods, including fine chemicals.[147] And, for another, the industry began to make efforts to improve its research and development capabilities. Two companies that increased their involvement in pharmaceutical research during the inter-war period and became highly successful decades later were Beecham and Glaxo. Beechams Powders, a proprietary Aspirin-based cold remedy launched in 1926, was a popular product for decades. Glaxo began life as a department of a company called Joseph Nathan that manufactured a dried milk product named 'Glaxo'. In 1924, the company negotiated a licence to extract vitamin D from fish oil using (and improving upon) a process patented by Columbia University. Glaxo Department subsequently produced a range of vitamin products and other dietary supplements, and it was turned into a private limited company in 1935.

The British pharmaceutical industry developed into a successful research and development-based one much later than that of the USA.

The country's early advances in synthetic chemistry did not, unlike the German case, lead to the development of new drugs. It cannot at all have helped that companies during the early twentieth century generally employed very few chemists. And, given the positive influence of drug safety regulations in the USA, the fact that they were virtually non-existent in Britain until as late as 1922, when the *Dangerous Drugs Act* was passed, to be followed in 1933 by the *Pharmacy and Poisons Act*,[148] was likely also to have hindered the development of a world-class pharmaceuticals sector.

Patent Controversies

As a relatively backward sector compared to its German counterpart, the US pharmaceutical industry favoured weakening protection in the early twentieth century. They justified this on the grounds that they were victims of unfair competition from abroad. In 1919, the American Pharmaceutical Association, an organisation founded in 1852 to represent pharmacists, publicly denounced the 'unfair monopolies on medicinal chemicals and dyes' held by German companies that they accused of abusing the US patent and trade mark systems. The Association alleged that they were doing this in two ways.[149]

The first was to deliberately miss out important information when disclosing their inventions to the Patent Office. Consequently, they could not be copied by others even after the patent (or patents) protecting the chemical product or process had expired. British companies were making similar complaints at this time. It is not as if such tactics were new. Richard Arkwright was also accused of writing dodgy specifications to give away as little information as possible over a century earlier. One of the more extreme cases was the famous Haber-Bosch nitrogen fixation process, arguably one of the most important single inventions in recorded human history,[150] which was protected by several US patents owned by BASF. It took many years of effort and millions of dollars in research expenditure for scientists to replicate it even after the patents had been expropriated by the government during the First World War. According to one account 'the Badische Company had effectively bulwarked this discovery with strong, broad patents which detailed meticulously the apparatus, temperatures, and pressures, but cleverly avoided particulars as to the catalysts employed or their preparation. This last information was the core of the process so far as its practical operation was concerned.'[151]

The second way, which is common today and is not usually considered any more to be wrong, was to secure indefinite control over trademarks covering the names of drugs. This was very beneficial to companies seeking to maintain as far as possible their monopoly control over drugs after the patents protecting them had expired. Such control of the name, in the rather bitter words of F.C. Stewart, Director of the Scientific Department of H.K. Mulford Company, then a successful producer of vaccines and serums,[152] and Chairman of the Committee on Patents and Trademarks of the American Pharmaceutical Association, 'practically enable[d] the commercial introducer to convert the entire educational machinery of the medical and pharmaceutical professions into a great advertising bureau for exploiting the sick room'.[153]

The Association advocated changes to the law allowing only chemical processes to be patented. If product protection continued to be permitted, the law should provide for compulsory licensing. With respect to trademarks on drug names, protection should expire at the same time as the patent. This is certainly not a position that the US pharmaceutical industry would hold today! It is interesting to note that the Association took a strictly utilitarian line on intellectual property rights:

> It should be understood that the patent and trademark laws, like all other laws, are primarily designed to benefit the public at large and only secondarily to benefit the individual… There are some who assume that the object of the Patent Law is to protect inventors in their so-called natural right to the exclusive manufacture and sale of their inventions and the object of the Trademark Law is to protect and foster monopolies. Nothing is further from the truth. The objects of the Patent and Trademark Laws are altruistic and not egoistic.[154]

This sounds all rather familiar. Such a view is quite common among generic producers and firms in today's developing countries that fear competition from wealthier and more technologically-advanced foreign companies better able to take advantage of intellectual property protection.

The Association failed to achieve reforms to the patent and trademark laws. It cannot have helped their cause that the changes they proposed conflicted with the interests of businesses in other sectors that had benefited greatly from the existing standards of protection and whose desire for reform was limited to improving their efficiency. It is interesting to speculate whether the changes they wanted to see would have been made if the USA had not decided to take part in the war and then to expropriate all those German-owned US chemical patents. As we will see, the British patent law *was* changed at this time to prohibit the patenting of chemical substances. As the US pharmaceutical industry began to develop its own products, its interests did become rather different.

Like the US system, the British patent system at the start of the twentieth century provided owners with stronger rights by the standards of the day. But, as will soon become clear, the historical development of the two systems took quite divergent courses so that for much of the century they varied quite widely, and offered quite different levels of protection for pharmaceutical inventions. Interest group politics provides at least part of the explanation.

As was explained earlier, the British pharmaceutical industry was a slow developer, and its economic importance prior to the First World War was thus quite small. Neither was it particularly innovative, so it had little use for the patent system. When it came to patent reform, while elements within the much larger chemical industry were very vocal and gained the ears of policymakers and politicians, the drug manufacturers had very little to say. Probably the most vocal and effective of these elements was Ivan Levinstein, who was mentioned earlier.

The first post-war legislative development in patent law that had a direct bearing on the interests of the pharmaceutical industry took place in 1919 with the passage of an amendment to the 1907 *Patents and Designs Act*. In response to wartime shortages of important products, the political establishment was ready to adopt a more mercantilist and defensive attitude towards strategic industries. The legislation reflected this attitude very strongly.

The 1919 amendment brought British patent law further into line with the law in most of Europe in that, while it extended the duration of patents from 14 to 16 years for the benefit of inventors who had been prevented from working their patents by the war, it singled out chemicals, foods and medicines for weakened protection. Patent protection was available only for those chemical substances produced by the particular process or processes claimed in the application. According to the Act,

> in the case of inventions relating to substances prepared or produced by chemical processes or intended for food and medicine, the specification shall not include claims for the substance itself, except when prepared or produced by the special methods or processes of manufacture described and claimed or by their obvious chemical equivalents.

In effect, then, the achievement of secure product protection required applicants to anticipate all possible ways of manufacturing the chemical. The main purpose of these measures was to make it easier for British firms to circumvent the patent monopolies of the German dyestuff firms while acquiring their own (process) patents into the bargain. But the law did not make it too easy for them either. In infringement cases concerning new chemicals protected by a patented process, the burden of proof was on the party whose manufacture of the chemical was alleged to infringe the patent.

Another measure affecting holders of patents for inventions 'intended for or capable of being used for the preparation or production of food or medicine', was that applicants for a licence could acquire one from the comptroller general (the head of the Patent Office). In settling the terms of the licence including royalty payments, the comptroller was required to take into account 'the desirability of making the food or medicine available to the public at the lowest possible price consistent with giving to the inventor due reward for the research leading to the invention'.

Clearly, the dyestuff industry was not the sole concern. The wartime shortage of drugs was obviously another factor in the wording of this section of the legislation. However, the government's interest was not primarily to increase the international competitiveness of the British pharmaceutical industry but to ensure greater self-sufficiency and create a level playing field for the country, bearing in mind that neither Germany, France nor Switzerland allowed chemical products to be protected except through the patenting of manufacturing processes.

It must be said that the pharmaceutical industry was not very influential in government or Parliament at that time. In fact, the industry did not even have a trade association to represent its interests until as late as 1929, when the Wholesale Druggists Trade Association (renamed the Association of the British Pharmaceutical Industry in 1948) was founded 'to advance the interests of its members through improved organisation especially regarding departmental or parliamentary legislation affecting the drug trade'.[155] Evidently, the government did not need to be persuaded by the industry that the measures it introduced were necessary for the country.

In 1930, the Board of Trade set up a committee under the chairmanship of Sir Charles Sargant to advise the government on possible reforms to the patents and designs law and on practices of the Patent Office.[156] In all, 53 individuals gave evidence including five from the Chartered Institute of Patent Agents, three from the British Medical Association, two from the Medical Research Council, and two from Joseph Nathan and Co. Nonetheless, the interests of the chemical industry were still given far more attention than those of the much smaller pharmaceutical industry. This may not have concerned the drug companies too much, though, as both sectors were primarily concerned to prevent foreign companies from using the patent system to dominate the domestic market. As it was, no substantial changes were made to the patent system during the inter-war era, which was a period of consolidation and gradual progress for the pharmaceutical industry.

Notes

1 Jones (2001). Like the word 'galaxy', Glaxo would appear to derive from γαλα (gala), the Greek word for milk. But why this word was coined is unknown.
2 Liebenau (1984), 330.
3 Stolz and Schwaiberger (1987).
4 Chapman-Huston and Cripps *op. cit.*, 17.
5 Liebenau *op. cit.*, 330.
6 Liebenau *op. cit.*, 330.
7 Gabriel *op. cit.*
8 Liebenau *op. cit.*, 336.
9 Church and Tansey (2007), 125.

10   This product was the subject of a well-known old English common law trademark case, which at the very least testifies to the early importance of branding in this particular line of business even before the introduction of trademark law: Singleton v. Bolton. See Bently (2014).

11   This product comprised extracts of the root of a Zulu medicinal plant (Pelargonium sidoides) used for treating coughs and known locally as Umckaloabo ('heavy cough') and another plant called chichitse. Charles Stevens, who was diagnosed with tuberculosis, was shown how to prepare the medicine by a traditional healer in South Africa who apparently saved his life. Stevens advertised the medicine thus: 'I do not say consumption is curable, but I say if you are consumptive I will guarantee to cure you or return your money in full'. The product was exposed by the British Medical Association as a quack remedy. Stevens sued for libel in 1912. The jury was unable to reach a verdict but a second trial in 1914 found in favour of the BMA. Newsom (2002).

12   Gabriel *op. cit.*

13   For the most comprehensive accounts of the synthetic dyestuff industry, see: Murmann (2003); Travis (1993).

14   Garfield (2001), 45.

15   *Ibid.*, 45.

16   Green (1915 [1901]), 190.

17   Haber (1958), 83.

18   Bensaude-Vincent and Stengers *op. cit.*, 183.

19   Originally known as Meister, Lucius & Brüning.

20   BASF stands for Badische Anilin- & Soda-Fabrik AG.

21   AGFA stands for Aktien-Gesellschaft für Anilin-Fabrikation.

22   Von Tunzelman (1995), 186.

23   Murmann and Landau (1998), 30.

24   Freeman and Soete. (1997), 297; Murmann and Landau *op. cit.*, 36–7.

25   Where they were able to exploit the relevant British patents (some of which were for their own inventions). *See* Bensaude-Vincent and Stengers *op. cit.*, 185.

26   Beer (1958); Freeman and Soete *op. cit.*, 106; Homburg (1992); Meyer-Thurow (1982).

27   Freeman and Soete *op. cit.*, 299.

28   This was the name given to the technology by Carl Duisberg, although Fritz Haber was really the discoverer of the process while Carl Bosch at BASF commercialized it. *See* Smil (2001).

29   Johnson (1992).

30   Murmann and Landau *op. cit.*, 40.
31   Murmann and Landau *op. cit.*, 32.
32   Murmann and Landau *op. cit.*, 40.
33   Chandler (1990).
34   Simon (1998), 17–8.
35   Homburg *et al, op. cit.*, 13.
36   Haber *op. cit.*, 119–20.
37   However, it should not be taken as a given that the financial success of domestic companies necessarily indicates enhanced net social and/or economic welfare of the citizenry; even more so in the case of the citizenry of foreign countries where these firms invest and/or to which they export.
38   Gaudillière (2008), 108.
39   M Horstmeyer (1998), 245.
40   Johnson *op. cit.*, 173.
41   Johnson *op. cit.*, 175.
42   Murmann (2003), 180–1.
43   Kronstein and Till (1947), 773–4.
44   Johnson *op. cit.*, 175.
45   Then known as Meister, Lucius & Brüning.
46   Kronstein and Till *op. cit.*, 774.
47   Bercovitz-Rodriguez (1990), 6.
48   Grubb (1999), 23.
49   Haber *op. cit.*, 203.
50   Hornix (1992), 90. On the other hand, in the United States publication of patents could be delayed for much longer. It has been suggested that German firms took advantage of this and of the possibility to use other legal means to restrain the leakage of valuable knowledge, and this gave them a competitive advantage over local firms. However, recent historical research suggests that domestic companies equally availed themselves of such opportunities to control access to knowledge and technology. Mercelis (2016).
51   Lord Mansfield may have been the first to articulate this view of patents as an information-for-monopoly transaction when he pronounced, in a 1778 case (Liardet v Johnson), that: 'the law relative to patents requires, as a price the individual should pay the people for his monopoly, that he should enrol, to the very best of his knowledge and judgment, the fullest and most sufficient description of all the particulars on which the effect depended, that he was at the time able to do'.
52   *See* Gispen *op cit.*, 265. Interestingly, from 1936, Nazi-ruled Germany rejected the long-established 'applicant principle' (*Anmelderprinzip*) in

favour of the 'inventor principle' (*Erfinderprinzip*). *See* Beier (1986), 322; Nicolai (1972), 109. The drafters of the law evidently considered it important to protect the interests of the individual while at the same time subordinating them to the interests of the State on behalf of the community. Otherwise there were no substantial changes to the patent system. *See* Klauer (1936).

53   For example, Homburg *op. cit.*, 110; Johnson *op. cit.*, 176; Murmann *op. cit.*

54   Murmann *op cit*, 29.

55   Wengenroth (1997), 143.

56   Murmann and Landau *op. cit.*, 31.

57   Wengenroth *op. cit.*, 144 [emphasis added].

58   Complaints about such practices were common and were made up to and during the First World War. For example, see Perkin (1915).

59   For a critical account of attacks on German firms' patent practices, see Wadlow (2011).

60   Similarly, inventions in the biotechnology field have tended to be treated by patent offices and the courts as if they were chemical inventions even though they differ in some fundamental ways.

61   Van den Belt and Rip (1989), 152.

62   Isomers are variants of a compound that contain the same atoms arranged differently. In other words, their ingredients are identical but their structures are different. The actual difference may be extremely trivial.

63   Van den Belt and Rip *op. cit.*, 152.

64   Murmann *op. cit.*, 156–8.

65   Van den Belt and Rip *op. cit.*, 154; also see Morris (2015).

66   Meyer-Thurow *op. cit.*, 378–9.

67   Maestrejuan *op cit.*, at 46.

68   Quoted in Owens (1991), 1081.

69   In Cuno Engineering Corporation v. Automatic Devices Corporation (1941) 314 US 84.

70   This was a common view in the courts during the 1940s. Indeed, during the Second World War period, the courts were hardly favourable to patent holders: 89 per cent of the patents involved in the cases brought before them were declared invalid. Killing the flash of genius concept in the USA was thus much longer in coming than in Germany, probably because of the individualist ideology which pervades American society. *See* Vaughan (1951), 782.

71   Dutfield (2013).

72   Johnson *op. cit.*, 177.

73 Gaudillière (2008) *op. cit.*, 110, 122. The reversal of the burden of proof onto the defendants in the case of process patents is now part of international trade law, being incorporated into the Agreement Establishing the World Trade Organization's intellectual property annex (that is, the aforementioned TRIPS Agreement).

74 Quoted in Bercovitz-Rodriguez *op. cit.*, 6.

75 Murmann and Landau *op. cit.*, 66.

76 Quoted in Noble (1977), 16.

77 Noble *op. cit.*, 105–8.

78 The following court case provides a useful history of and background to Section 1498: Zoltek Corp. v. United States, No. 09–5135 (Fed. Cir. 2012).

79 Silverman and Lee (1974), 186–7.

80 The Knowledge Ecology International website provides excellent resources on Section 1498. https://www.keionline.org/cl/28usc1498, visited 12 March 2020.

81 Simon (1998), 17.

82 Farrar (1974).

83 Due in large part to lobbying by the timepiece industry.

84 Penrose (1951), 17.

85 Penrose *op. cit.*, 123.

86 Haber *op. cit.*, 119.

87 For background, see Chachereau (2015).

88 Travis *op. cit.*, 43.

89 Murmann *op. cit.*, 90.

90 Murmann and Landau *op. cit.*, 40.

91 Haber *op. cit.*, 200; Wengenroth *op. cit.*, 144.

92 At the second reading of the Patents for Inventions Bill, as reported in *Hansard* (1883) 16 April, 360, 363.

93 United Kingdom Board of Trade (1901).

94 Reed (1992), 117.

95 *Source:* Green *op. cit.*

96 Reed *op. cit.*, 118.

97 Murmann *op. cit.*, 191.

98 Haber *op. cit.*, 112.

99 Aftalion (1991), 39.

100 Van den Belt (1992), 62.

101 Simon (1998) *op. cit.*, 17.

102   Simon (1998) *op. cit.*, 63.

103   Bensaude-Vincent and Stengers *op. cit.*, 184.

104   Penrose *op. cit.*, 155.

105   The novelty test does not require that inventions be new in any absolute sense, but that they not have previously been available to the public. If a patented chemical was later found lying undisturned for billions of years in a mineral, this would not destroy the invention's novelty.

106   Cochrane v Badische Anilin & Soda Fabrik (111 US 293, 1884) [emphases added].

107   For well-researched and convincing evidence to support this view in the UK context, see Dutton (1984).

108   Porter *op. cit.*, 333–4.

109   Duffin (1999), 107.

110   Wimmer (1998), 287–8.

111   Stolz and Schwaiberger *op. cit.*, 195.

112   Bynum (1994) *op. cit.*, 167; Porter *op. cit.*, 450.

113   Wengenroth *op. cit.*, 144.

114   Phenacetin can have some serious side-effects. In the 1890s Bayer made and tested the therapeutically active part of the compound, acetaminophen (or paracetamol) but found it to be unsafe as well. As we saw, it was tested again many years later, found to be safe enough to be commercialised, and marketed under the trade names Panadol and Tylenol as well as paracetamol. *See* Stone and Darlington (2000), 88–9.

115   Dormandy (2006), 350; Jeffreys (2004).

116   Stone (1763), 53.

117   Dormandy *op. cit.*, 354.

118   Maclagan (1876).

119   Dormandy *op. cit.*, 359.

120   Kobrak (2002), 120.

121   Jeffreys *op. cit.*, 96

122   This was discovered in 1874 at St Mary's Hospital in London by a team led by Frederick Pierce. It turned out to be 'one of the first drugs ever produced by modifying a natural molecule'. *See* Stone and Darlington *op. cit.*, 93.

123   Sneader *op. cit.*, 359–60.

124   Armstrong *op. cit.*, 1024.

125   Smith and Barrie (1976).

126   Vane (1971, 1994); also, his Nobel Lecture — http://nobelprize.org/nobel_prizes/medicine/laureates/1982/ vane-lecture.html. Also: Ferreira, Moncada and Vane (1971); Smith and Willis (1971).

127 O'Callaghan (2014).

128 At the end of the Second World War, I.G. Farben was broken up and Hoechst and Bayer were revived as separate companies. For much of the second half of the century, both were among the world's biggest pharmaceutical companies. However, in 1999, Hoechst merged with Rhône-Poulenc to form a new company, Aventis.

129 This section is based largely on information on the history of these companies available on the websites of Novartis (http://www.novartis.com) and Hoffman LaRoche (http://www.roche.com).

130 Achilladelis (1993), 283.

131 Liebenau *op. cit.*, 339.

132 Liebenau *op. cit.*, 341.

133 Liebenau *op cit*, 341.

134 Chandler (1990), 164.

135 *Ibid.*, 169–70.

136 This company was acquired by Glaxo in 1958.

137 Slinn (1995), 174.

138 Slinn *op cit*, 184.

139 Slinn *op cit*, 174–5.

140 Kobrak *op. cit.*, 44.

141 Lesch (2007) *op. cit.*, 26.

142 Greenberg (1926), 23; Lesch (2007) *op. cit.*, 26–7; Roe (1943), 702; for an extended discussion on these events see Wadlow (2010).

143 Moser and Voena (2012). Germany behaved quite differently to the US and Britain. 'In July 1915, the *Bundesrat* had passed a law guaranteeing that foreigners would keep their patent rights. Only in some cases, in which the national interest was clearly at issue, would foreigners lose their patent rights for the duration of the war.' *See* Kobrak *op. cit.*, 60.

144 This was a subject of a court case in 1920. The famous American judge Learned Hand ruled that aspirin was a generic term for the purposes of sale to the public, but that for sales to wholesalers and pharmacists, Sterling's trademark rights remained in force. *See* Jeffreys *op. cit.*, 145, 151–2.

145 Steen (1995).

146 Parascandola (1985), 17. See also Steen (2014).

147 Abraham (2002), 233; Owen (1999), 363.

148 Slinn *op. cit.*, 172.

149 American Pharmaceutical Association (1919), 77–9.

150 Smil (2001); Mann (2018).

151   Haynes (1945), quoted in Mowery and Rosenberg (1998), 74. It may conceivably have been true that the problem was less that the disclosure was deliberately insufficient than that it was just so technically complex to reproduce and practice.
152   Mulford went into decline after the First World War and was bought up by Sharpe & Dohme in 1929, which merged with Merck in 1953. *See* Galambos with Sewell (1995).
153   Stewart (1919), 75.
154   Stewart *op. cit.*
155   Abraham (2002) *op. cit.*, 232.
156   United Kingdom Board of Trade (1931).

Part 3

Science, Business Strategy, and Growth

Chapter 6

Making Hormones

From Origins to Growth

In the early decades of the pharmaceutical industry, which as we saw emerged largely in Germany, the first products tended to be painkillers, fever-reducers or anti-infectives whether for patients in that country or others, or in the colonial tropics. However, progress was initially quite slow. In a brief article published in 1900 called 'What is a disease', which very succinctly describes the knowledge of the day regarding disease, its author, a physician in Britain felt moved to close it with the following rather negative statement: 'Medicine is a science without a method, and until our leaders adopt one we shall not take the place that belongs to us.'[1] As we will see it took more time for the foundational biomedical discoveries and the first new modern medicines to become available to be supplemented by a sufficient quantity of pharmaceuticals to say that things were really getting better.

The period from 1900 marks the beginnings of a departure from the industry's dual roots in dyestuff chemistry and plant or mineral-based product pharmacy — not that these ceased to be important especially the former. Hormones were an important factor in this transformation, being natural products of human and mammalian origin that could be prepared in isolated (and increasingly pure) form or synthetically.

The 1920s to the 40s were a crucial period for the industry. Until the mid-1930s, the number of effective new chemical entities was small, the research-based pharmaceutical industry remained quite limited in size, especially outside Germany, and most of the drugs available would be considered primitive to today's doctors, pharmacists and patients. According to the medical journalist James Le Fanu,

> The newly qualified doctor setting up practice in the 1930s had a dozen or so proven remedies with which to treat the multiplicity of different diseases he encountered every day: aspirin for rheumatic fever, digoxin for heart failure, the hormones thyroxine and insulin for an underactive thyroid and diabetes respectively, salvarsan for syphilis, bromides for those who needed a sedative, barbiturates for epilepsy, and morphine for pain. Thirty years later, when the same doctor would have been approaching retirement, those dozen remedies had grown to over 2,000.[2]

One should not be too negative. Undoubtedly, there were therapeutic advances before the end of the 1930s from the antipyretics to the antitoxins, serums, vaccines, the hormones and, perhaps most outstandingly, insulin, some of which are mentioned in the quote; indeed sufficient to some historians to refer to these treatments as forming a 'therapeutic revolution'.[3] However, excepting the antipyretics, much of the discovery and initial production took place outside industry in such locations as state research laboratories and universities. Arguably that hasn't changed as much as many in the industry today would like us to assume. But the lack of success spelt out by Le Fanu, such as it was, probably had much to do with the continued lack of knowledge about the intricacies of cell function. This meant that discovering compounds affecting the functioning of target cells was of necessity heavily dependent on serendipity.[4] Once cell function was better understood, researchers became less dependent on good fortune. Admittedly, good luck continues often to be an essential condition for success and not every drug even today has a well understood mode of action.

In the meantime, a lot of money was made in the interwar period from vitamins. Somewhat belatedly perhaps given all the advances in other life science fields, food and nutritional science had begun to advance in the early part of the century. It became increasingly apparent that several diseases, especially those mostly afflicting the poor and undernourished were linked to deficiencies in substances normally present in the bodies of healthy and well nourished people. Several diseases including scurvy, rickets and pernicious anaemia became linked to the lack of availability of what became known as vitamins either because they are not consumed in sufficient quantities or because individuals are unable to absorb them from food. Vitamins are a class of micro-nutrients essential to human health that are consumed as nutrients in the food we eat as part of a well-balanced diet.[5] Thus, the way to treat such diseases was by replacing or supplementing these chemicals. It did not take long from their discovery — it was only in 1911 that Casimir Funk coined the word vitamin (or to be precise 'vital amines' or 'vitamines') — until it became a lucrative business to 'pharmaceuticalise' part of the deficiency response by providing these 'foods' in the form of *quasi*-medical products. In due course, as over-the-counter pills they became popular not just with vitamin deficiency victims but also with the worried well. In time such products included multivitamins which, as the name suggests, comprise vitamins bundled together — typically with minerals added — into a single pill. However, we devote the chapter to a class of products of far greater long term importance for the industry: hormones.

Hormones and their Challenge for Science, Business and the Patent System, and the Continuing Relevance of Natural Products

In a sense, living things are highly ingenious chemical factories. Among the most intriguing types of chemical manufactured by multicellular organisms are the hormones. Hormones, produced in certain organs called endocrine glands, are chemical messengers that perform a range of regulatory functions relating to growth, development, metabolism, and general well-being including immunity. They are delivered to where they are needed not down specific passageways or ducts, but through the bloodstream, which is why they were originally referred to as 'internal secretions' in contrast to the duct-transported 'external secretions' before Ernest Starling at University College London gave them the name 'hormones' in 1905.[6] This of course means that they may operate at some considerable anatomical distance from their place of manufacture. Hormones include adrenaline (epinephrine), insulin, erythropoietin (EPO) and steroids. Steroids include the corticosteroids and sex hormones like the oestrogens and testosterone. Hormones promote some activities and inhibit others depending on the context. For example, those elements of the endocrine system which make reproduction possible also ensure that women are infertile during pregnancy. Consequently, sex hormones can aid conception and contraception. A large number of ailments, some of which are fatal, are related to the inability of the body to produce them in sufficient quantities. However, hormone treatments can provide beneficial results even in people whose bodies can produce them normally, though harmful side-effects are also possible.

Aside from the fact that hormones were not cures but treatments that needed to be used continuously — something obviously good for business — the expertise required to both discover and mass-produce these products could not be satisfied alone by the synthetic chemistry that German scientists and firms were so much more advanced in during the first decades of that century than the British, French and Americans. As natural products, the initial challenge with hormones was to isolate and purify them, both at that time immensely difficult tasks. Synthesis in those early days was not a feasible option.

The relationship between hormones and health is highly complicated and it is impossible to do justice to its complexity in such a book as this. However, a chapter on hormones can still be instructive in terms of our coevolutionary perspective on science, business and patents. As historian of science Nicolas Rasmussen explains:

> Present fashion must not make us forget that in the first half of the twentieth century, hormones took pride of place as life's master molecules, and the endocrinologist took precedence over the geneticist as the scientist offering the means to control life. For such are the inherent implications of master molecules: to discover and manipulate these substances is to acquire the means to control the vital processes and phenomena governed by them. The master molecule thus constitutes an intersection between intellectual, therapeutic, and commercial interests, naturally attracting the most ambitious participants in biomedical science and industry.[7]

For science, the first set of tasks was that of how to isolate and purify these chemicals, and to identify and secure biological sources of the active principles of extracted hormones or of suitable raw materials for synthetic ones. As we will see, their sources were quite various including animal glands, plant sapogenins and human and animal urine.

The second challenge was that of how to relate these hormones to function and therapeutic use. Characterising them chemically was hugely difficult, especially with large molecules like insulin, which is also a protein. Thus the early hormone patents described how to prepare substances, but tended to have much less to say about their chemical characteristics. Obviously, though, they had to describe their use or industrial applicability. Much of the work was carried out by academic scientists, frequently ones who were consulting for drug companies.

After that, the biggest difficulty became that of how to standardise and mass produce them on a commercial scale, and then provide them in a form suitable for delivery to patients. Deciding whether to follow the extraction or the chemical synthesis routes depended largely on which was most scientifically feasible and the most economic given the expertise, facilities, finance and raw materials available to a firm or institution. While chemical synthesis, pioneered largely by German scientists and firms, seemed self-evidently more advanced than extraction, it was not necessarily more efficient or commercially successful. How to mass-produce hormones entailed also a consideration of what was patentable. Biosynthetic methods became crucial, and this usually required commitment from the private sector. For business, competition was intense, the risks were great, and the research was expensive. Aggressive and strategic patenting was considered necessary, just as it is today.

Academic scientists and their university employers also used the patent system, either for financial reasons or, on occasions, to protect the interests of patients in safe and accessible treatments. In the commercial world, patent ownership and licensing was used to dominate and divide up markets, block new entrants and force out existing ones. With so much patenting going on, non-owners and those refused licenses had little space left in which to innovate and get patents or even just to avoid getting sued. But patents were also sources of scientific information and commercial intelligence, and as such could be beneficial to all market actors and aspirant ones too. Such high-volume usage of the system and the patent documents themselves undoubtedly influenced the structure of the market in hormonal products and the identities of the actors. But their influence went further than this, including the trajectories that commercially oriented scientific investigation followed. If it was patentable it was likely to be commercially interesting. If it was not patentable, or the patent situation was more uncertain, it became much less interesting.

For an increasingly patent based industry, the question raised by new types of product is that of whether the existing rules allow them to be protected. In fact the legislation and case law of at least some turn of the century jurisdictions were fully capable of envisaging substances extracted from, copied from or otherwise modelled on nature being treated by patent offices and courts as inventions. Nonetheless, such things were not commonly patented in most countries before hormones. Once hormones emerged as products, though, we find that granting offices and courts were favourably disposed towards hormone-related patent claims and routinely allowed them whether or not chemicals and therapeutic products per se were protectable. But whether they and other products were patentable as exact synthetic copies of natural products or as preparations extracted from body tissue or fluid was not something to be taken for granted, as we will see. In countries where only chemical processes were patentable the question arose of whether the products made through such processes could be indirectly protected. As we saw, in the German case it turned out that they could but the situation was initially uncertain.

The patent situation in the United States was especially uncertain in the early years of hormones. Since the country's first genuine pharmaceutical products were not, as in Germany and Switzerland, synthetic chemicals but were of natural origin, the question arose quite early of whether purified hormone extracts could, as so-called products of nature, be protected. If natural, they were surely not new; neither were they manufactures. Or were they?

Adrenaline, Insulin and Cortisone

The first hormones, particularly adrenaline, presented particular challenges for the patent system, at least in some countries. The way these challenges were met has had long term repercussions in terms of determining how far patenting should be allowed to go in molecular biology and biotechnology. If such drugs comprise nothing more than naturally-occurring chemicals separated from their surrounding tissue and prepared in concentrated form, how can they be patented as new inventions? And if they could not be, would this not be an area of medical science that the industry would seek to avoid? As we will see, these 'natural products' were an early demonstration of how patent law from an early time in the industry's history was fully able to scoop up such 'inventions' and place in that category of things we call patentable inventions.

In Europe, such conceptual difficulties were also 'solved' in favour of allowing hormones to be patented. Thus, 'the patents on hormones that the Reich [German] patent office accepted in the 1920s and 1930s established precedents that were used to consolidate the notion that purified biological products in general should become proprietary'.[8] Britain was hardly a follower of German legal precedents but patent law there was just as amenable to such expansiveness, at least in this particular respect.

Two other important points to note here are, first, that innovation in hormones was largely about coming up with new, efficient and cost-effective processes. The products tended either to be isolated and purified natural substances, synthetic copies that were based on natural product precursors, or chemically-related variants or analogues. Consequently, the fact that chemicals per se were not patentable in much of Europe was not really a problem, and for most of the period covered there was little in the way of industry-sponsored lobbying for the inclusion of chemical substances as patentable subject matter. Second, international competition among steroid producers became intense and patent strategy including the establishment of cartel-like arrangements became a key factor in asserting and maintaining market power.

Adrenaline and the patenting of natural products

Inspired in part by some experiments on extracts from the adrenal glands carried out in the 1890s at University College London, John Jacob Abel at Johns Hopkins University in the United States produced a relatively pure form of the active principle of part of the gland called the adrenal medulla,

(*Continued*)

(Continued)

which he called epinephrin.[9] A few years later, Jokichi Takamine, a US-based Japanese scientist, came up with an extract of sufficient purity to display some of the effects of the hormone as it functioned in the body — not that the function of adrenaline was understood at the time except to a rudimentary degree. He filed two patents in 1903 and 1904 for a glandular extractive product claiming purified forms of adrenaline, as it was also called,[10] and for this compound in a solution with salt and a preservative.[11] Takamine licensed the patents to Parke Davis & Co. Around this time, a number of adrenaline-based products were sold in the US and Germany, where Hoechst marketed a product called Suparenin, among other countries for a wide range of ailments for which they were not always effective. But Parke Davis's trademarked Adrenalin products became market leaders on account of their relative purity, safety and efficacy. Takamine's work was very much commercially orientated. Previously he had patented a process of making a fungal enzyme which claimed a number of different preparations of the enzyme itself.[12]

Takamine's two patents were the subject of a 1911 court case in which Parke Davis successfully sued H.K. Mulford & Co. for infringement. The litigants were primarily concerned about priority and not really about sub-ject matter including the issue of whether isolating or purifying a natural product made something that was new. According to precedent it did not. Accordingly, the court established that the novelty of such extracts was not necessarily destroyed by the prior existence of less pure extracts if the differ-ence was of kind rather than of degree.[13] Regarding the first of the two patents, Judge Learned Hand, who later became a very famous jurist in the United States, held that

Takamine was the first to make it available for any use by removing it from the other gland-tissue in which it was found, and, while it is of course possible logi-cally to call this a purification of the principle, it became for every practical purpose a new thing commercially and therapeutically.[14,15]

However, like a fool rushing in where angels fear to tread (if that isn't too harsh), the judge went further than this — and much further than he needed to do to settle the case. He denied that there was any rule to prevent the patentability even of natural products merely extracted from living things if to do this made them 'available' for the first time. Thus

(*Continued*)

patentability may be extended to *an otherwise unchanged naturally occurring substance*, as long as the active principle in its original surroundings is not also claimed: 'But, even if it were merely an extracted product without change, there is no rule that such products are not patentable.' By saying this, he misunderstood legal precedents that sought to impose stricter novelty requirements in respect of natural products. Nonetheless, despite this ruling coming from a district court, this statement has had enduring legal influence in the United States affecting judgements regarding patentability of types of invention that could reasonably be considered more natural than artificial.[16]

A little footnote to add to this case is that research around this time by Abel, who years later produced a crystalline form of insulin, proved that Takamine's Adrenalin products were not so pure after all, containing another hormone, noradrenaline. One wonders what Abel thought about Takamine at this time. Takamine had visited Abel's laboratory and had had the benefit of reading his publications. Takamine published nothing on his adrenalin work until he filed his patents. 'Takamine was accustomed to commercial practice with its patents and registered trademarks, and he kept his experience to himself. Abel, accustomed to academic practice in which information was frequently freely exchanged, laid all his data before Takamine.'[17] Nonetheless, had Hand been aware that Takamine's invention was not quite what it claimed to be, it does not automatically follow that he would have considered the patent to be any less valid given his reliance on 'the common usages of man'. As a legal pragmatist, he was more concerned with practicalities than with strict scientific accuracy which in any case for courts was hard to attain at the time — and sometimes continues to be today.[18]

Evidently, in the USA at least, the extent to which a product is novel does not correlate by necessity with the extent of the artificiality of its construction. If the form of the substance is original, that is, novel, it does not matter if the chemical it comprises is not. In Europe, a similar point can be made. That said, in European not allowing the patenting of chemicals *per se*, the conceptual difficulties highlighted by the present case were resolved in favour of allowing hormones to be protected, albeit through the patented processes used to prepare them. In the United Kingdom, though, Takamine's adrenaline inventions covering the preparations themselves were patented without challenge or controversy.

Insulin is a hormone produced in the pancreas that enables cells to metabolise glucose and the body to store sugar in the form of glycogen. Diabetes is caused either by the inability of the pancreas to produce insulin at all or in sufficient quantities or by the body's 'refusal' to use it when it can be produced. Insulin was named, patented and made available to diabetics for the first time in the early 1920s. Coining a name and getting it accepted does lend it scientific legitimacy, apportion credit to the discover-namers, and offer potential commercial advantages to those first to place it on the market. This is nowehere truer than in the case of insulin. This was despite the fact that it took four more decades before its complex chemical composition was worked out. This situation has been rather common. Often drugs were patented before scientists knew how they worked (this is often true today), or even, in the case of large molecules like insulin, *what* they were.

The discovery of insulin

The relationship between diabetes and something in the pancreas was discovered in 1889 by Oskar Minkowski who found that a dog whose pancreas had been removed suffered the effects of diabetes. To Minkowski, it followed that the loss of the pancreas actually caused diabetes. In the following years, he and others conducted experiments to find out more about the relationship between the pancreas and sugar metabolism. By 1910, around 400 individuals had tried out their pancreatic extracts on animals and even humans. One of the most promising experiments was carried out in 1906 in a Berlin clinic by Georg Ludwig Zuelzer, who injected his extract into a patient. The man showed signs of recovery but Zuelzer had run out of extract and he died. Later tests with his extract showed that it produced harmful side-effects that could not be eliminated.

In October 1920, Frederick Banting, a doctor and surgeon trained at the University of Toronto, came across an article by a pathologist called Moses Barron entitled *The relation of the islets of Langerhans to diabetes with special reference to cases of pancreatic lithiasis*. He determined immediately to

(*Continued*)

find this nameless pancreatic internal secretion. He approached Professor John Macleod at University of Toronto, who offered him laboratory facilities. In time, the insulin team grew with the addition of Charles Best and James Collip.

In May 1922, the discovery of insulin, as the group decided to call it, was announced at a meeting of the Association of American Physicians. What remained was the daunting challenge of producing pure insulin in sufficient quantities to treat more than a handful of patients. Following the announcement, the demand for insulin grew tremendously as did the pressure to meet it. To increase their anxiety, they were advised that failure to patent the discovery could result in competing patent claims that might even force them to halt their work.

Putting to one side their concerns about the ethics of patenting medical discoveries, the group discussed the possibility of filing a Canadian patent that would be assigned to the University. But they had no experience in this, nor did they have much idea about what was patentable. 'To reach their decision and build their strategy for administration of a medical patent, the discoverers of insulin studied precedents.[19] These included Takamine's patents and also the patenting some years earlier of another hormone, thyroxin, by an academic scientist called Edward Kendall, about whom we will learn more later. Kendall wrote to Macleod advising him to file a patent. Kendall was mindful of the fact that while the Toronto group knew insulin was a single chemical substance they were unable to say what it actually was. They did isolate and purify insulin, but only to the extent that it could be administered to patients and keep them alive and well indefinitely. They could not patent insulin *per se*, but only their own preparation of something they had a name for but knew very little about, including how it worked. In his letter, then,

Kendall suggested defining it in the patent in terms of its physiological and clinical effects: 'in regard to the patent, you will of course be unable to patent the substance as yet, but you should have no trouble with patenting the process, and you can make this very broad, so broad that I feel sure you can safeguard the preparation. The substance can be defined in your case by its physiological action, as nothing similar exists.'[20]

(*Continued*)

(*Continued*)

A Canadian patent was filed and granted. Banting, Best and Collip were named as the inventors. Patents were subsequently filed in 25 countries, suggesting there were few concerns as to the inherent patentability of the inventions disclosed in all of those jurisdictions.[21]

The US application, assigned to Toronto with Collip and Best but not the reluctant Banting named as inventors, was initially rejected but not because there was anything inherently unpatentable about the product or the process. One reason was that Zuelzer had been granted a patent in 1912 on his extraction process. The application was amended, showing that the Toronto method was substantially different and more effective. Banting's name was added as co-inventor, and the patent was then granted. A deal was struck with Eli Lilly, an Indianapolis-based drug company. Decades later, Eli Lilly marketed a new form of insulin by a very different method: genetically engineered human insulin using the patented recombinant DNA technology.

While not usually considered to be as significant in the commercial sense as the antibiotics, cortisone and its steroidal relatives and derivatives were hugely important for the pharmaceutical industry. Indeed, cortisone's seemingly miraculous therapeutic effects could not have been predicted by pharmaceutical chemists. In fact, they could only have been discovered by individuals who were in regular contact with patients. To be fair, though, Merck understood this point very well and acted accordingly (see box).

Cortisone and the evolution of patent strategy

In 1948, Merck organized a conference of endocrinologists to discuss clinical use of a synthetic version of a hormone from the adrenal gland which it called Compound E. Merck had produced small quantities and was willing to distribute it among clinical researchers for testing.[22]

One of the recipients was Philip Hench at the Mayo Clinic in Rochester, Minnesota. Hench decided to experiment by treating a rheumatoid arthritis sufferer with Compound E, which he later named cortisone.

(*Continued*)

The result was a spectacular improvement in the patient's condition. During the following months, similar results were obtained with other patients. Although cortisone turned out to have some unpleasant side-effects, the drug version of cortisone and its derivatives (collectively known as the corticosteroids) had a major health impact since they successfully treated a tremendous range of hitherto untreatable diseases that were not obviously related and whose causes were hardly understood.[23]

Why did Hench decide to try this particular compound? First, he had previously observed that the condition of rheumatoid arthritis sufferers improved when they were pregnant or had jaundice.[24] This led him to speculate that a hormone might be responsible. Second, he was fortunate enough to work at the same establishment as the previously mentioned Edward Kendall, an experienced and entrepreneurial endocrinologist who had been studying the adrenal hormones, and who was a consultant to Merck. Merck had in fact been interested in the adrenal gland steroids including cortisone for some time.

Kendall had isolated some of the adrenal hormones, including one with the chemical name 17-hydroxy-11-dehydrocorticosterone, or Compound E for short, which with other Merck chemists he had been trying to synthesize. The Second World War was underway and there was a growing expectation that the US would have to enter it. With rumours that the Germans had found a way to enable their pilots to fly at extraordinarily high altitudes through injections of an adrenal hormone, the US government saw it as a priority to promote and coordinate research on the corticosteroids, especially Kendall's Compound E. In October 1941, two months before the Pearl Harbor attack, a conference was organized bringing together Kendall and university and corporate scientists.[25] Weeks later, Kendall was able to make sufficiently good progress to file a patent and was encouraged to approach Research Corporation, a non-profit foundation formed to handle patents arising from collaborations between academics and industry as a way to support academic research. According to the deal that was struck, 'Research Corporation would apply for and manage Kendall's patent (which was to be kept secret in the interest of national defence) in exchange for assignment of the patent and half of any royalties'.[26] In total, Kendall assigned 12 US patents to Research Corporation, which from 1950 entered a patent pool

(*Continued*)

(Continued)

(see below). Merck licensed these patents, and agreed to work with Kendall in synthesizing Compound E. Use of the rest of Kendall's research was also exclusive to Merck as he adopted a practice of keeping it secret from the other academic scientists and companies working on Compound E, including those granted government contracts to do this work; contracts which, as it happened, required the academics (other than Kendall) to waive any intellectual property rights arising from their research. The companies, which by 1942 comprised Parke Davis, Merck and the US Schering,[27] were under no such constraints though.[28]

By 1943, there were serious doubts as to whether the corticosteroids could do much for altitude tolerance after all. Nonetheless, the government continued to treat this work as a priority, possibly because similar work was going on in Europe by Tadeus Reichstein of the University of Basel, then collaborating with Ciba. Competition became intense to come up with new synthetic and biological processes for producing cortisone in abundant quantities, and as part of such efforts, to identify suitable intermediates. Later on, firms competed to make more potent analogues. In 1944, Merck's Lewis Sarett synthesized cortisone using deoxycholic acid in ox bile as the starting material.[29] This was not particularly efficient, and work went on to try to improve the process. The basic challenge was to shift oxygen atoms to the right location in the molecule. Doing so required multiple chemical steps that were expensive to do and yielded minuscule amounts. Sarett's improved (and patented) method of 1948 and other enhancements at Merck certainly helped, but there was much to do. Whittling down the number of steps to fewer than 30 did not improve yields all that much.

It turned out that synthetic chemistry could not do the job by itself, and once the technical obstacles became ever more apparent, the number of competition entrants shrank.[30] Key to success, it transpired, was the development of biosynthetic processes integrating use of micro-organisms as chemical reagents with synthetic chemistry. It is worth mentioning here that such technologies benefited from the penicillin experience (and in turn facilitated the development and production of new antibiotics later on).[31] The companies that remained or decided to get involved when others fell by the wayside included Ciba, Upjohn, Glaxo, Schering, Roussel-Uclaf and Organon, a Dutch firm co-founded by an abattoir owner.[32] Russell Marker,

(*Continued*)

an American scientist at Syntex, a Mexican company he co-founded, had previously identified diosgenin, a chemical found in Mexican yams, as an abundant and suitable precursor for progesterone, a sex steroid, which could in turn be converted into other steroids. Syntex's Carl Djerassi managed to synthesize cortisone from diosgenin, though this did not lead to any industrial application.

In the early 1950s, Upjohn's Herbert Murray and Durey Peterson figured out that the female hormone progesterone was a suitably abundant precursor for the much rarer cortisone and for other corticosteroids, especially since Syntex had found a way to produce large amounts cheaply, and that a mould called *Rhizopus* could by fermentation be used to introduce oxygen atoms into the progesterone molecule at the right location, turning it into cortisone.[33] In 1952, they announced a successful biosynthesis of cortisone, and the process was later successfully applied to the production of other naturally-occurring anti-inflammatory steroids and some new analogues. These were important as cortisone's various harmful side-effects became more evident. In all, 'seventy-four patents were issued and 54 scientific articles published on the extensions of this work.'[34]

Syntex came back with a better biosynthetic process, this time using a byproduct of sisal called hecogenin that was also known to the UK National Institute for Medical Research.[35] This process was licensed by Syntex to Glaxo, which had access to sisal cultivated in Kenya. Glaxo, an increasingly science-based company by then, and one well-connected with public sector medical research establishments, did generate some important know-how in this area too, and this was licensed back to Syntex.[36] Ciba also got engaged in hecogenin biosynthesis after giving up on ox bile in the mid-1950s.[37] The US Schering company also came up with a biosynthetic process for making cortisone, and in 1954 invented cortisone analogues called prednisone and prednisolone while trying to find a new way to synthesize cortisone.[38] Due to priority challenges from five other companies, it took 10 years for Schering to be granted a US patent on prednisone, still the most commonly prescribed anti-inflammatory steroid drug.[39,40]

With all the patenting activity going on, companies sought to access patent specifications as soon as they were published anywhere in the world in order to find out what their rivals were doing and also to seek gaps in the

(*Continued*)

(*Continued*)

patent claims that they could fill. For example, Syntex acquired the specification of Upjohn's South African patent application on its new process just as soon as it was published. Organon examined Schering's Belgian patent application on prednisone on the very day it was published and, finding that 'some potential chemical routes to the novel compounds had not been claimed', came up with a new process which it patented.[41]

As might be expected, potential freedom-to-operate difficulties were immense, even for the pioneering Merck, and some cooperation was felt to be necessary. Even in his 1950 Nobel Lecture, Edward Kendall felt compelled to mention patent problems: 'the patent situation which eventually would control the manufacture of cortisone by Merck and Co., Inc. and three other companies was complicated, confused and to many it seemed hopeless'.[42] In response, in 1950 the Cortisone US Patent Pool was set up by Research Corporation. Initially this comprised Merck and the Mayo Clinic, which had an interest in Kendall's patents, as well as Ciba, Organon and Schering, each of whom had less closely-related patents that nonetheless had the potential to block further commercially-orientated work. Upjohn joined later. Elsewhere, there was a Cortisone and Related Compounds Agreement. The parties to this were Merck, Ciba, and Organon.

This 'provided mutual licenses and options for licenses on future research results.'[43] Patent pools and such inter-corporate research and marketing arrangements are of course controversial in that they can be seen, at least in many cases, as privileging existing market entrants that have acquired enough intellectual property for admission to the club. It is likely that intended market entrants were kept out as a result. It has been suggested, for example, that 'the complexity of the patenting seems to have played a part in ICI's decision not to enter the steroid field' during the 1950s.[44]

The Sex Hormones

The sex hormones were a subject of similarly intense business and academic rivalry over several decades, beginning before the discovery of cortisone and continuing for some time after cortisone's star had already waned. So we must now go further back into the past, in fact to the late 1920s when the sex hormones were beginning to be isolated.

The sex hormones are produced in three glands, mainly the gonads (ovaries or testes) but also in the pituitary and adrenal glands. Alternatively, they may be produced by conversion from other hormones in other parts of the body. They are responsible for the development of primary and secondary sex characteristics. Female sex hormones comprise the oestrogens and progesterone. Androgen is a collective term for the natural and synthetic male sex hormones. Probably the best known one is testosterone.

Urine was often the most convenient source of naturally-occurring sex hormones. But since the concentration of the desired hormone is normally extremely low, synthesis was attempted from quite an early stage. The first oestrogen to be isolated, from pregnant mares' urine, was oestrin in 1929 by Edward Doisy at Washington University in St Louis. Patents were licensed to Parke Davis, which marketed it as Theelin.[45] The feat was repeated during the following months at Göttingen University in Germany using urine supplied by Schering, and then (presumably not personally) by Ernst Laqueur at University of Amsterdam. The next one to be isolated was oestriol in 1930, this time by Guy Marrian at University College London. Progesterone, which is produced in the ovary, was isolated in 1934 almost simultaneously by Adolf Butenandt at Göttingen and groups working at Columbia University, Vienna University and at Ciba. Shortly after, Butenandt figured out its chemical structure. The first patents went to Schering.

The first male sex hormone to be isolated and then synthesized was androsterone in 1931 and 1934 respectively. Butenandt was the isolator, using extracts supplied again by Schering from the vast quantities of urine generously donated by the Berlin police force: 25,000 litres, from which he was able to obtain 50 mg of crystalline androsterone, as he called it.[46] Butenandt's purified androsterone was tested by Schering who patented the process without even naming Butenandt as co-inventor.[47] The synthesiser was Leopold Ruzicka at Ciba.

Testosterone was discovered and isolated in 1935 by Laqueur's Organon funded team at Amsterdam. Ruzicka and a colleague at Ciba, Albert Wettstein who had earlier been one of the first to isolate progesterone, synthesised testosterone from cholesterol, worked out its structure and filed a patent that same year. Competition was intense, innovations were going on in different places almost simultaneously, and it is not always clear who were the pioneers and who were the followers.

Schering and Ciba found themselves in control of key patents relating to the sex hormones and were keen to take full commercial advantage. However, a few other European firms were also in possession of important patents and some cooperation was thus necessary. The main ones were Organon, Böhringer Mannheim and Roussel. Schering secured patent licensing deals, first a very favourable one with Organon, and then with Ciba. In May 1937, these companies formed the European Hormones Cartel with the latter three firms being the junior partners. Accordingly, members 'granted each other the right to use their inventions and experience for the furtherance of common interests of the parties in the commercial exploitation of their therapeutic preparations.'[48] The Second World War changed the situation of course. For one thing, the Nazis placed Organon under the control of Schering. Also, in 1941 the US Justice Department stopped the American branches of Ciba, Organon and Schering from behaving as a cartel.[49] For another, ways were found to circumvent the cartel by finding alternative means of synthesizing sex steroids other than by the cholesterol route employed by all these firms.

By the 1950s, after 30 years of patenting activity in the field of sex hormones, considerable change had taken place in their status from crude glandular extracts to industrial products and this was reflected in the patent system. As Gaudillière explains:

> Steroids had become drugs manufactured by industry in (relatively) large quantities, and were now biochemical substances defined in terms of structure and metabolism rather than anatomical origins and mode of action. In other words, the sex hormones had become biotechnological 'goods'. The management of intellectual property played a critical role in these processes of industrialization and molecularization, because it helped align sex hormones with chemicals and chemically constructed therapeutic agents.[50]

Not just a pill: 'the pill'

The story now turns to sex hormones as oral contraceptives, something that most companies were at first deeply reluctant to have anything to do with due to moralistic opposition. This situation made private non-commercial sources of research funding especially important. Initial interest in practical

(*Continued*)

uses of progesterone in relation to fertility concerned not how to make women temporarily fertile but how to help the infertile to get pregnant.[51]

A physiology professor at the University of Innsbruck called Ludwig Haberland has been cited as the one who first came up with the idea for a hormonal contraceptive.[52] In a 1919 experiment, he found that a female rabbit with ovaries implanted from a pregnant rabbit could not get pregnant despite regular bunny-propagating activity. However, a concept was one thing and a product quite another. Even with the isolation and purification of progesterone, much more needed to be done. One obvious problem is that being a natural hormone, progesterone cannot possibly pass through the digestive system intact. An additional steroidal ingredient was essential to help it along its perilous journey. Identifying and adding that ingredient would take two more decades. There were three other difficulties to be overcome.

The first was to find a suitably abundant raw material. Russell Marker solved that one thanks to Mexico's wild yams, of which barbasco turned out to be the best diosgenin provider. The second was to discover an effective process to partially synthesise the precursor and intermediate chemicals. After Marker left Syntex, his replacement, George Rosenkranz, learned to use diosgenin to partially synthesize both progesterone and testosterone — cheaply and on a large scale. This led to a lowering of international prices and broke the market power of the European steroids cartel.

The third difficulty was that of how to synthesize a derivative that was potent *and* capable of getting from the mouth to the bloodstream intact. At its most simplistic, this involved a procedure for removing a methyl group at position 19 on the carbon backbone of the progesterone molecule. The result was a substance called 19-norprogesterone, that is, progesterone without the methyl group attached to carbon atom 19.[53] The process employed was based on a modified application of the so-called Birch reduction, named after Arthur Birch, then at Oxford University. It was freely available because Birch's request to patent it had effectively been refused — something he was not happy about complaining that as a result "Britain lost any rights to work that it initially funded".[54] The feat also benefited from related work done by Max Ehrenstein at University of Pennsylvania.

(*Continued*)

(*Continued*)

But they did not stop there. Having climbed on the shoulders of Birch and Ehrenstein to see further, they found another useful pair of shoulders to stand on. These belonged to Hans Inhoffen at Schering. Djerassi and Rosenkranz applied a discovery made by Inhoffen at the German Schering company. This was to add a pair of triple-bonded carbon atoms (an 'acetyline group') to position 17 on the testosterone molecule. This gave rise to a chemical with mild progestational activity that could be taken orally: ethisterone. Again, there was no patent on this technique in Mexico, though there was one in the United States.[55] What remained was to put together these various insights provided by others and marry them to the advanced chemical arts being performed by the Syntex team. As Djerassi himself explained, 'on the reasonable assumption that removal of the 19-carbon atom increases progestational potency and addition of acetylene confers oral efficacy, Rosenkranz and I put both these observations together.'[56] In October 1951, one of Djerassi's assistants at Syntex, Luis Miramontes, 'completed the synthesis of . . . 19-nor-17 -ethynyltestosterone or, for short, "norethindrone" — which turned out to be the first oral contraceptive to be synthesised.'

In November 1951, Syntex filed a patent. Syntex were in fact looking for a treatment for menstrual disorders, not an oral contraceptive. At the time, there was no market for oral contraceptives and the industry was hesitant to face the anticipated condemnation including from the Catholic Church.[57] Up to the 1970s, contraception was illegal or severely restricted in several American states and also in several other parts of the western world. Nonetheless, research on the female sex hormones went on as commercial possibilities were very much present even without contraception. Furthermore, rich individuals and private donors like the Rockefeller Foundation were willing to take up the slack. Norethindrone (or norethisterone) was approved by the United States Food and Drug Administration (FDA) in 1957, marketed under the name Norlutin, and indicated for menstrual and gynaecological problems.

Syntex was not without rivals. In 1953, Frank Colton of G.D. Searle,[58] then a small Chicago-based company, who had worked on cortisone at the Mayo Clinic, synthesized norethynodrel for which a patent was filed in August of that year. This was in fact an isomer of norethindrone, which is to say that it is built of the same atoms but with a different architecture. In

(*Continued*)

this case the structural differences were very slight. Indeed, norethyndrodel pretty much becomes norethindrone once it has passed through the digestive tract,[59] though it displayed none of the androgenic effects sometimes experienced with norethindrone.

Syntex encountered delays in getting norethindrone to market as a contraceptive. It had a contract with Parke Davis in which the latter firm undertook to secure FDA approval and to market the product in the United States. But Parke Davis got cold feet and Syntex had to find another partner. It was not until January 1962 that it was approved as an oral contraceptive. The following year it was marketed by licensee Ortho Pharmaceutical as Ortho Novin, a combination of norethindrone with oestrogen mestranol.[60]

In the meantime, Searle had stolen a march on Syntex. First, although its patent was filed 21 months later than Syntex's, it was granted five months earlier, on 29 November 1955 as opposed to 1 May 1956 for norethindrone. Second, while its FDA approval for norethynodrel (Enovid) as a treatment for gynaecological and menstrual problems came around the same time as Norlutin, it beat the latter product to market as an approved oral contraceptive by 19 months. FDA consent for 'ovulation inhibition' came in June 1960, a time when the social and political climate was more morally accepting towards contraception.

The first total synthesis of an oral contraceptive that was cost-effective was achieved in 1960 by Herchel Smith, a former student of Arthur Birch's. Norgestrel, sold as Ovral, was a close derivative of Djerassi's and Miramontes's norethindrone but was more potent. It came on the market in 1968 and was sold by Smith's employer Wyeth, and the German Schering. During that decade a range of contraceptive products came on the market produced and sold by companies from the US, the UK, Germany, the Netherlands and France. Patenting was of course technically possible thanks to earlier precedents as discussed about. But by now it was also morally acceptable.

It is interesting to note that moral opposition to contraception was in some part reflected in the patent system, at least in Britain. In 1927, the Solicitor General refused a UK patent application on a contraceptive device. He would not be drawn as to whether such an invention was immoral or not; nonetheless, he was not prepared to exercise the Crown's discretion in favour of granting a patent on such a product despite its fulfilling all the technical requirements.[61] In due course, the morality of contraception was no longer an issue for patent examiners or courts. In 1971 the Patents Appeal Tribunal held that methods to prevent conception are not *per se* methods of treatment by therapy, and are therefore not subject to the statutory exclusion from patentability of such methods.[62]

What we Have Learned so Far

The development and commercialization of therapeutic hormones shows that the origins of the modern pharmaceutical industry do not lie only in the (mostly German) former dye-makers and chemical synthesisers like Bayer, BASF and Hoechst which were first to become expert chemical synthesisers and drug-makers and arguably 'invented' in-house research and development a few years before Thomas Edison. Natural product-based companies, often American, represent another pillar. With hormones, vitamins and later on penicillin and the antibiotics, which we cover in the next chapter, the best of these companies began to compete for size with the big German firms once they learned how to do two things well. The first of these was to integrate the disciplines of natural product chemistry, fermentation, endocrinology and synthetic chemistry. Companies in various countries, but especially in the US and Britain, with varied expertise and able to take advantage of the many physiological insights coming out of universities and medical research establishments during the early decades of the twentieth century also came to the fore, a point the next chapter will reinforce. By the 1930s, interdisciplinarity was becoming increasingly important. That would prove important when it came to the antibiotics and, somewhat later on, biotechnology. The second was to adopt the kinds of patent and market control strategies pioneered by Bayer and the other German firms. These strategies could be offensive and aggressive, but when the need arose they were defensive and cooperative. Importantly, British and American scientists contributed much during this period. Certainly, the competitive position of companies outside of Germany was much improved by operating outside of the afore-mentioned synthetic dyestuff paradigm. According to medical historian John Lesch:

> In areas of drug innovation that were not so dependent on medicinal chemistry in the sense of molecular synthesis and molecular modification, but rather on the isolation, purification, and chemical and physiological characterization of naturally occurring compounds such as hormones and vitamins, much important work was done outside of Germany between 1900 and 1935.[63]

Nonetheless, the picture is a complex one. Much progress was undoubtedly made by the isolators. Insulin stands out here as the strongest evidence. Yet the European synthesisers were able for a time to take control of the steroids market from the 1930s, establishing a global cartel that proved very difficult to break. Nonetheless, the industrial chemical expertise of the Americans began to match that of Germany, as is well exemplified by the biosynthesis of cortisone and its very close relative hydrocortisone, achieved by a number of North American firms in fairly quick succession. This helped US firms and the US industry more generally to become dominant in pharmaceuticals from the 1950s — though the main German and Swiss firms continued to be major leading-edge firms as some of them still are.

Today, we are living with the legacy of the hormones era. As stated earlier, once hormones emerged as products, patent granting offices and courts were generally quite favourably disposed towards hormone-related patent claims. In countries allowing chemicals to be patented, hormones were inherently patentable whether as synthetic chemicals or as preparations extracted from body tissue or fluid. On the basis of similar rationales, genes, microbes, plants and animals are now patentable too, as we will see in more detail in Chapter 9.

Notes

1 Macilwaine (1900).
2 Le Fanu *op. cit.*, 206.
3 Marks (1997), 17–18.
4 Le Fanu *op. cit.*, 206.

5   Of course, the idea of a well-balanced diet is hardly new. But what has changed, and continues to, is medical opinion, followed by companies when it suited them, as to what such a diet should comprise. The present author well remembers the advertising slogan "Six slices a day is the well-balanced way" for a brand of tasteless white bread sold in a plastic bag.

6   'The chemical messengers .... Or "hormones" (from ὁρμάω, I excite or arouse), as we might call them, have to be carried from the organ where they are produced to the organ which they affect by means of the blood stream and the continually recurring physiological needs of the organism must determine their repeated production and circulation through the body.' *See* Starling (1905), 340

7   Rasmussen (2002).

8   Gaudillière (2008), 125.

9   Rubin (2007), 292.

10   US Patent no. 730,176 ('Glandular extractive product'), issued on June 2 1903.

11   US Patent no. 753,177 ('Glandular extractive compound'), issued on February 23 1904.

12   US Patent no. 525,823 ('Process of making diatastic enzyme'), issued on September 11 1894.

13   Takamine had originally claimed the natural substance itself but this was refused by the examiner.

14   Parke Davis and Co. v. H.K. Mulford and Co., 189 Fed. 95 (S.D.N.Y. 1911) affirmed, 196 Fed. 496 (2nd Cir. 1912).

15   Since Parke Davis registered 'Adrenalin' as a trade mark in the United States, the natural substance is referred to as epinephrine in that country, and this is becoming international practice.

16   For a detailed analysis of the case and its implications see Harkness (2011).

17   Davenport (1982), 80.

18   For Judge Hand this was something to be regretted. As he stated at the end of his judgement: 'I cannot stop calling attention to the extraordinary condition of the law which makes it possible for a man without any knowledge of even the rudiments of chemistry to pass upon such questions as these ... How long we shall continue to blunder along without the aid of unpartisan and authoritative scientific assistance in the administration of justice, no one knows; but all fair persons not conventionalized by provincial legal habits of mind ought, I should think, unite to effect some advance.'

19   Cassier and Sinding (2008), 154.

20   Cassier and Sinding *op. cit.*, 154.

21 Cassier and Sinding *op. cit.*, 153.

22 Lloyd (2002), 583.

23 Le Fanu *op. cit.*, 25

24 Glyn (1998).

25 Rasmussen (2002), 315.

26 Rasmussen (2002) *op.cit.*, 315

27 The German company Schering's United States branch split from the parent company during the Second World War when the US subsidiary was confiscated by the government and later became a separate firm.

28 This shows how academics could sometimes be more concerned to restrict access to knowledge than companies. Indeed, it illustrates how 'collaboration with industry threatened, ironically, to facilitate an informational communalism that the academic moral economy was traditionally more inclined to resist than the diffusion of medical inventions.' Rasmussen (2004), 177.

29 Hirschmann (1992).

30 Peterson (1985), 6.

31 Bud (1993) *op. cit.*, 106; Peterson *op. cit.*, 9; Quirke (2005), 646–7.

32 As elsewhere, there was a shortage of animal glands for academic research into hormones in the Netherlands. Since there were no pharmaceutical companies at the time, Ernst Laqueur at University of Amsterdam concluded that it would be necessary to form a hormones business. He approached the abattoir owner, Zaal van Zwanenberg, who was looking for customers for the huge amounts of animal waste being produced, and together they set up Organon. Laqueur became scientific consultant to Organon and was able to ensure his university had access to a good supply. *See* Oudshoorn (1990), 14–5.

33 Syntex received a massive order for progesterone from Upjohn, and suspected this must be due to some novel chemical process. It managed to discover what the process was, as mentioned in the main text, by reading a published South African patent filed by Upjohn. *See* Hogg (1992), 594; Peterson *op. cit.*

34 Peterson *op. cit.*, 8

35 Most probably Syntex discovered this application of hecogenin just before NIMR.

36 Djerassi (1984), 355; Quirke (2005) *op. cit.*, 665–6.

37 Heusler and Kalvoda (1992), 493.

38 Heusler and Kalvoda *op. cit.* It later turned out that prednisolone is the active metabolite of prednisone.

39 Sneader (1984), 208.

40   Herzog and Oliveto (1992), 619.

41   Szpilfogel and Zeelen (1996), 485.

42   *See* http://nobelprize.org/nobel_prizes/medicine/laureates/1950/kendall-lecture.pdf. The other winners of the Nobel Prize in Physiology or Medicine that year were Hench and Reichstein, whose team had managed to identify and isolate 27 cortical-steroids, and was also a key player in the international race to synthesize cortisone in collaboration with Ciba (during wartime) and Organon.

43   Heusler and Kalvoda *op. cit.*, 493.

44   Slinn (2008), 196.

45   Rasmussen (2004) *op. cit.*, 176.

46   Oudshoorn *op. cit.*, 19.

47   Gaudillière (2008) *op. cit.*, 114.

48   Szpilfogel and Zeelen *op. cit.*, 483.

49   Laveaga (2005), 745 (fn.6).

50   Gaudillière (2008), 126.

51   Porter (1997) *op. cit.*, 569.

52   Djerassi (2001), 16–9.

53   Miramontes, Rosenkranz and Djerassi (1951).

54   Birch (1992), 372.

55   A United States patent for this was filed in 1939 by Hans Inhoffen and assigned to Schering. It was granted in 1944: US Patent no. 2,358,808 ('Valuable compounds of the pregnane series and a method of producing the same'), issued on September 26 1944.

56   Djerassi *op. cit.*, 47. See also Djerassi *et al* (1954).

57   Marks (2001), 31–4.

58   Colton (1992).

59   Djerassi *op. cit.*, 54.

60   Marks *op. cit.*, 76.

61   *A & H's Application* [1927] 44 RPC 298.

62   *Re Schering Ag's Application* [1971] RPC 337.

63   Lesch (2007) *op. cit.*, 5.

Chapter 7

The Anti-infectives: Sulphonamide, Penicillin, and the Antibiotics

You will recall Perkin's famous discovery in 1856; in reality an attempt to make a drug (quinine) that resulted in a dye, that kick-started a new industry making one type of fine chemical: a dye, and then adding a related type to its portfolio: drugs. Eight decades later, the most important pharmaceutical 'moment', and perhaps the most significant up to that time, at least with respect to that particular evolutionary pathway if not to the industry more generally, was the discovery of a dye that turned out itself to be a drug. This was sulphonamide, a discovery of corporate lab origin, which marked the first chemotherapeutic revolution envisaged by Paul Ehrlich. It would go too far to suggest that the pharmaceutical industry up to the Second World War was German. But neither is it all that inaccurate especially in respect of medicinal chemistry. The discovery of the sulphonamide anti-bacterials in the 1930s could only have been made in Germany and by a German company, one steeped in the traditions of dye chemistry but sufficiently organised scientifically to be able to bring together highly trained individuals from a wider range of disciplines. And yet, the sulfa drugs were a short-lived triumph for the German company involved, I.G. Farbenindustrie, which was formed in 1925 by the merger of the main German chemical firms, and indeed for Germany. Foreign companies were able to catch up on I.G. Farben very quickly. This time, Bayer's long experience in strategic intellectual property strategy was of no use in defending the company's lead.

According to medical historian John Lesch, 'the sulfa drugs ... stand at a pivotal moment in the history of twentieth-century medicine. They are at once the culminating event of the first major phase of the industrialization of pharmaceutical innovation, and the initial event of the second great phase of that process, the therapeutic revolution that continues in our time'.[1] He could have added that trade in a sulphonamide product led to a disaster that decisively change the course of pharmaceutical regulation (see box).

The sulphonamide revolution was founded on the working hypothesis first formulated by Paul Ehrlich, the great German chemist and immunologist, that the ability of dye chemicals, some of which were already shown to have analgesic and antipyretic properties, to stain microbes and tissues selectively might enable them to affect the metabolism of disease-causing microbes without destroying human tissue. Just as dye chemicals bind to fabric and then stain it, Ehrlich, as we saw earlier, believed that certain chemicals, dyes or otherwise, could be found with a selective affinity for specific infective agents and containing a toxic part to immobilize them.

The discovery of the sulfa drugs

The sulphonamide story begins in the late 1920s, when Heinrich Hörnlein, a senior researcher at an I.G. Farben research facility originally part of Bayer, brought together a team comprising Gerhard Domagk, a biomedical researcher, and two chemists, Fritz Mietzsch and Joseph Klarer. The idea was to follow Ehrlich's example by testing azo dyes for therapeutic effects against bacterial agents. Published research suggested that some azos had antibacterial effects. Moreover, azos were susceptible to molecular manipulation, allowing for lots of variants to be tried out.[2] Mietzsch and Klarer would provide the dyes and Domagk would test them both *in vitro* and *in vivo*. This turned out to be very wise. In 1932, on the basis of successful earlier work overseen by Hörlein on sulphonamide-containing azos for dyeing textiles, Klarer synthesized a compound of this kind for Domagk to test. While it failed to display any effect *in vitro*, it did show action in mice infected with streptococci. Klarer produced another variant that was even more effective *in vivo*. On December 25 1932, a German patent was filed on the process for making this red crystalline powder, which had the chemical name of 4-sulfonamido-2, 4-diaminoazobenzene but became better known as Streptozon or Prontosil.[3] Three years later Domagk described the discovery in a German journal article.[4] While the mode of action was unknown, a considerable amount of chemical and biological insight and

(*Continued*)

skill went into the discovery. This was rational drug design 1930s style; Ehrlich's concept of chemotherapy in action. As Lesch explains, 'whereas the medical researcher took the variability given in nature, tried to analyse it in detail, and identified points where chemical therapy might find a purchase, the chemists produced variability by synthetic manipulation.'[5]

Meanwhile, France had over a period of 70 years reverted from being an industrial chemistry leader to a copier, and, to the great irritation of the German chemical industry, had patent practices to match. From the First World War onwards, French businesses had few qualms about copying German pharmaceutical products, and like the United States and the United Kingdom, France had expropriated German patents and trademarks. Hörlein complained about this situation in 1926: 'in the pharmaceutical field a circumstance prevails that is not all that different from that of the robber knights of the Middle Ages'.[6] Prontosil was patented in France but this did not do I.G. Farben any good at all. First, French patent law allowed chemicals to be protected but not medicines. In effect this meant French companies could copy the invention *as a drug* safe from being sued for patent infringement, which, to Hörlein's chagrin, they did. In very short time, Roussel was selling a copy which it called Rubiazol. Second, scientists at the Pasteur Institute studied the patent and synthesized several other dyes which were then tested following the methods described in Domagk's article published earlier that year (1935). In doing so they discovered that part of the Prontosil molecule, later known as sulphanilamide, was responsible for the therapeutic effect and this was not the dye part.[7] This simpler compound was easier and cheaper to make and did not have the side effect of turning some patients red. To make matters worse, Bayer had patented a process for making this same chemical three decades earlier as an intermediate in dye-making unaware of any therapeutic action. The patent had now expired meaning the chemical was in the public domain and fully available for any scientist or company to modify it and improve its effectiveness for the same infective agents and for others too. While Prontosil was patented in the UK and the US, this did not prevent anybody from using sulphanilamide.

As a consequence of all this, the sulphonamide revolution was unaffected by any patents on the original drug, not just in France but elsewhere too, and its onset was all the rapider for it. By the end of the 1930s numerous companies in Britain, France and the United States were selling

(*Continued*)

(*Continued*)

sulphonamide drugs. One of the most successful of these was M&B 693. It was discovered by a British company called May & Baker, by that time owned by the French firm Rhône-Poulenc. M&B 693, which entered the market in 1938, was more effective against streptococci as well as other organisms including pneumococci, and was also less toxic.[8] This was probably Britain's first internationally-important pharmaceutical product. Other similar substances were subsequently synthesized and found also to have therapeutic effects against a range of infectious diseases, including leprosy. These became known collectively as the sulphonamides, or sulfa drugs.[9] It is noteworthy that 'the companies that rushed to ride the [sulfonamide] bandwagon, and did so successfully, were predominantly *chemical companies with strong R&D expertise in dyestuffs*: Ciba, Geigy, Sandoz, Hoffman LaRoche, as well as ICI, American Cyanamid, Rhône-Poulenc/May & Baker'.[10] Merck and Sharp & Dohme (which merged in 1953), which were also involved, were among the few exceptions to this rule.

Unfortunately, there was at least one tragic incident, and this had some far-reaching consequences. In 1937, 76 people in the USA lost their lives after taking the highly toxic Elixir of Sulfanilamide made by a company called Massengill. An editorial in the *Journal of the American Medical Association* lamented that:

under our present laws the responsibility for protection of the public rests on the Food and Drug Administration, which is as efficiently armed as a hunter pursuing a tiger with a fly swatter. Under our present laws there is nothing to require S. E. Massengill Company or any other firm to divulge the formula or to make adequate pharmacologic or clinical tests before placing a hazardous 'medicine' or proprietary preparation on the market. Ironically the label for Elixir of Sulfanilamide-Massengill carried the recommendation 'continue at this dose till recovery'![11]

In a letter to a doctor who had lost a patient to the drug, S.E. Massengill callously denied responsibility saying that 'we regret exceedingly this unfortunate occurrence, but as we violated no law and made no error in our manufacture, I do not think that we should be blamed by the unlooked for action of this product'.[12] The government responded by introducing regulations requiring that drugs be tested for safety before they could be sold to the public.[13] These measures were subsequently adopted elsewhere. Allowing drugs to be sold without safety testing is of course unthinkable now.

The sulfa drugs, despite that disaster, were undoubtedly a tremendous boon for the many patients who might otherwise have lost their lives. They also contributed to future drug discovery. Research into the bacteriostatic action of sulphanilamide, most notably by Paul Fildes and Donald Woods, led to the formulation of a new working hypothesis that guided scientists in their design of new drugs for specific microbial targets: competitive antagonism. The idea is that certain chemicals play a vital role in metabolic processes that are specific to particular species of microbe. The possibility arises that structurally related chemicals can be designed which 'trick' the target microbe into taking them up and using them in place of the real substance. But since they do not perform the same role, the process cannot take place, and the microbe is weakened or destroyed.[14] Adoption of this principle did not bear any immediate fruit but has led to the development of several important drugs over the years. These include para-amino salicylic acid (PAS) a treatment for tuberculosis discovered in 1946 by the Danish doctor, Jorgen Lehmann; azathioprine, an immuno-suppressive drug developed in a US lab of Burroughs Wellcome by George Hitchings and Gertrude Elion; and the beta-blockers such as propranolol, that were developed in the 1960s by James Black, then at ICI. A decade later, a team led by Black was responsible for another triumph of rational drug design, the anti-ulcerant cimetidine sold under the name of Tagamet (see Chapter 9).

In Germany, synthetic chemistry was from the start the basis for most pharmaceutical discovery with much of the research done by industry itself. North America and the United Kingdom were rather backward in this regard for much of the first half of the twentieth century. The focus continued well into the twentieth century to be on the isolation of chemicals found in living things.[15] At first, these were phytochemicals like alkaloids and glycosides. But such 'backward' approaches turned out to provide advantages once therapeutic interest shifted to chemicals found in humans and animals, such as hormones, and of course microbes. The balance of industrial power began to shift away from Germany and in a westward direction from the late 1930s, and moved more decisively after the Second World War. Whereas 'in the late 1930s German pharmaceutical sales claimed approximately forty-three percent of the world market', world leadership 'passed to the United States, where the war had accelerated an expansion of research, development, and production of pharmaceuticals already under way by 1939.'[16] Antibiotics were a large part of the reason for this.

Penicillin: From mould to antibiotic medicine

Penicillin, the first antibiotic, is a story in three acts.[17] The first begins in 1928 when it is initially discovered and some early experiments are carried out suggesting therapeutic possibilities. It takes place mostly at St Mary's Hospital Medical School in London, and centres mainly on one person, Alexander Fleming, who was subsequently cast as a hero of science. Act two commences ten years later. The story shifts to Oxford University, where small-scale manufacturing is carried out and the first experiments demonstrating its therapeutic effects on animals and later humans and confirming its non-toxicity take place. Act two is about a team of people located in one place. The third act starts in 1941 when Florey and Heatley go to America and methods are developed in that country to produce penicillin in industrial quantities. Starting with those two protagonists, eventually the story tells of a vast network of individuals working in many places the majority of whom probably have never been named in any historical account.

As is well known, Alexander Fleming, a bacteriologist at St Mary's Hospital, returned from holiday and came across a mouldy dish in the lab (still preserved as it was as a museum). Noticing a sterile area between the mould and a bacterial colony, and informed by earlier research on the anti-bacterial qualities of natural substances, especially lysozyme, he reasoned that the fungal mould exuded a substance that was affecting bacterial growth. Fleming's main contributions to science were, first, to publish his observations in the *British Journal of Experimental Pathology* describing the liquid's selective inhibition of bacteria and suggesting its possible use as an antiseptic, and second to give the name 'penicillin' to the filtered liquid in which the mould was grown so as 'to avoid the rather cumbersome phrase "Mould broth filtrate"';[18] and third, to distribute samples around Europe and the United States for others to experiment on.[19]

The fungus was subsequently identified as *Penicillium notatum* but further work was for a time hampered due to what historian Robert Bud calls 'the fragmentation of science' in which bacteriologists and chemists were failing to work together. This situation began to change in the 1930s.

(*Continued*)

As Bud explains, 'biological scientists in leading universities were increasingly consulting with companies and collaborating with industry. Interdisciplinary teams were being established. The experiences of the work on vitamins, insulin, and plant steroids were providing precedents for the successful collaboration of academic and industrial researchers'.[20]

This was definitely true for Oxford where a new science area was established that included the Sir William Dunn School of Pathology and its neighbour on South Parks Road, the Dyson-Perrins Laboratory which was the university's organic chemistry department. In 1935 Australian-born Howard Florey was appointed Professor of Pathology. Florey was able to establish a team of talented scientists trained in different but complementary disciplines. Most important of these, though, were two biochemists, Ernst Chain, a Jewish immigrant from Germany, and Norman Heatley.

Florey and Chain decided to work on penicillin, not at first, as they admitted, to save people's lives, but because they thought isolating the highly unstable active principle would be an interesting challenge that other groups had failed to overcome. This is not to say they were ever indifferent to the humanitarian aspects of their work. With funding from the Rockefeller Foundation, Chain, who thought incorrectly that the active compound was a protein, and the team Florey had assembled succeeded in isolating a powder that turned out to contain 1 percent of penicillin. Given the original solution contained one part in a million of penicillin, this was some achievement. Norman Heatley, whose role has over the years tended to be overlooked, also contributed decisively at this stage, suggesting a way to extract and stabilize the penicillin. This proved to be quite effective. In March 1940, Chain had enough to test on two mice and realized by their lack of reaction it was a small molecule and not a protein. Later on that year, they tested their substance on infected mice and published their highly promising results in *The Lancet*.[21]

It should be mentioned that the Oxford group used the word 'penicillin' to refer to the active principle and not, as Fleming had done, to the liquid in which it resided. According to one account, 'Florey often said later that had he and his group applied a new name to the active material, it would have avoided much confusion and conflict over credit for the drug.'[22]

The first attempt to inject penicillin into patients suffering bacterial infection took place in New York in October 1940. But the quantities

(*Continued*)

(*Continued*)

available were too small to make a difference. Far more promising results were achieved by the Oxford group in February 1941 when they injected penicillin into a dangerously ill policemen suffering from horrific bacterial infections that were 'eating him like a worm in an apple'.[23] Initially, results were spectacular — he made a dramatic recovery. Unfortunately, they ran out of penicillin, the infections returned and he died a month later. In August 1941, a detailed article was published in *The Lancet* that described methods to grow the mould, and methods of assay, production, purification and extraction. It also reported some highly promising test results against several bacterial species, and therapeutic trails conducted on animals using different delivery methods, and on ten individuals including the aforementioned policeman.[24] The problem was that they were unable to produce enough to treat and cure large numbers of people and without being able to do so it was proving extremely difficult to attract the attention of an industry reluctant at this stage to take the risk of investing funds and effort in developing what was still an unproven substance, and in a wartime situation.

In early 1941, Florey had come to the conclusion that the United States was the only hope. He persuaded the Rockefeller Foundation to fund his travel to the US on the basis that he would reveal everything the Oxford group knew about penicillin to date in exchange for commitment from a US company to scale up production and one kg of powdered penicillin to be used for further human trials. In June 1941, Florey left for the United States with Norman Heatley. Chain had already fallen out with Florey and the medical establishment, including the Medical Research Council, over the question of patenting. To German scientists, patenting in this situation was perfectly normal practice. But in Britain it was considered to be indecent. Even in the United States, where the scientific culture was supposedly more commercially-minded, health-related patenting by universities was not a universally admired practice, though it could certainly generate a decent amount of funds, at least for some, and undoubtedly could serve some useful public purposes such as regulating the quality of medicines made available to the public.[25] At the time, the Principles of Medical Ethics of the American Medical Association stated that 'it is unprofessional to receive remuneration from patents for surgical instruments or medicines; to accept rebates on prescriptions or surgical appliances, or perquisites from attendants who aid in the care of patients.'[26] Despite this, the University of Wisconsin gained

(*Continued*)

considerable royalties from the late 1920s onwards thanks to the assertiveness of the Wisconsin Alumni Research Foundation (WARF), which was set up to maximize the University's income from its patents (some of which were health related). The University and the Foundation continue to be criticised by those who feel that universities should not be associated with such behaviour.[27] Steenbock's inventions related to production of vitamin D, a steroid derivative whose wider availability helped to eradicate childhood rickets,[28] raised particular concerns. They were patented between 1928 and 1936 by WARF in the US and the UK, and were attacked on both sides of the Atlantic.[29] The Medical Research Council (MRC) actively opposed them on public interest grounds.[30] Bud believes that the strength of the MRC's resistance to the patenting of penicillin was a consequence of the vitamin D controversy. But in any case, the *Lancet* article probably put paid to any possibility of patenting, at least in the United Kingdom.

Perhaps the most important advance — in the sense of turning penicillin the natural phenomenon into penicillin the health product available to millions — took place at the US Department of Agriculture's Northern Regional Research Laboratory in Peoria, Illinois, which Florey and Heatley visited for its expertise in deep fermentation methods. Heatley agreed to stay on there, where he worked with a scientist called Andrew Moyer. It was suggested that a locally-abundant waste product called corn steep liquor might be a productive addition to the culture medium and this turned out to be completely correct. In the meantime, Florey was actively promoting industrial interest in penicillin production. In this effort he got support from the right places, and as a result the four most interested companies, Merck, Squibb, Pfizer and Lederle, were given assurances that penicillin's immense importance to the national interest at a time when the US was drifting towards war meant that their sharing of research results would not lead to antitrust investigations.

In 1943, the US was fighting in the Pacific and demand for penicillin became overwhelming. The War Production Board offered financial assistance and more than 20 more companies began to produce it. In the UK a few companies got involved but productivity gains were modest unlike in the United States, where they were spectacular. Pfizer was most successful of all. At the end of 1945, it was producing more than half of all penicillin being made and prices were falling drastically.[31]

(*Continued*)

(*Continued*)

Heatley was very free with his knowledge, not just at the NRRL but also on visits to some of the companies. The same was true for Florey. However, such openness was not always reciprocated. Moyer in particular was less than candid. Not only did he publish under his name a joint article with Heatley, but he was also granted patents in the UK and US on his production methods — though he made no efforts to enforce the three British ones he owned.[32] Florey became frustrated by the practice of companies on both sides of the Atlantic of keeping their research secret and he never did receive the hoped for one kg of penicillin. Nonetheless, the popular complaint that the United States 'stole' penicillin from Britain does not really hold water. The Rockefeller Foundation had funded much of the Oxford team's work. This was at a time when Florey was constantly struggling, usually with limited success, to bring in funds from domestic sources like the Medical Research Council where it was felt perhaps that the recently-discovered sulfonamides signalled the final victory of the 'synthesisers' over the 'isolators', that is, synthetic organic chemicals over biologicals. The latter now appeared to some, mistakenly as it turned out, as rather passé.[33] It is true that UK firms after the war had to pay not inconsiderable fees to US firms in order to use their production know-how, but that's business. Florey went to the US in a wartime situation with the objective of getting penicillin produced in sufficient quantities to test on and treat patients, not to defend the interests of British industry. He proved to be a highly effective catalyst. In any case, the lesson was learned and the UK government (and Oxford University) subsequently took a much more pro-patent line when other antibiotics were discovered later such as cephalosporin as it did over public sector inventing more generally — though not in all cases, such as the aforementioned Birch reduction and monoclonal antibodies (Chapter 8).

Actually, the assumption that British industry sat still while American firms did all the running in the 1940s would not be fair. A recent history of Glaxo reveals that the company made efforts to contact Florey expressing interest in penicillin, but he did not reply to the two letters sent to him. To the author of this history, 'these events contrasted with Florey's later assertion that he had contacted several British pharmaceutical manufacturers without success'.[34] In fact, at least three British companies — ICI, Glaxo and Kemball-Bishop — produced increasing quantities of penicillin from the early 1940s using surface fermentation. But neither the existing

(*Continued*)

technologies, nor minor improvements to them, were sufficient for mass production on anything like the scale achieved soon after in the USA.

Who discovered penicillin? And who deserves the credit? And what does penicillin tell us about drug discovery that the earlier stories may not do? The first question is difficult to answer. Fleming was first to make it known to the scientific community and to give it a name. But he was not the first to be aware of its antibiotic qualities. Fleming, crucial as he was, probably received too much credit compared to Florey, Chain and Heatley who with their other colleagues achieved — under extremely difficult wartime conditions — the highly taxing tasks of isolation, purification, production (albeit not on a large scale) and demonstrating effectiveness on sick patients. Heatley's contribution was especially underrated. At least the other three received a share of the 1945 Nobel Prize for Physiology and Medicine. He received very few accolades in his long life, which ended in 2004, though he had the good grace not to express any bitterness he may have felt.

Perhaps the biggest achievement, though, was that in a few short years, it became possible to treat not just a handful of people but millions. By 1944, 19 American companies were producing penicillin.[35] In time the market became less concentrated as more companies entered it and the price fell. By 1950, 21 million people around the world were being treated every month.[36] For this, we have mostly the countless unheralded (mostly US-based) scientists working in government and corporate laboratories to thank. Of course, these people depended ultimately on the earlier research done in Britain and the free sharing of what scientists in that country had learned.

There were no real geniuses or heroes. It was good science, good management and a great deal of effort and determination by people on both sides of the Atlantic that turned Fleming's initial discovery into the extraordinary life-saving drug penicillin truly was. Penicillin never did become the anticipated victory for the 'synthesisers'. It was synthesized in 1957 but fermentation was and remains more economic. Admittedly, as we will see below, the synthesis of penicillin did give rise to immense possibilities in terms of discovering semi-synthetic derivatives.

Aspirin was a triumph of good marketing, insulin of sheer determination and of the emerging 'industry-university complex'. Both involved

(*Continued*)

(*Continued*)

clever intellectual property strategy, which took advantage of the opportunities the law provided, whether in the pursuit of profit or for utilitarian reasons. Penicillin was itself not patented but there was of course plenty of patenting relating to the methods of producing it, methods which evolved rapidly as part of the war effort. The penicillin story reinforces a persisting view, admittedly somewhat contestable in light of the sulphonamide discovery discussed earlier, that those observations and insights leading to revolutionary new treatments have tended not to come from corporate research and development labs. It underlines also that true scientific achievement viewed at a distance is almost always collective, though at closer distances and at earlier stages of the discovery to development process, individuals can be decisive. As Sir Henry Harris, Florey's successor as Professor of Pathology at Oxford put it, giving Heatley his due but completely overlooking act three, 'without Fleming, no Chain or Florey; without Chain, no Florey; without Florey, no Heatley; without Heatley, no penicillin'.[37]

Penicillin also demonstrates the importance of bringing together and effectively managing researchers from a wide range of disciplines within research teams and of collaborating between such teams. It reminds us too that commercial innovation is so often not about bringing new substances into existence but about finding ways to maximize the production and standardization of those that already exist. Hence the importance of process innovation and the commercial interest in the patenting of industrial processes where product patents are unavailable or the product is not new anyway. This might seem a rather old-fashioned view, but it is becoming pertinent again with biopharmaceuticals like human insulin and erythropoietin where intellectual property and drug regulation 'conspire' to provide long-term monopoly protection of substances that can hardly be said to be new, if they ever were new.

The penicillin story doesn't really end anywhere near here. Confirming the chemical structure of the molecule, including its so-called 'beta lactam ring structure', admittedly a rather purist view of what discovery should mean, was achieved in 1945 by Dorothy Hodgkin by means of the X-ray diffraction technique. Penicillin was chemically synthesized in 1957 by John Sheehan at MIT, whose work was funded by Bristol.[38]

This was a very big deal. Sheehan's synthesis made it possible to efficiently produce a key intermediate for a whole range of semi-synthetic penicillins, called 6-aminopenicillanic acid (6-APA). This offered an attractive alternative route to the discovery of new penicillins to the expensive searching and screening of new micro-organisms. As with the synthetic dyestuffs, a patent covering key antiobiotic intermediates, sometimes the core of the original compound, potentially had enormous commercial value and was very much desired. Sheehan's US patent, filed in October 1959 and granted in April 1962, actually mentions that this compound 'has great commercial value as a starting material in the production of natural and synthetic penicillins'.[39] But competition in the early 1960s was intense. Numerous companies from around the world filed patents related to 6-APA, including American Home Products, Astra, Ballerup, Banyu, Bayer, Beecham, Lepetit, Olin Mathieson, Pfizer and Smith Kline & French. The most serious competitor was Beecham, an old company you read about earlier, that had just moved into pharmaceutical research and was determined to stop missing the penicillin gravy train. This time it caught the train *and* became one of its main drivers.

Two young Beecham scientists, George Rolinson and Ralph Batchelor, then working under Ernst Chain who had moved to the Istituto Superiore di Sanita in Rome, applied some quite ingenious analysis to independently arrive at 6-APA.[40] Beecham filed patents on this discovery as early as August 1958. However, Beecham was still dependent on Sheehan's method of turning 6-APA into other penicillins and to Bristol for know-how in terms of fermentation facilities. Beecham, Sheehan and Bristol agreed temporarily to collaborate. Bristol assisted Beecham in starting up a new antibiotics factory in Worthing, England, Beecham licensed its patents to Bristol and allowed it to sell outside the British Commonwealth for a 5 percent royalty.[41] Nonetheless, patent disputes were not entirely resolved, and the one between Sheehan and Beecham concerning who was first to invent was not finally settled in the United States until 1979.[42] Sheehan won, but by then the commercial stakes were no longer so high. Beecham had become very successful at developing semi-synthetic penicillins, starting in 1959 with phenethicillin (marketed with Bristol under the name Broxil) and following up, most notably, with methicillin (Celbenin), ampicillin (Penbritin) and amoxycillin (Amoxil).

All of these presented technical challenges. In the case of methicil-lin, Beecham succeeded in overcoming the difficulties by licensing discoveries made elsewhere. One can argue that this is the patent system working as it should, that is to say, not so much as an incentive to innovate, which is simply an after-the-event rationalization dreamed up by economists, business gurus and corporate lobbyists, but by creating a market in technology and providing an organized source of commercial intelligence. As Bud explains:

> Methicillin did require a new production technology. The first semisynthetic penicillin, phenethicillin, could be made without accomplishing the difficult step of isolating 6-APA. Making methicillin, however, required the pure core compound by itself. In principle, this isolation had been achieved at Beecham, but in practice their process was laborious. How much easier if an enzyme could just snip off existing side-chains from ordinary penicillin to reveal the core! In October 1958, Beecham managed to find an E. coli bacterium that made an enzyme able to produce 6-APA from the penicillin V that had been developed in Austria. Going one better, however, within a few months, the Bayer Company in Germany found how to do the same from the cheaper relative, the original Penicillin G. This technology was in turn licensed by Beecham, who were able to develop it further. The chemists were therefore given a cheap source of reactive 6-APA on which they could build to assemble new penicillins. The dream of chemical control which had inspired the wartime synthetic enterprise had now been partly realised.[43]

Thanks to its rather quickly acquired record of innovation and ability to work the patent system to its advantage, Beecham did very well out of the antibiotics revolution. Between 1960 and 1970, the company's pharmaceutical sales increased nearly 16-fold. However, as we will see below, the antibiotic producers also found ways to abuse the patent system in ways that were both detrimental to the interests of consumers and also to innovation and fair competition.

Patents and the Antibiotics Revolution

'Fleming's' penicillin was no one-off. Penicillin, the first antibiotic, set in train a commercial and therapeutic revolution. Penicillin was not patented, as aspirin should probably not have been on account of its already being known about. But, as we saw, the industrial processes to mass produce it were as were the derivatives and the methods of producing them. Most subsequent antibiotic drugs have been patented despite their natural origins. Various types of penicillin and semi-synthetic analogues came on the market during the following decades, including those effective against resistant strains of disease-causing microbes like staphylococcus. And while its discovery was accidental, penicillin inspired scientists to search for other microorganisms producing substances that are toxic for other microbes but harmless to humans. The result was the discovery and development of such antibiotics as streptomycin (1943) cephalosporin (1945) and tetracycline (1953), the first two of which are discussed below. Many of the antibiotics came from the soil, but there were a range of interesting sources including a chicken's throat (streptomycin) a sewage outlet (cephalosporin) and monkey dung (fusidic acid).[44] It was largely out of the investment of profits from the antibiotics revolution into research and development that today's research-based pharmaceutical industry emerged, especially in the USA and Britain.

The patent system, however, presented something of a challenge, at least in the United States. The emergent American pharmaceutical industry could see the possibility of making unprecedented profits from antibiotics screened through increasingly routine screening of microbial samples. What they sought was blanket patent coverage. But it was uncertain that the patent system including the courts could deliver what they wanted in this respect. There was in fact very little creativity in what they were doing and the products themselves were basically gifts of nature. But as William Kingston has revealed, successful lobbying by the American pharmaceutical industry, along with efforts of others supportive of a more patent friendly law, achieved the incorporation in the 1952 Patent Act of helpful language in order to ensure that antibiotics discovered through techniques of systematic mass screening and processes to manufacture them could be patented. As Kingston explains, 'on behalf of their pharmaceutical industry clients, New York Patent Bar Association members drafted a Bill and were able to get it introduced in Congress, and this, supplemented by other Bills and pressures, brought about the changes they wanted.'[45] Essentially, the non-obviousness criterion was incorporated into patent law in a particular way that meant 'patentability shall not be negatived by the manner in which the invention was made.' This phrase was intended to keep the invention threshold from drifting too high. According to its underlying purpose it was successful.[46] Subsequently, albeit not necessarily as a consequence, the US pharmaceutical industry, previously somewhat backward compared to its German and Swiss counterparts, became the world's biggest on the strength of antibiotics.

Streptomycin and Vitamin B12 — Two stories in one

In 1944, scientists headed by Selman Waksman at Rutgers University in the United States announced their discovery of a new antibiotic called streptomycin.[47] It came from a micro-organism called *Streptomyces griseus* which had been known about for around 30 years before being screened for antibiotic activity. This became the second antibiotic to come to market and the first to be effective against tuberculosis.

The discovery of streptomycin and its activity against TB was achieved by a team of scientists led by Waksman with collaborators from the Mayo Clinic who suggested to Waksman that he test the substance against the tubercule bacilli, and later on carried out the animal tests and human clinical trials.[48]

In 1948, two US patents relating to streptomycin were granted. The earlier patent that was filed covered methods of extraction and production. Filed in February 1945, it was granted in September 1948. The inventors were Selman Waksman and his student Albert Schatz, who assigned it to the Rutgers Research and Endowment Foundation even though the work was financially supported by Merck.[49] The second patent to be filed, in August 1945, was granted two months earlier than the first one.[50] The inventor was Merck's Robert Peck. This one, obviously a later invention, covered not just various processes but also several crystalline salts of the streptomycin itself. Although streptomycin was a natural product that could hardly have been invented by any of the three scientists, the patent claimed to the satisfaction of the examiner that 'for the first time, streptomycin is available in a form which not only has valuable therapeutic properties but also can be produced, distributed, and administered in a practicable way.'

(*Continued*)

While Waksman received most of the credit including a Nobel Prize, as with penicillin, industry was largely responsible for finding how best to mass-produce it. As for which person was responsible for the discovery, Albert Schatz claimed that he deserved a bigger share of the credit on the basis that he was the one who actually isolated the chemical in 1943, in fact just four months after Waksman had taken him on.[51] This issue has become quite controversial, with both individuals having their advocates.[52]

Leaving matters of credit and personal financial gain aside, Waksman arranged with Merck that royalties from any patents would go to the university. There was of course no certainty that any discoveries would turn out to be patentable anyway, but of course they were, and these were enormously lucrative. Nonetheless, Waksman managed to persuade Merck, concerned perhaps not to be seen to be exploiting what had recently become a state university, to transfer patent ownership to the Rutgers Research and Endowment Foundation so that production could be licensed to as many manufacturers as possible. Not surprisingly, while the university earned millions of dollars, the price of streptomycin fell during the following decade as competition increased and production methods improved.[53] From 1946 to 1950 alone, it dropped seventy-fold.[54]

Subsequently, the regulatory environment, and corporate business models along with them, changed in ways that made the drug firms more determined to keep price levels high by preventing competitors from entering the market for their drugs. Most of the reforms were introduced after the war and had to do with safety and efficacy testing, but an important early change in the United States came in with the 1938 *Food, Drug and Cosmetic Act*, which divided drugs into over-the-counter drugs and prescription (or 'ethical') drugs. The latter could only be sold with a doctor's prescription. While prescription drug sales promotion was aimed at the doctors, the actual buyers were wholesalers, pharmacies and hospitals. Doctors generally had no particular reason to treat price as a factor in determining which drugs to prescribe. Therefore, the demand for drugs was more price-inelastic than it would have been if the buyers and the prescribers were the same people, or indeed if there were a single buyer for the whole country able to negotiate price from a stronger bargaining position.[55] The streptomycin patent was in itself an important new regulatory development since it clarified to the industry that the new antibiotics were patentable despite being 'products of nature'.[56]

(*Continued*)

(Continued)

In this context, a rather significant event was the extraction of a pure substance that was not an antibiotic but a vitamin. Even so, given its identical microbial source, it merits coverage in this chapter. In December 1947, scientists at Merck headed by Karl Folkers isolated a pure cobalt-containing substance from liver.[57] This substance, which was useful in treating pernicious anaemia, was christened cyanocobolamin but became much better known as vitamin B_{12}. Important as it is physiologically, plants and animals cannot produce vitamin B_{12} themselves; only micro-organisms have this particular ability. Four years later, scientists from Oxford and Cambridge Universities and from Glaxo elucidated its rather complicated chemical structure.[58] In early 1973, Robert Woodward and Albert Eschenmoser completed, with the help of a huge team of assistants, the total synthesis of vitamin B_{12}, widely recognised as an extraordinary achievement.

While eating liver or liver extract had been the only way for people suffering from deficiency-related illnesses such as pernicious anaemia to acquire the substance, this was not ideal from the commercial point of view or for patients. While the pure form discovered by Merck was a major discovery, the ideal approach was to go to a microbial source. After all, some microbes can actually make it, besides which thanks to the antibiotics revolution fermentation technology had reached a level to enable the mass production of many microbial products. Months later, Merck scientists discovered one such source, 'a mould found in the fermenters that produced streptomycin'. This was of course *Streptomyces griseus*.[59] This additional substance from the same source was subsequently protected in the United States by two US patents that turned out to be the subject of litigation.[60] Although the product claims of the second one were invalidated by a district court in 1957, they were reinstated on appeal. Both patents were the subject of another court case in 1967. The court upheld the first patent entirely, stating:

The patentees of the '794 patent have given to the world, for the first time, a medicine that can be used successfully in treating all patients suffering with pernicious anemia, a medicine that is subject to accurate standardization, and avoids the unfavorable reactions of the earlier liver extracts. It did not exist in nature in the form in which the patentees produced it, and nothing in the prior art either suggested or anticipated it.[61]

Although five of the 12 claims in the second patent were invalidated, the principle that a 'composition of matter' consisting of a purified form of a natural product could be patented subject to passing the tests of non-obviousness and utility was not called into question.

In the United Kingdom, when it came to publicly funded research outputs popular resentment about 'the loss of penicillin to the Americans' translated into a more pro-patent stance. Having failed to gain financially from penicillin, Oxford University was in no mood to miss out next time either. Research on cephalosporin gave Oxford the opportunity to generate considerable wealth from patent-protected drug discovery and the government to establish a new institution to commercialize inventions arising from publicly funded research for the benefit of the nation.

Cephalosporin: Discovered in Sardinia, invented at Oxford University

Ironically, just as penicillin was discovered in Britain but with the profits made in America, cephalosporin was discovered in Italy but developed in Britain which was where most of the money was made. This was thanks not only to the ingenuity of the remaining Oxford penicillin team members, but also to use of the patent system and the 1948 establishment of the National Research Development Corporation (NRDC), a kind of national WARF, which managed the cephalosporin patent portfolio on behalf of Oxford and the nation.

In 1945, Giuseppe Brotzu, working in Sardinia, discovered a mould with antibiotic properties called *Cephalosporium acremonium* and carried out some promising *in vitro* and clinical tests. This discovery was no fluke but was based on some keen observation. As recounted by a former colleague of his:

In the dark, sombre years of the second world war, Brotzu, with the help only of A. Spanedda, in a Cagliari half deserted and devastated by the bombing, devoted his efforts to establishing, why, despite the habit many young people had of going swimming, at Su Siccu, where the local sewage system drained into the sea, there were no outbreaks or cases of typhoid fever related to bathing.[62]

Like Fleming before him, he was unable to go further, but was nonetheless eager to attract attention to his promising discovery. He published his findings in an in-house journal that he apparently set up for the purpose,[63] and sent a sample to Oxford.[64]

Research at Oxford in collaboration with the Medical Research Council's Antibiotic Research Station at Clevedon turned out to be extremely fruitful even though success was not achieved without time and effort. It became apparent that Brotzu's mould yielded several antibiotics related to penicillin, sharing the latter's beta lactam ring structure, with variable activity against different infective agents, and different abilities to

(*Continued*)

(Continued)

> withstand growing resistance of these agents to penicillin. The most promising of these was isolated in 1955 by Edward Abraham and Guy Newton and was named cephalosporin C.[65] Mass production through fermentation was much more difficult than with penicillin and greater biochemical expertise proved to be vital. In time the technical obstacles were overcome and patents covering the production of cephalosporin C were filed. Licensing revenues were substantial because cephalosporin C turned out to be a key precursor for the manufacture of a range of semi-synthetic cephalosporins. The patent position became especially strong once the compound's core could be described chemically. This was announced in 1961,[66] with proof provided soon after through Dorothy Hodgkin's X-ray analysis.[67] The core was 7-aminocephalosporanic acid (7-APA for short), which was claimed in a number of patents filed in the UK, USA and various European countries. These were to the tremendous financial benefit of Oxford University.[68]

Controlling the Antibiotics Market

By the late 1940s, American companies were starting to become a victim of their immense scientific and commercial successes. As they began to discover and market increasing numbers of effective but interchangeable antibiotics, the threat of price-reducing competition became a reality in the case of both penicillin and streptomycin. In the USA, the price per dose of penicillin fell from \$20 during the Second World War (when the government purchased all penicillin produced) to \$1 in 1946, and to 10 cents in 1949. Between 1948 and 1955, the price of streptomycin plunged from \$20 per gram to only 15 cents.[69]

The companies did not accept this situation passively. They responded by striving not only to improve their competitiveness as individual firms, but also by cooperating with others to reduce competition and its harmful effects on profitability.[70] Accordingly, first, they adopted strategic intellectual property policies. For example, they protected their drugs by a combination of patents and trademarks, and asserted their rights aggressively in the courts. Ironically, as we saw earlier, the German companies who pioneered this tactic earlier in the century had been condemned for doing so by the American firms of the time. Second, those companies that developed new drugs but did not market their own products (such as Merck and Pfizer) set up large sales teams or acquired or merged with companies that already had them. Third, they sought to keep competitors out and prices high for as long as their patents remained in force.

Three options were available to them that could under certain circumstances be adopted simultaneously. One way was to restrict patent licensing.[71] Among the first companies to adopt this tactic in a collective way were the five that cornered the market in broad spectrum antibiotics. Companies that continued to license their patents to all-comers found out in time that this was not a profitable way to do business. This was the experience of Ciba, with its plant-derived drug reserpine (Serpasil),[72] and with isoniazid, a tuberculosis treatment that had been developed independently by Hoffman LaRoche and Squibb.[73] The second option was to license patents using highly restrictive provisions that, for example, prevented licensees from supplying foreign markets, and required them to purchase the intermediate chemicals from the licensors, or that retained the rights of licensors to follow-on innovations by licensees. The third option was to cooperate in certain ways with competitors selling similar products, for example by sharing patents and fixing prices.

One of the most controversial instances of the use of patents to support anti-competitive behaviour by the industry took place during the 1950s when five companies formed an international antibiotics cartel. The story begins with the introduction of the broad spectrum antibiotics, whose chemical structures were unknown when they first came to market, but turned out often to be extremely similar to each other. The earliest of these products were Lederle's Aureomycin (introduced in 1948) Parke Davis' Chloromycetin[74] (1949) and Pfizer's Terramycin (1950). The similarity of these products stimulated intense competition which was reflected not just in increased marketing and advertising expenditures but also in a determination to elucidate the chemical structures of these drugs and to develop portfolios of related compounds. Pfizer's research proved the close affinity of Aureomycin and Terramycin and resulted in a very similar but more effective new substance, which was the first ever semi-synthetic antibiotic. This was patented and given the name tetracycline. Lederle also discovered tetracycline by the same method and filed patent applications. Subsequently, Bristol and Heyden Chemical Corporation came up with tetracycline by another method and also applied for patents. Pfizer's and Bristol's patents were granted in 1955 after being initially rejected.[75] The other companies' patent applications failed. However, it was extremely doubtful that either Pfizer's or Bristol's patents should really have been awarded. Indeed, the companies themselves were apparently fully aware that they were vulnerable to legal challenge.[76] But by agreeing to respect Pfizer's patent and to limit competition, a group of five companies — Pfizer, Cyanamid (Lederle's parent company) Bristol, Squibb and Upjohn — cornered the tetracycline market and managed to ensure that the price of their closely related products remained high and almost equal for about a decade.

According to regulatory scholar John Braithwaite, the situation suggested that the patent was providing 'a cover for conspiratorial behaviour to partition a market which in the absence of the patent would have been clearly illegal'.[77] The prices did begin to decline from the early 1960s, though. This was during the US Senate's investigation of anti-competitive behaviour by the pharmaceutical industry, and afterwards when McKesson & Robbins, an old drugs wholesaler and distributor business, entered the market and stayed there by convincing Pfizer that it was willing to face a patent infringement suit with confidence that the court would find in its favour. Although the government failed — despite its determined efforts — to prove that the companies had violated antitrust law or had defrauded the Patent Office, they had to pay hundreds of millions of dollars in legal settlements. Nonetheless, the profits the five companies made not just in the USA but worldwide through their control of tetracycline were enormous, helping turn them into major pharmaceutical corporations.[78] One can only speculate about how many people's lives might have been saved if prices had been allowed to fall earlier.

Backlashes

Unsurprisingly, such behaviour provoked a backlash on both sides of the Atlantic. In the United States, politicians responded by subjecting the industry to very close scrutiny. From 1959 to 1962, the Senate Subcommittee on Antitrust and Monopoly, under the chairmanship of Senator Estes Kefauver, carried out an inquiry into the pharmaceutical industry. After three years of hearings, the Subcommittee concluded that the drug companies were charging too much for their drugs and making excessive profits. Through patenting and branding, Kefauver and the subcommittee believed, they were free to charge as much as they liked, and were using this freedom to excess. Yet many of these companies were spending more money on sales promotion than on research. Moreover, many seemed more interested in developing modified versions of existing drugs (nowadays referred to as 'me-toos') than in trying to achieve genuine therapeutic advances. The subcommittee believed that the patent system encouraged such 'inventing-around' owing to the fact that chemical substances were protectable, and not just processes.[79]

Some of the subcommittee's findings were subsequently discredited, such as the claim that countries without patents produced a higher quantity of therapeutically advanced drugs than those with patents. In fact, the breakdown of important drugs (as listed by the subcommittee) that were discovered by countries allowing product patents, only process patents, and no patents at all for drugs, was 94:82:0 respectively.[80] Nonetheless, the subcommittee made a strong case that many companies had indeed been indulging in profiteering and anti-competitive behaviour with the help of the patent system, and that the public was ill-served by such practices. Even so, attempts to introduce legislation to drastically weaken patent rights failed, and the industry managed to get away with its profits intact, albeit with a tarnished reputation.

Around the same time, the climate in Britain also became a little more hostile towards 'Big Pharma', especially foreign pharma. In 1961, the government decided to confront the broad spectrum antibiotics cartel by authorizing the National Health Service (NHS) Hospital Services to purchase imported (mostly Italian) generic versions of several of these drugs whose patents were still in force. This action saved the NHS £4 million. Generic producers were encouraged by this and began to apply for compulsory licenses. Consequently, 50 so-called Section 41 applications, named after the relevant part of the statute, were submitted to the comptroller during the 1960s. Before 1960, no applications at all had been submitted. However, of the 50 applications only four were allowed, most of the rest being withdrawn. This situation was due to the difficult legal procedures that applicants needed to comply with. Even so, the very possibility of compulsory licences probably encouraged the patent-holding firms to be more cooperative about prices than they would otherwise have been.

Pfizer was not at all happy with this situation and decided to make a stand by taking the Ministry (now Department) of Health to court for infringing its patent on tetracycline. In 1965, the House of Lords decided that the Ministry was acting within the provisions of the 1949 Act that permitted use — but not sale — of inventions by 'services of the Crown' subject to payment of royalties to the patentee. Although the decision did not allow the General Medical and Pharmaceutical Services, through which 80 per cent of NHS-provided drugs were consumed, to do the same thing, 'the pharmaceutical companies were aghast at what they felt to be abrogation by the State of the fundamental principle of patent rights. Prophecies were made that the British industry would wind up its drug research and become totally dependent on foreign developments'.[81]

As it turned out, such prophesies were unjustified. This was so despite the fact that worse was to follow for the industry. In 1967, the Sainsbury Committee, set up to investigate the relationship between the pharmaceutical industry and the NHS, published a report which recommended that the General Medical and Pharmaceutical Services also be treated as a service of the Crown with authority to acquire generic versions of patent-protected drugs.[82] The government was initially reluctant to implement this, owing no doubt to pressure from the industry. But the provision was incorporated through an opposition amendment into the 1968 Health Services and Public Health Act.[83]

On the other hand, Section 41 compulsory licences were abolished as recommended by another committee established by the Board of Trade to examine the patent system and the patent law ('the Banks Committee') whose report was presented to Parliament in 1970.[84] The government of the time was reluctant to act upon the recommendation, but in 1977 another government did so through legislation incorporating the European Patent Convention into UK law. Its decision to do so was part of a negotiation with the industry in which the latter agreed to cooperate on the introduction of advertising regulations.[85]

Antibiotics and Hormones — Similarities and Differences

Must of what was concluded about the patenting of hormones and the triangular relationship between patents, business and science in that particular context could be said about antibiotics. The antibiotics era was likewise characterised by close but occasionally antagonistic relationships between universities, hospitals and companies, increasingly sophisticated patenting strategy, and resort by industry to behaviour verging on the anticompetitive in cases where they were encountering freedom-to-operate problems or if there was a danger of severe price reductions caused by the existence of competitors seeking to place similar products on the market.

Concerning the academic-clinical-corporate nexus, both hormones and antibiotics evidenced a kind of division of labour in which industry built on discoveries, sometimes patented and sometimes not, made by universities and clinical research laboratories, and turned them into a range of mass-produced commercial product families with a fair amount of variability within these families. Such variability could be commercially important but therapeutically negligible. But in other cases, improved variants were genuine and worthwhile for patients and not just of benefit to market-savvy companies. To be fair, industrial research and development often entailed considerable effort and ingenuity. Rarely was anything handed to them on a plate. Consequently, one can argue that the pursuit of profit based on patent-protected innovation did help to advance scientific progress, especially on the practical therapeutic side, though the abuse of patents would likely have had the opposite effect.

One difference between hormones and antibiotics is that the latter drugs had the potential to save millions of lives and, despite the problems of resistance, undoubtedly did succeed in doing so. The public health impacts of hormones, with the exception of insulin, were on a relatively smaller scale during the periods covered. Consequently, involvement by the State in ensuring that drugs were available to the public was likely to be more present in the case of antibiotics than with hormones. This does appear to be the case, with instances of at least one government challenge to a cartel, and the invocation of public interest limitations to patent rights. Furthermore, the profits from antibiotics were especially large as compared to hormones, and this increased industry's industry in influencing patent law, as it did do in one particular case. Apparently, the hormone makers were less inclined to invest in efforts to challenge the status quo. Either the stakes were not so high, or the law already gave them pretty much what they wanted.

Thus far, we can see that during the sulphonamide revolution the future looked synthetic. And yet, from the 1940s to the 1960s, many of the most important new drugs were based not on synthetic chemistry as one might have expected, but on the discovery of substances found in nature, such as microorganisms and hormones. This situation favoured companies whose expertise lay in natural product research and fermentation science, especially when they became more adept at synthetic chemistry as well. Since many of these companies were American or British, these two countries became relatively more innovative than the German, Swiss and French firms whose scientific and technological traditions were more on the side of synthetic chemistry. By the mid-1960s, it was becoming apparent that the balance of industrial power was shifting somewhat from the chemical-pharmaceutical giants like Bayer, Hoechst, Du Pont and ICI to those firms whose backgrounds were related more closely to the biological sciences.[86]

But above all, this seemed very much like progress, and it must have seemed to many people that the good times would just keep on rolling. From the 1950s, cell biology, human physiology and our understanding of disease causation advanced considerably. Drug discovery and development continued to be empirical endeavours involving failure most of the time. But such undertakings were undoubtedly more scientific than ever before. The early 1950s discovery of the double helical structure of DNA led to much excitement. These advances, achieved by public sector scientists, many working in universities, and funded by taxpayers and non-profit foundations, appeared to fully justify optimism that the boom would just go on and on. With enough money spent US President Nixon's 1971 declaration of war on cancer which precipitated massive funding commitments to cancer research would lead to victory. Like other metaphorical 'wars on' (e.g. drugs, perhaps a bit less metaphorically, that Nixon also launched in the same year), it was tremendously expensive and more of a defeat than a victory even if some of the basic research it supported was valuable in the long term.[87] Scientists became ever more optimistic, despite the fact that modes of action of many drugs were not fully understood (and are still not today), that drugs could be designed rationally from the bottom up as it were. The next chapter brings us up to the present as regards new and emerging technologies and how they relate to business, law and regulation.

Notes

1 Lesch (2007) *op. cit.*, 5.
2 Ibid., 59.
3 Ibid., 60–1.
4 In doing so, he did of course make it known to the world. In 1939, Domagk was awarded a Nobel Prize, which he collected after the War. Mietzsch, Klarer and Hörlein received no share. To Lesch, this exemplified the way that 'in its allotment of credits to individuals, the Nobel Prize tends to efface the roles of colleagues and supporting institutions. This distortion is especially egregious in a case such as Domagk's'. Similar criticisms have been made of patents. *See* Lesch (2007) *op. cit.*, 289.
5 Lesch (2007) *op. cit*, 64.
6 Quoted in Lesch (2007) *op. cit.*, 156. France was not the only country he was referring to.
7 Sneader (1985) *op. cit.*, 287.
8 Sneader (1985) *op. cit.*, 288.
9 Weatherall *op. cit.*, 152.
10 Achilladelis *op. cit.*, 285.
11 Journal of the American Medical Association (editorial) (1937), 1544.
12 Quoted in JAMA *op. cit.*
13 Mann (1999), 35.
14 Weatherall *op. cit.*, 152–4.
15 Sneader (2005) *op. cit.*, 356.
16 Lesch (2007) *op. cit.*, 291.
17 For authoritative accounts of the penicillin story see Brown (2004); Bud (2007); Hare (1970); Lax (2004); Macfarlane (1979, 1984).
18 Fleming (1929), 227.
19 Bud (2007) *op. cit.*, 26.
20 Bud (2007) *op. cit.*, 27.
21 Chain *et al* (1940).
22 Lax *op. cit.*, 110.
23 Lax *op. cit.*, 195.
24 Abraham *et al* (1941).
25 For an illuminating contemporary discussion on the issue, see Fishbein (1937).
26 Quoted in Fishbein *op. cit.*, 1539.
27 Weiner (1989). The most recent controversy about WARF's patenting activities concerns its patents relating to stem cells.

28 Vitamin D was originally referred to as the 'antirachitic vitamine'. Steenbock's process offered a more palatable alternative to cod liver oil, then known to be an abundant source of the vitamin.

29 Apple (1989); Mowery and Sampat (2001), 788.

30 Bud (2008) *op. cit.*, 178.

31 Lax (2004) *op. cit.*, 284.

32 Robert Bud, pers. comm., 29 May 2008. Moyer's US patents were assigned to the US government's Secretary of Agriculture.

33 Medawar (1996), 166.

34 Jones (2001), 64.

35 Temin (1979), 435.

36 Bud (1993) *op. cit.*, 104.

37 Quoted in Lax *op. cit.*, 112.

38 Sheehan (1957).

39 US Patent no. 3,028,379 ('Process for the production of 6-amino-penicillanic acid'), issued on 3 April 1962.

40 Ballio *et al* (1959).

41 Lazell (1975), 150.

42 Sneader (2005) *op. cit.* For a personal account of his almost interminable patent dispute with Beecham, see Sheehan (1982).

43 Bud (2005) *op. cit.*, 128–9.

44 Le Fanu *op. cit.*, 13. Another promising place to look is the oral cavities of animals which can be very rich sources of promising microbiota. Terekhov *et al* (2018).

45 Kingston (2004a), 310.

46 Rich (1964), 860. It should be mentioned that this was not the view of the Supreme Court, which in 1966 considered that the 1952 Act did not change 'the general level of innovation necessary to sustain patentability'. At the same time, though, the Court admitted that the intention of 'the last sentence of §103' was 'to abolish the test … announced in the controversial phrase "flash of creative genius"'. *Graham v. John Deere*, 148 USPQ (BNA) 459 (1966).

47 Schatz, Bugie and Waksman (1944).

48 Amyes (2001), 45–9.

49 US Patent no. 2,449,866 ('Streptomycin and process of preparation'), issued on 21 September 1948.

50 US Patent no. 2,446,102 ('Complex salts of streptomycin and process for preparing the same'), issued on 27 July 1948.

51 Ibid., 44–5.

52 Wainwright's (1990) account as does Pringle's (2012) thoroughly researched one both favour Schatz and criticise Waksman, while Kingston (2004b) has defended Waksman.

53 Sneader (1985) *op. cit.*, 325; Temin *op. cit.*, 436.

54 Weatherall *op. cit.*, 181.

55 Steele (1962), 139–43; Temin *op. cit.*, 434–5.

56 Steele *op. cit.*, 136; Temin *op. cit.*, 436.

57 In doing so, Merck beat Glaxo by five months. However, Glaxo soon went over to Merck's method of production. *See* Jones *op. cit.*, 121; Rickes *et al* (1948a); Smith (1948).

58 Bonnett *et al* (1955); Hodgkin *et al* (1955).

59 Jones *op. cit.*, 121; Rickes *et al* (1948b).

60 US Patent no. 2,563,794 ('Vitamin B-12'), issued on 7 August 1951; and US Patent no. 2,703,302 ('Vitamin B-12 active composition and process of preparing same'), issued on 1 March 1955.

61 Merck and Co., Inc. v. Chase Chemical Company *et al* (1967) *United States Patent Quarterly* 155:152.

62 Scarpa (1998). Downloadable from http://pacs.unica.it/brotzu/.

63 Brotzu (1948). Downloadable from http://pacs.unica.it/brotzu/brotzu.pdf. English translation: http://pacs.unica.it/brotzu/brotzuen.pdf.

64 In 1971, Oxford University did the decent thing and conferred on Brotzu an honorary doctorate in science. The following year he was awarded a diploma by NRDC.

65 Newton and Abraham (1955), 548.

66 Loder, Newton and Abraham (1961). Also, Hale, Newton and Abraham (1961).

67 Hodgkin and Maslen (1961).

68 *See* Sneader (2005) *op. cit.*, 296–7. Patents include UK Patent no. 953695 ('Derivatives of cephalosporin C'); and US Patent no. 3,207,755 ('Transformation products of cephalosporin C and derivatives thereof'), issued on 21 September 1965.

69 Achilladelis *op. cit.*, 287.

70 Achilladelis *op. cit.*, 288.

71 Licensing nonetheless had its uses as it does today. For example, it may have been useful to patent-holding companies unable to meet a large international demand for a product. In addition, licensee companies may be better equipped than the patent holders to market the product. And small

companies discovering a new chemical entity but lacking the funds to cover the research, development and marketing may have had no alternative. Such is the case for many present-day start-up pharmaceutical and biotechnology firms.

72 It is possible that Ciba's decision to license reserpine came about because it was uncertain about the validity of its patent, since the compound was the isolated active principle of an Indian medicinal plant used for centuries in traditional medicine. *See* Steele *op. cit.*, 159.

73 Frost (1963), 97.

74 Chloromycetin, or chloramphenicol (by its generic name) turned out to have harmful side-effects. The resultant decline in sales was a factor in Parke Davis' decline and 1959 merger with Warner Lambert. However, sales of the drug enjoyed a revival in the 1960s because the company's sales representatives were able to reassure physicians that, with care, the drug could be used safely. *See* Achilladelis *op. cit.*, 288; Kefauver (1966), 88.

75 Sneader (1985) *op. cit.*, 327.

76 Braithwaite (1984), 184–5.

77 Braithwaite *op. cit.*, 184.

78 Braithwaite *op. cit.*, 176; Temin *op. cit.*, 441.

79 Kefauver *op. cit.*, 29–99.

80 Cooper (1966), 160.

81 Taylor and Silberston (1973), 237.

82 United Kingdom Ministry of Health (1967).

83 Hancher (1990), 321.

84 United Kingdom Board of Trade (1970).

85 Hancher *op. cit.*, 323.

86 Thomas (1994), 478.

87 Kevles (1993).

Chapter 8

Biotechnology, Personalisation, Precision, and the Digital Turn

The previous chapter closed with a few words on scientific progress and business change from the 1950s. Molecular biology advanced a long way from when little was known about genetics to after the structure of DNA was discovered and the chemical's role in inheritance, cell function and dysfunction became ever better understood. But medical applications were not immediately apparent.

This one takes us up to the present day looking into three new areas of medical scientific and technological development. The first is based on molecular biology, and includes recombinant DNA and monoclonal antibodies, and gene and cell therapies. In respect of genetics, it was learned that some 4,000 diseases are associated with single-gene defects and it became easier to identify the specific gene at fault. Additionally, numerous health disorders have polygenic (involving more than one gene) and multifactorial causes in which genes, lifestyle and environment are implicated in varying proportions. These include diabetes, heart disease, cancers and hypertension. But identifying relationships between these more comple diseases and 'bad' inherited DNA sequence regions on the vast human genome comprising six million bases was, and remains, an immense task besides which identifying correlations and causations does not lead inexorably and speedily to medical products.

Alongside a better understanding of human genetics and the health-related implications which we are still learning about, a range of molecular biological techniques were devised that had major biomedical applications. Some of these lead to commercially successful treatments. Two that have been especially transformative for the industry and for the legal-regulatory complex are recombinant DNA and the production of monoclonal antibodies using hybridomas. Both of these were discovered in the 1970s and together precipitated the development of a type of medicine very different from the traditional small molecule drugs that hitherto dominated the pharmaceuticals market from its nineteenth century beginnings. Biologics are very large molecule products that are hard if not impossible to synthesise and are produced in living organisms, initially genetically engineered bacteria using rDNA, but nowadays typically in eukaryotic cells of mammalian origin that are able to handle the production of very large and highly complex molecules. Despite their recency, biologic drugs have quite quickly emerged as some of the biggest selling medicines in the history of the industry. Their introduction has had tremendous impacts on the industry — including how it is structured, and the division of labour from discovery to marketing. It has also affected, and been affected by, regulation and intellectual property, and of course politics.

The second new area comprises technologies enabling and enhancing the collection, storage, exchange, analysis and utilisation of data in digital forms. These latter technologies, which are converging with biological ones, are increasingly being seen as health relevant. They are contributing to our ability to tailor healthcare and medical products to individual patients on the basis of specific molecular and other information. Accordingly, we focus on both biological technologies ('biotechnology' for short) and digitalisation and digital technologies, including digital medicine. Admittedly, this is a somewhat artificial distinction given the undeniable trend of what we might call 'biodigital convergence'. Before going further, we need a few words on what I mean by this and why it seems to be incredibly important.

Digital technologies are used in the production, analysis and use of molecular biological data such as genomic sequences, and are seen by many as permitting a full comprehension of how cellular and subcellular processes work, and of how they can be manipulated. Accordingly, living things themselves are being treated as human-made technologies,[1] ones that are substantially digital in nature and susceptible to human control, design and enhancement. Subcellular structural and functional elements are increasingly described in terms of information and computer science analogies, metaphors and definitions.[2] The complexity of biology is thus facing rapidly expanding micro-processing power and information management solutions accompanied by compatible modes of scientific and business communication. To many commentators, this confluence promises to radically change our world.

So what *is* 'biodigital convergence'? I take it to refer to the treatment of molecular biology (including genomics and the other 'omics' disciplines such as proteomics and transcriptomics, bioinformatics, systems biology and synthetic biology), whether for the purpose of science communication, legal practice or of policymaking, as branches of information technology. Much of the rhetoric of science communication in this field is affected by data science and technology and 'information talk'. These phenomena are drastically changing scientific and commercial practices and discourse in the life sciences. For many adherents, it follows that regulatory and policy 'solutions' devised for existing and earlier digital/information technologies can be applied to all emerging ones along the spectrum of sciences and technologies sharing an essentially informational nature. This goes for intellectual property law, and technology and product regulation. One practice that is tied to biodigital convergence is genetic data mining, which 'entails the analysis of large amounts of genetic data to identify proclivities to disease and potential diagnostics and therapeutics.'[3] There are increasing numbers of patents relating to data mining methods using artificial intelligence, robotics and data science: a sign of things to come.[4] Concerns have been raised about the possible impacts such patents have on openness (in the sense of free availability) and specifically on the free flow of data that competing researchers should ideally have access to.[5] Patents, paradoxically, are supposed to enable inventors to be anti-competitive in the short term by enabling them to own a legally enforceable right to exclude others in exchange for openly disclosing the invention. This is supposed to be a good thing because the 'carrot' of a patent award is supposed to stimulate competitive behaviour and to create a market in inventions as disclosed in and claimed by patents. As property, patents can be bought, sold and licensed. But in recent years, the United States has become concerned about stopping 'pre-emption', that is, ensuring patent law doesn't inhibit future discovery by tying up laws of nature, natural phenomena, abstract ideas or mental steps which form the 'basic tools', or 'building blocks', of human ingenuity, science and technology. Legally, then, the situation is a little uncertain in the United States as to what can be protected and how enforceable already-granted patents are.

Personalisation is also enhanced by a third development which overlaps very much with the above two: the discovery and optimisation of highly sophisticated precision medicines for dangerous diseases like the various cancers. Some of these are designed to act like guided missiles or smart bombs that hit only the enemy cells, leaving surrounding ones unaffected. Others are aimed at disrupting harmful cellular processes that if unchecked will destroy 'good' cells such as with Parkinson's disease, or turn good cells into bad ones such as with cancer. Of the first kind, such life-saving precision medicines include large molecule drugs like antibody-drug conjugate drugs (ADCs). ADCs are a prime example of multispecific drug design so-called because different parts of the active chemical enable it to bind to more than just a single drug target. These have become more common and are considered by some in industry to represent an 'incipient fourth wave',[6] coming after traditional drug discovery as represented by the hormones and antibiotics, rational drug design, and recombinant DNA products. Of the other kind, a cancer small molecule medicine called Glivec stands out. Glivec was in many ways a scientific breakthrough that — and this is also very important — made evident to industry that a targeted threatment for a relatively small number of patients could nonetheless be highly profitable (see below). One reason for current excitement in industry is their potential to overcome the undruggability problem, which is that 98 percent of human proteins have not thus far proved susceptible to binding to a lab-produced chemical.[7]

We will also look at a few other emerging biotechnological developments including regenerative medicine using pluripotent stem cells, and some highly promising cell therapies becoming available including for cancer. These include most recently chimeric antigen receptor T cell (CAR-T) immunotherapy and stem cells. New and emerging technologies such as gene editing (CRISPR), nanotechnology, synthetic biology, artificial intelligence and robotics have so far largely untapped medical potential but could become transformative. CRISPR is especially promising given the possibility to 'fix' those many single-gene defect diseases.

But first, let us put the science and technology to one side for a moment and take stock of the industry. According to *GlobalData*,[8] the world's top-twenty pharmaceutical corporations comprise the following (Table 8.1). At first glance, the structure of the pharmaceutical industry, especially at the top, has changed surprisingly little given all the changes of recent decades. There is still a group of global corporations holding dominant positions that were established a long time ago, or whose roots go back over a century, in the case of Bayer to the industry's very beginnings.

This is not surprising. Monetary, technical and regulatory barriers to entry have become unprecedentally high. Nonetheless, these barriers are not insurmountable. A small number of firms founded as late as the 1980s have found their way through, growing into large corporations, remaining independent by avoiding takeover, and now becoming important global players. The biggest of these are Amgen, Celgene and Gilead. AbbVie goes back only to 2013 but it was spun off Abbott which has of course been around for a very long time. CSL will be unfamiliar to many. It started life as an Australian government vaccine and insulin manufacturer founded in 1916 that was privatised in 1994. It has since become a highly successful biotechnology company, making such products as vaccines, antivenoms (clearly important in a country like Australia blessed with a wealth of highly toxic snakes, spiders and sea creatures), and pharmaceuticals.

Table 8.1.   The world's top-twenty by market capitalisation in the first quarter of 2019

1. Johnson & Johnson
2. Roche
3. Pfizer
4. Novartis
5. Merck
6. Eli Lilly
7. Novo Nordisk
8. AbbVie

(Continued)

Table 8.1.   (*Continued*)

9. Amgen

10. Sanofi

11. GlaxoSmithKline

12. AstraZeneca

13. Gilead Sciences

14. Bristol-Myers Squibb

15. CSL

16. Takeda Pharmaceuticals

17. Bayer

18. Celgene*

19. Merck KGaA

20. Allergan**

*As of January 2019, part of Bristol-Myers-Squibb
**As of June 2019, part of AbbVie

The biggest pharmaceutical companies in 2020 have never been bigger than they are now. One might suppose this to be a natural consequence of decades of growth on the basis of increasing success in converting research dollars into an ever larger and better portfolio of medicines whose sophistication surely improves unidirectionally over time. But this is worse than simplistic: it is fundamentally wrong.

The 1930s to the end of the 1950s are widely considered to be the Golden Age of pharmaceutical discovery, the time of plenty one might even say. The 1960s and 70s bring less precious metals to mind. Those decades experienced a sharp fall in the number of new drugs placed on the market, and lead to change in the structure of the industry and how it did its business. In the United States, the number of new single chemical entities fell from 63 in 1959 to 11 in 1968. In the same period the number of firms introducing these products fell from 43 down to 9.

Between these two same years, average R&D expenditures per new chemical entity, which had been quite flat during the 1950s, shows a substantial increase especially from 1962.[9] According to another study, between 1969 and 1989 the number of new chemical entities launched per year on the world market fell from over 90 to under 40.[10] And increasingly the 'new' chemical entities were so-called me-too drugs, which are patentable modifications of existing treatments that may or may not be significant improvements. This was recognized early on by the pharmaceutical industry. In a study published in 1973, the authors were told by several industry representatives 'that the end of the first chemotherapeutic revolution is almost in sight'.[11] The situation had reached the stage where 65 per cent of 'new' drugs approved by the Food and Drug Administration for sale in the USA from 1989 to 2000 contained active ingredients found in existing products. Of these newly approved drugs, 54 percent 'differed from the marketed product in dosage form, route of administration, or were combined with another active ingredient', while 11 percent 'were identical to products already available on the US market'.[12]

Two explanations seem especially plausible for this productivity plunge. The first was the massively increased development costs of medicines. In the United Kingdom, for example, 'by 1978 the "development time" for each new drug had increased to around 10 years, while the "development costs" had escalated from £5 million in the 1960s to £25 million in the mid-1970s to a staggering £150 million by the 1990s'.[13] Nowadays these are far higher, though how much is a contentious issue depending as it does on the methodology adopted, and — arguably — who is paying for the research.

All new regulations and reforms of existing ones are likely to affect how businesses make money from health, probably none more so than those requiring the submission of increasing volumes of clinical trial data. There does indeed seem to be an unmistakeable correlation between these expensive to comply with regulations being introduced and the number of new drugs introduced per year falling in the years after. Is there a causal relationship between these heightened costs and the new safety and efficacy regulations? There is little doubt that there is. But does this fully explain the fall in new products? This sounds intuitively plausible especially given that such regulations increased the risk that a drug candidate could fail during the later stages of development after substantial amounts of money had been spent and time consumed. Such sunk costs could never be recouped — although failures can provide lessons having subsequent commercial benefit. Unsurprisingly, some within the industry have indeed taken this view that, in short, any failure lays not with them but elsewhere.[14]

The argument that regulators are the cause of reduced productivity, and that this is a bad thing, requires one to treat the latter as measurable solely by the quantity of medicines that are approved, and that the regulatory regimes introduced in the 1960s that required strong standards of safety and efficacy were excessive or even unnecessary. If we see these modified regulatory regimes instead as a necessary means to impose quality control, it seems more likely that they would stimulate *more* productivity — even with the added research and development costs — in terms of the quality of medicines actually placed — eventually — on the market. That said, the large proportion of me-too medicines implies this did not ensue either. It is unclear whether the most recent trend is more favourable or not. Either way, this lack of clarity underlines the importance of studying the relationship between the two closely in order to see how positive synergies between them can be enhanced for the public benefit.[15]

The second explanation relates to increasing difficulties in translating improvements in the production and utilisation of new knowledge and technologies, some of which were extremely radical, into ground-breaking new products. It may be that much of the low-hanging fruit had already been harvested, and the desire to find more such fruit to gather persists for being cheaper and easier than the alternatives. This may in fact be a more important factor than just the challenges of the era of new and stronger regulation. Either way, one manifestation of the industry's difficulties is the preponderance of me-toos and an increased dependence on a small number of so-called blockbuster drugs (see below).

The shift from randomness to rationality in drug design based on advances in molecular biology was only partial, and insufficient to have more than occasional successes. This is not to say that science and technology came to a standstall. Far from it, in fact, but it took some time for progress in the underlying science to translate into groundbreaking new medicines. Indeed, from the standpoint of 2020, it is very much evident that since the mid-1970s, the various biomedical sciences, and technologies both biological and digital, have each advanced tremendously as we have seen. They are converging more than ever and we are only beginning to tap into the tremendous synergies of this biodigital convergence alongside better knowledge of cell biology, and techniques like solid-phase synthesis, combinatorial chemistry enabling the development of massive compound libraries for screening, and large molecule drugs.[16]

Decline is not necessarily easy to trace in time or place, if for no other reason than that the word can be applied in several possible ways; nor are explanations necessarily obvious ones. Decline can be assessed solely by number of products or their quality, but not necessarily. Another logical measure of success or decline is the number of medicines per dollar of research expenditure, although this would keep quality out of the equation. In an influential article published in *Nature Reviews Drug Discovery*,[17] the authors find that the decline actually began around 1950. 'Decline' in this article is explained by factors that include but go a little beyond the conventional explanations as discussed above. The authors posit that from that year onwards the number of medicines approved per billion dollars spent on research and development has on average halved every nine or so years. The fall is quite modest during the 1950s but then steepens from 1960. They call this phenomenon Eroom's Law (which is the famous and much more optimistic Moore's Law written backwards). They claim four causes as follows: the 'better than the Beatles' problem; the 'cautious regulator' problem; the 'throw money at it' tendency; and the 'basic research–brute force' bias.

The first cause is that to be successful new drugs should be better than the old ones that still work; otherwise the older ones will still be prescribed or purchased over the counter — which they often are. Whereas Ed Sheeran (for example) doesn't have to better at writing songs or performing than Paul McCartney to make a very good living despite the music marketplace being so crowded with great music from the past and classic old rockers still touring, it is a lot harder to come up with a sellable medicine where there are lots of effective tried and tested generic alternatives. This pushes companies to go for more complex and harder to treat diseases which hardly lead to quick and easy results. In their opinion, this cause is likely to matter more than the low-hanging fruit one.

To me this is not correct, failing to take into account factors covered in this book. Clinical trials of new medicines compare efficacy with an existing standard product or a placebo if there isn't one (otherwise it would be unethical given the latter contains no active ingredient). All new medicines must undergo these trials but companies may sponsor them for existing medicines for the purpose of expanding the label for further indications and types of patient. With comparative trials, the expectation is that if they are better than existing ones they will get marketing approval. And if they are found to be, they may replace the existing product as the standard treatment which is of course the ideal situation for the trial sponsor. It is fair to say that approval of a new medicine is not a guarantee that physicians will prescribe it unless they are obliged or strongly recommended to do so. However, there are serious doubts as to whether the new medicines necessarily really are better.

According to a recent German study:

> research covering drug approvals since the 1970s suggests only a limited number of new drugs provide real advances over existing drugs. Most studies put the proportion of true innovation at under 15%, with no clear improvement over time.[18]

Overall, more than half of new medicines introduced into the German healthcare system have no added benefit.

In the United States, there have been some trenchant criticisms about approved cancer drugs having marginal benefits despite their enormously high prices. As one recent study has claimed:

> The use of expensive therapies with marginal benefits for their approved indications and for unproven indications is contributing to the rising cost of cancer care. We believe that expensive therapies are stifling progress by (1) encouraging enormous expenditures of time, money, and resources on marginal therapeutic indications and (2) promoting a me-too mentality that is stifling innovation and creativity. The modest gains of Food and Drug Administration–approved therapies and the limited progress against major cancers is evidence of a lowering of the efficacy bar that, together with high drug prices, has inadvertently incentivized the pursuit of marginal outcomes and a me-too mentality evidenced by the duplication of effort and redundant pharmaceutical pipelines.[19]

One should not of course downplay the value to an individual suffering a terminal disease of a medicine that prolongs her life for a few more months. But the question of whether these medicines can justify the allocation of scarce research funds and scientific capabilities especially when the high prices restrict their availability is a valid enquiry.

And once these non- or barely-superior products get approved, the 'problem' such as it is can be — *and is* — overcome by branding and marketing, and not just in those countries where advertising of prescription medicines is permitted.

The second cause is something that we have already considered: that regulatory hurdles have increased over the years. The reporting demands of regulators are ever more rigorous. The article tellingly cites the Chief Scientific Office of Novo Nordisk concerning FDA requirements for two new insulin therapies: 'If printed and stacked, the many million pages of documentation, with a total of 9 million electronic links, [would] exceed the height of [the] Empire State Building.'

The throwing money tendency is clearly based on an expectation, or maybe just a hope, that monetary expenditure will inexorably lead to good results — which turn out to be ill-founded. As for the last cause, this is likewise a consequence of over-optimism — hopes that were dashed about the time it would take to translate basic research in molecular biology into medicines and about high throughput screening generating new products more quickly. Having said that the emergence of biologic drugs may represent a reversal given the growing proportion of new medicines of this category.

Sustained productivity decline is hugely disappointing from a public health perspective. But was the pain shared by the industry? Overall, the answer is a fairly resounding 'no'. From 1950 to 1972, the US pharmaceutical industry's research and development costs increased significantly, from US$39 million to US$728 million.[20] But despite this, global annual sales jumped from US$1.4 billion to about $US8 billion. Net profits showed a similar level of growth, from US$129 in 1952 to US$734 in 1972. How do these profits compare to those of other industries? Average net profits after tax as a percentage of net stockholders' equity rose from 17 percent in 1960 to 18.3 percent in 1972. This looks very healthy for the pharmaceutical industry when we compare the average for US manufacturers as a whole between the same years: 9.3 percent in 1960, to 10.6 percent 12 years later.[21] This ability to remain highly profitable however well or badly the industry performs is certainly striking. Clearly, the industry managed to find ways to cope.

In fact, the situation precipitated change in how the industry did its business that was in many ways highly successful, if not necessarily optimal in terms of social welfare. Success was assisted in no small part by the phenomena introduced earlier of medicalisation and pharmaceuticalisation, which means more prescriptions for more people, especially in the United States, the world's biggest national drugs market.

If we accept that the period of lowest productivity measured by quantity is — approximately speaking — the mid-1970s to the mid-1980s, this coincides with the beginnings of the blockbuster drugs era. Blockbuster drugs are those that hit the sales figure of one billion dollars a year and are, or at least were then, targeted at a large patient population. The population was large either because it was clearly of benefit to many people or, which may have been just as likely, because pharmaceuticalisation led to them being prescribed to huge numbers. Note here that pharmaceuticalisation doesn't really work for cancer where death will likely ensure if left untreated and, even with surgery or radiotherapy, pharmaceuticals are likely to be indispensable. But for many chronic conditions which do not necessarily cause life-threatening diseases if untreated, the avoidance of medication and/or resort to other risk-mitigating non-medical practices may often be just as effective if not more so.

The blockbuster *era* is one characterised by huge profits alongside increased vulnerability. Companies become so dependent on such medicines that their quests for the next blockbusters came to be an essential element of their business models; as did their efforts to delay generic competition for their existing ones. The first of these drugs was cimetidine (Tagamet), which reached $1 billion per year in sales in 1979. Of course, important drugs, including treatments for HIV/AIDS, continue to be developed and manufactured and the turning of AIDS from death sentence to treatable condition, albeit thanks to massive external research and funding, is without doubt a magnificent achievement.

It is a fact of economic life that the most profitable medicines are not necessarily the ones that save the most people's lives or even that save any lives at all. These may well improve peoples' lives but they are not exactly lifesavers and may well be administered to large numbers of people who do not really need them, or who could achieve the same quality of life enhancements by other means such as more exercise, reduced consumption of unhealthy foods among other products, or professional counselling to enhance self-image. Only one of these costs money, and the others are either free or will save money. This might be a cynical view but what we can see is that there was a massive shift towards non-communicable conditions rather than curable infectious diseases, and towards the low-hanging fruit rather than the medicines needed to treat complex diseases which, as we will see in the next part of the book, have proved to be very tough nuts to crack. And it is hardly surprising than in a period of generally rather low returns from R&D investment, the incentive to spend vast amounts of money on marketing products that *did* make the cut was very hard to resist at least in a country like the United States which is the world's largest national drugs market and one which permits advertising of prescription drugs to the general public, as well as the selling of sickness itself. The well-informed physician is likely to become aware of a highly original first-in-class medicine or a first treatment for a previously pharmaceutically-untreatable condition. On the other hand, a me-too drug seems more likely to require aggressive marketing for it to be successful.

The downside of dependence on the revenues from one or a few blockbuster drugs is potentially a massive fall in overall income for a company when patents expire with no blockbuster drugs coming up to mitigate the potential revenue collapse. Falling off the so-called 'patent cliff' can be a painful experience. This is where lifecycle management comes in and the patent and trademark rules can be extremely helpful in extending marketplace monopolies on extending medicines, as well as shifting patients onto follow-on products, an activity nowadays referred to as 'product-hopping'.

Underlying Trends Driving Change

The relationships between biomedical science and technology, innovation, regulation and the law are dynamic and arguably changing faster now than ever before. Even so, there is continuity too. Here as elsewhere there is a tendency to overuse the word 'revolution'. To understand what is going on and why things are happening now, and to provide context for the technological advances of recent decades as covered in this chapter, we need to take account of three major drivers of change. These drivers are not all new but their prominence has become more noticeable since the beginning of the modern health biotechnology era in the early 1980s, a time when the pharmaceutical industry was, as we saw, in the midst of a slump with fewer genuinely original drug products entering the market. These are: (i) internationalisation, (ii) complexity, and (iii) fragmentation. Our co-evolutionary approach is very relevant to the discussion here, as elsewhere.

Internationalisation

Internationalisation is manifested in several ways. Emerging economies such as China and recently developed ones like Singapore and South Korea are either producing health innovations of the kind they were not doing earlier, or they are making large investments in the life sciences which will bear fruit sooner or later. This expansion in the geography of expertise and investment has entailed an increase in international research and commercial collaborations. It has also vastly increased the interest of pharmaceutical companies in the intellectual property rules of other countries, especially those that are markets, or potential markets, for their products — or which are large producers and exporters of generic drugs like India.

Many developing countries, especially in Asia, have become wealthier, with rapidly expanding middle classes. This has several important consequences. First, the number of consumers of health products due to increased health spending and enhanced purchasing power is rising worldwide. This is of course a very good thing for industry. Second, the disease profiles of many developing countries are become more similar to those of the developed countries. This is not just because wealthier people anywhere in the world live longer than the poor, and diseases that tend to affect the elderly most are broadly similar everywhere: non-communicable ones like cancer, cardio-vascular diseases, Alzheimer's, etc. It is also because there is a certain amount of uniformity in the lifestyles including diets of people having similar levels of income and purchasing power *wherever they happen to live*. As people get richer, for example, they tend to consume more meat products and processed foods. This means diseases affecting people are become more and more the same wherever they live. This prospect for industry of the global similarity of disease profiles and life expectancies with their attendant market and economies of scale opportunities appears to be quite new. You have to go back to before the end of the nineteenth century to return to such a situation. This was a time when populations in Western Europe and North America became much wealthier than in the rest of the world, and public health and hygiene had improved dramatically leading to a big fall in outbreaks of infectious diseases that were continuing to decimate populations in other parts of the world. Admittedly, tropical disease research institutes were being set up in Europe then to find cures for diseases affecting people in the colonies but not in Europe, but these were mostly for the benefit of settlers and expatriates.

Of course, we are talking about trends and there is no suggestion that even in the more successful developing countries, health problems, many of which are avoidable, do not continue to affect many people that even the least wealthy Europeans and North Americans need not fear. This explains current interest in the issue of neglected diseases. Moreover, Africa remains an exception to this, as do failing states and war-torn countries elsewhere. Admittedly, the adoption of unhealthy diets from other countries is not just due to prosperity, but also effective marketing and sheer convenience, cheapness and ubiquity. Hundreds of millions of people around the world can afford a regular cheeseburger. For example, Mexico is experiencing an explosion in diabetes incidences. This has coincided with the increased consumption of fast food instead of more balanced and nutritious diets having fewer carbohydrates. Again, this is potentially quite advantageous for the pharmaceutical industry. Finally, as the industry increasingly looks to the world as a whole for potential consumers and faces local firms whose ability to copy can, in some countries at least, be quite sophisticated, it becomes ever more assertive about being able to avail itself of intellectual property protection in every market it seeks to enter.

Complexity

A trend towards further complexity is evident in a number of ways, beyond the adage that the more one knows about something, the more one realises how much more there is out there that we do not or cannot know — true as that is.

For one thing, understanding at the molecular level of specific malfunctions which lead to disease has increased dramatically, for example in cancer. However, this does not lead automatically to cures. Indeed, insights into disease causation are the start and not the end of a journey that may be long indeed. The likelihood is that it will engage the expertise of many individuals from numerous disciplinary fields not all of whom are likely to be working in the same laboratory, company or place of employment. There is still room for individual brilliance but teamwork (or better said teamswork because there may be many teams involved) is all. Innovation has always been primarily collective, even if certain individuals may stand out for making decisive contributions, but it is especially so in the life sciences of the present day.

Another area of complexification is in relation to the drug itself. Until quite recently drugs were almost by definition small molecule products. Historically, these were typically isolated plant metabolites or microbial products, or synthetic versions, perhaps with modifications, made in a lab. Others were synthetic without being modelled on ones found in nature. There were also animal products such as hormones. As we have seen, and will see in further detail below, in recent decades there has been a big growth in biopharmaceuticals (or 'biologics') including therapeutic proteins like insulin, erythropoietin, and various monoclonal antibodies (MAbs). These now make up about a quarter of global pharmaceutical sales.

Fragmentation

Fragmentation follows from the point made earlier that the discovery and development of drugs and other health products such as vaccines and diagnostic tests increasingly requires the expertise of numerous individual scientists and teams having quite diverse disciplinary backgrounds that are unlikely to be found under the same roof. Indeed, they may be spread across countries and continents and work in companies, universities, hospitals, government health research institutes, and health charities. Apart from these entities, organised patient groups are sometimes actively engaged in the search for new treatments as well. These are likely to have different missions, interests, and ways of getting their work funded. And increasingly, the private sector side contains not just the traditional giants ('Big Pharma') but highly specialised small firms, often spun out of universities who have useful services and possibly quite unique skills to offer, and perhaps a few highly valuable patents, but who have no products at all to sell. Building networks that satisfy all parties is no easy task. Intellectual property rights can help or get in the way, depending on who acquires them and how they are managed. The aggressive assertion of rights can be highly divisive and counter-productive in terms of stimulating innovation and ensuring that products are made available to all of those who need them and under fair terms and conditions. This in turn raises questions about the imperative to maximise taxpayer value (as opposed just to shareholder value) where much of the work is government supported, and the availability of public interest safeguards in patent law.

The rest of the chapter explains how we got here, and what happened along the way, focusing on science, technology and business. The following chapter completes the story by covering the evolution and globalisation of intellectual property law during the same period.

From Molecular Biology to Biotechnology

The 1980s saw the emergence, most noticeably in the United States, of a new pharmaceutical subsector comprising small firms, often start-ups spun out of universities, seeking to exploit promising new technologies discovered in those universities and adopting commercialisation approaches quite different from the more conservative established corporations. One stimulus in the United States was the passage in 1980 of the Amendments to the Patent and Trademark Act, commonly known as the Bayh-Dole Act. The Act was intended to encourage universities and public research agencies to file patents they were permitted to own on inventions arising from government- (that is, of course, taxpayer-) funded research as a means of facilitating technology transfer to the private sector. In part the legislation reflects a shift in government and societal perceptions about the role of the university, one that continues to this day, and certainly not just in the United States. Whereas the contribution of universities to national prosperity through progress in science and technology was assumed as a given, universities found themselves pressured to demonstrate relevance and accountability and continued financial support on the same scale as previously was no longer to be assumed. Blue skies research was valued less than high impact research having practical applications.

Previously such institutions had to assign patents to the government, a requirement that seems perfectly right and proper if one inclines to the view that taxpayers should be the ones to acquire or otherwise gain from what they have paid for. The belief that taxpayers have legitimate interests that intellectual property rights and the way that they are managed and asserted fail to fully reflect, if at all, is a powerful one that is held, as it happens, by the present author.

Be that as it may, and we cannot really avoid confronting such an argument, the development of commercial biotechnology was driven mostly by discoveries coming out of universities arising usually from research funded by the state rather than by the private sector. With universities owning these patents, and for the first time managing them themselves rather than leaving this task to outside or affiliated but independent entities like Research Corporation and WARF,[22] they became licensors seeking to maximise returns from their patents. This also triggered the formation of countless new companies as entrepreneurs and university scientists with the support of venture capitalists and other investors rapidly started to build businesses around patented technologies based on these discoveries once commercial possibilities had been identified. This trend affected the direction and progress of the life sciences in far-reaching ways for the pharmaceutical industry. This was not just because of the increasing amount of in-house science being carried out by firms thanks to this wave of investment and the migration of top scientists to the private sector; there has also been a growing tendency, especially evident today, for research funding criteria to include economic relevance and to entail some degree of 'knowledge transfer' for the benefit of national industry and the university itself through patent licensing revenues. This is not of course specific to the life sciences, though, but as one of the most rapidly advancing and strategically important fields of knowledge, the life sciences exemplify this better than almost any other.

Biotechnology, like so many other words with the 'bio' prefix, sounds like a neologism. In fact, it was coined early in the twentieth century by a Hungarian agricultural engineer called Karl Ereky, who included within its meaning 'all such work by which products are produced from raw materials with the aid of living organisms'.[23] Over time it has acquired a confusing variety of definitions. It may be defined quite broadly or much more narrowly. Typical of a broad definition is that of the (now defunct) US Office of Technology Assessment: 'biotechnology, broadly defined, includes any technique that uses living organisms (or parts of organisms) to make or modify products, to improve plants or animals, or to develop microorganisms for specific uses'.[24]

Alternatively, biotechnologies may be classified by generation. Thus, the first generation includes traditional technologies like beer brewing and bread making. These go back at least to the Sumerians of ancient Mesopotamia and of course they can be practiced in any domestic kitchen with easy to find ingredients and a few inexpensive pieces of equipment. The second begins with the microbiological applications developed by Pasteur and continues with the mass production by fermentation of the antibiotics. Tissue culture and modern plant and animal breeding also fall within this generation.

The third generation includes techniques like recombinant DNA, monoclonal antibodies, polymerase chain reaction (PCR), animal cloning, and stem cells, all of whose emergence was triggered by post-Second World War advances in molecular biology. Most innovation in these new fields takes place in the USA, Western Europe and Japan though countries like South Korea and China are increasing their involvement. Nowadays, biotechnology is often treated as being synonymous with the third generation of biotechnologies. This is how the word is used here. As such, biotechnology is an interdisciplinary enterprise, a scientific melting-pot centred on molecular biology, whose main language of communication and expression is chemistry,[25] but which draws not only upon a wide range of life sciences, but also on other less obviously related fields like computer science and chemical engineering. Biotechnology also brings together a diversity of industrial sectors that benefit from using it, not just health.

For Arthur Kornberg, a Nobel laureate for his pioneering research on DNA synthesis, 'the most rational understanding of life' is 'its reduction to the molecular details of chemistry'.[26] This conceptualisation of life as essentially chemical, embodied in — and promoted through — the discourse of biotechnology, is undoubtedly appealing to those who esteem modern science for its progressiveness and rationality. Using this way of imagining life to base arguments for extending protectable subject matter to microorganisms, plants, and animals played a significant role in the evolution of patent law in various countries from the 1980s, and ultimately in the global regime too.

The uniqueness of modern biotechnology lies, in the words of anthropologist Paul Rabinow, 'in its potential to get away from nature, to construct artificial conditions in which specific variables can be known in such a way that they can be manipulated. This knowledge then forms the basis for remaking nature according to our norms'.[27] That is one way of looking at it. But it is of course a highly anthropocentric view. We are part of nature ourselves. We synthesise, but so does the rest of nature, including our own bodies which without our say-so biologically manufacture a whole host of complicated chemicals out of other ones. Evolution itself is the greatest force for artificiality and invention, not the human brain. For over three billion years, the living world has evolved amazingly practical chemical reactions and contrivances that humans had nothing to do with. Single-celled organisms came up with aerobic respiration, nitrogen fixation and photosynthesis. Bacteria even invented the wheel as an aid to locomotion long before humans.[28] Nonetheless, it is true that in this human-centred world of ours, a semblance of intervention in and control over natural forces is a prerequisite for any plausible claim to have made a biotechnological invention, as it should be.[29] Otherwise it is a product of nature (under United States patent law doctrine) or a discovery (under European patent law), and not a human artefact.

While modern biotechnology is very much a late twentieth century phenomenon, it is the result of scientific advances that go back well over a century. In brief, the basic rules of heredity had been worked out in the 1860s by Gregor Mendel, whose findings were rediscovered in 1900 and then applied to crop improvement[30] rather than medicine. Chromosomes had been discovered, also in the 1860s, and were found to behave in a systematic manner during cell division. Why they did this and for what purpose were barely understood. Nucleic acid had also been identified in cells and was isolated in 1869 by Friedrich Miescher who called it 'nuclein'. He found it unique and definitely not a protein, but it was not considered by him or anybody else at the time to play any role in heredity.[31] The so-called modern synthesis of evolution and genetics along with the adoption of mathematical methods was certainly a major development much written on by historians of science, but this came much later and even with it, our knowledge of genetics and of how to harness genetics to improve health remained quite rudimentary up to the mid twentieth century. It consisted of some basic, albeit important, rules and bits of information, and some interesting experimental work.

Molecular biology emerged in the early-middle part of the twentieth century.[32] The term was actually coined by a scientist working at the Rockefeller Foundation, an important source of research funding and scientific guidance in this area from as early as the 1930s.[33] According to a historical account by French scientist Michel Morange:

> molecular biology is a result of the encounter between genetics and biochemistry, two branches of biology that developed at the beginning of the twentieth century. These two disciplines had each clearly defined the object of their research: the gene for genetics, proteins and enzymes for biochemistry. Molecular biology emerged when the relation between these two objects became clearer. Scientists identified the gene as a macromolecule (DNA), determined by its structure, and described its roles in protein synthesis'.[34]

Molecular biology offered what Lily Kay called, to borrow one of her book titles: 'the molecular vision of life'. However, since the term's coinage by Warren Weaver in 1938 its meaning underwent a shift towards one more focused on DNA — perhaps inevitably once it was identified chemically — and in time genes were regarded more and more as reservoirs of coded information, an insight often attributed to Schrödinger.[35] Indeed, this dual nature of DNA: as being both 'stuff' and a source of information some of which will have medical implications for scientists to discover drove much research and its dominant discourses, whilst provoking confusion in the minds of courts deciding on the patentability of genes.

In terms of chronology, Morange helpfully divides what he calls the 'molecular revolution' into two parts: 'The new conceptual tools for analysing biological phenomena were forged between 1940 and 1965. The consequent operational control was acquired between 1972 and 1980.' Table 8.2 presents most of the major breakthroughs in medical biotechnology to date. An immediately apparent observation is that industry contributed very little as compared to universities. It starts with a major early advance, when three researchers at the Rockefeller Institute in New York — Oswald Avery, Colin McLeod and Maclyn McCarty — following up on an experiment carried out in 1928 that found virulent but dead *Streptococcus pneumoniae* injected into mice along with a non-virulent but living type of the same species still caused infection. The earlier scientist, Frederick Griffith, concluded that the former type had transformed the latter type rendering it pathogenic. But what was the transforming principle? The article's one sentence conclusion stated thus: 'The evidence presented supports the belief that a nucleic acid of the deoxyribose type is the fundamental unit of the transforming principle of Pneumococcus Type III.'[36] This might seem rather explicit, but its significance might have been clearer had they also used the word gene — which continued to be more of a concept than a 'thing'. Apparently Avery was cautious to go too far even though he did believe it was a gene that caused the transformation.[37] Despite much hesitation from many in the scientific community, scientists came to accept that it must be DNA, and not proteins as many of them had thought, that provides the chemical language of instruction for the transmission of genetic traits in all organisms and that genes are made of DNA.

Table 8.2.   Scientific breakthroughs in molecular biology and biotechnology: 1953–2001[38]

1944	Oswald Avery, Colin McLeod and Maclyn McCarty publish results of experiment in which virulent but dead and non-virulent but living *Streptococcus pneumoniae* injected into mice still caused infection — and that the 'transforming principle' making the bacteria harmful was DNA and not protein
1951–3	George Gey and colleagues at Johns Hopkins University establish first 'immortal' human cell line, named HeLa after the patient whose tumour cells were cultured (Henrietta Lacks);[39] used in the development of the polio vaccine; first human cells to be successfully cloned at University of Colorado; in time many uses found as research tools

Table 8.2.   (*Continued*)

1953	James Watson and Francis Crick at University of Cambridge discover double helix structure of DNA
1961–66	Marshall Nirenberg, Heinrich Matthaei, Severo Ochoa, Gobind Khorana and others decipher genetic code for the 20 amino acids involved in producing proteins
1973	Stanley Cohen and Herbert Boyer demonstrate gene splicing (recombinant DNA) technique
1975	Georges Köhler and Cesar Milstein produce monoclonal antibodies using their hybridoma technology
1977	Genome of NX174 virus sequenced by Frederick Sanger using his dideoxy sequencing method New biotech company Genentech clones human gene, causing a human protein (somatostatin) to be expressed in bacteria
1978	Genentech clones human insulin
1981	Leroy Hood and colleagues at California Institute of Technology invent automated gene sequencing machine
1985	Invention of polymerase chain reaction (PCR) at Cetus Corporation, attributed to Kary Mullis
1995	Genome of first free-living organism (*H. influenzae*) sequenced by Craig Venter and Hamilton Smith at The Institute of Genome Research using 'whole-genome shotgun sequencing' technique
1996	Dolly, the first mammal cloned from an adult cell, born in Scotland
1998	Genome of first animal (*C. elegans*) sequenced by Robert Waterston, John Sulston and colleagues of Washington University and the Sanger Centre
2001	Human genome sequenced in draft form by the Human Genome Project and Celera Genomics

Subsequent to Avery, McLeod and McCarty's discovery, groups of researchers undertook to elucidate the structure of the DNA macro-molecule.[40] The competitors included Linus Pauling, the renowned American biochemist, working at the California Institute of Technology, Maurice Wilkins and Rosalind Franklin at King's College, London, and James Watson and Francis Crick at Cambridge University. As is now well known, Watson and Crick were first to come up with the double helix model, which they announced in May 1953 in a brief article in *Nature*.[41]

The Business of Biotechnology

The biotechnology revolution has its roots in an invention and the setting up of a company to exploit it. The invention is recombinant DNA (often shortened to 'rDNA'). It is normally attributed to Stanley Cohen and Herbert Boyer whose names are on the patent. However, arguably it is invidious to attribute the invention solely to these two persons. Historian of science, Doogab Yi, refers in reference to this invention and the era more generally, to 'the uneasy disjuncture between scientific authorship and legal invention in the history of recombinant DNA technology'.[42] This disconnection, which is not always controversial, is the case for many inventions in the life sciences and beyond. Polymerase chain reaction (PCR) is a good example (see box below).

In some cases, it could be argued that *no* single individual or group deserves legal recognition or property rights, including those with their names on the patent, since the invention was so incremental; in others, the number of deserving people may be more numerous than would be prudent for a patent application to accommodate. In an article about rDNA, which was actually developed by a group of scientists, Smith Hughes seeks to explain the logic of patenting while showing how it may clash with established scientific norms about credit:

> Although the patent application procedure requires citation of the research upon which an invention is based, it also aims to reduce the number of inventors to the one or few deemed responsible for the conceptual, rather than merely technical, contribution. Singling out one or a few inventors from a scientific team, as patenting protocol requires, diverged from the custom in scientific publications of assigning individual credit through coauthorship to everyone who had directly contributed to the research being reported. Moreover, compared to scientific convention, the legal definition of inventorship seemed to slight the full dimensions of a scientific discovery, leaving out some collaborators, institutional and personnel resources, and the background of research upon which a discovery is based.[43]

As we will see, the anti-cancer drug Glivec ('Gleevec' in the United States), a genuine biomedical success, demonstrates perfectly the validity of such criticisms. In this case the number of inventors was reduced to those responsible for the technical contribution of coming up with the right chemical, whereas the foundational and conceptual research and the empirical 'leg-work' was done by others not named on the patents. Some of them, however, were credited albeit in other ways than through being named on patents.

The PCR story

Polymerase chain reaction is a revolutionary gene technology for amplifying small pieces of DNA *in vitro*.[44] It is not so much a product or a process as a research tool that has multiple applications. It is popularly regarded as a true invention that can be traced to an individual, Kary Mullis, to a time (albeit approximate) according to his own version of the story: Spring 1983, and to a highly specific place, again by his own account: in the car he was driving at mile-marker 46.58 on Highway 128 in California.

PCR uses a naturally-occurring enzyme called DNA polymerase to amplify sections of DNA rapidly, precisely and in staggeringly large quantities. DNA polymerase, a chemical well known at the time, performs various roles in the cells of living things including in the copying of DNA. Previously, the method used by scientists to copy DNA was cloning, basically to insert the desired piece of DNA in a microorganism and then to 'harvest' increasing quantities of the copied DNA as the microbes with the added DNA reproduced themselves, something they do quite enthusiastically under the right conditions. Mullis's main contribution was to conceive of a way to control the action of DNA polymerase so that only selected pieces of DNA were copied, and then to launch and manage a cycle of repeated and exponential copying. As Paul Rabinow explains in his ethnographic study of Cetus Corporation, *Making PCR*, the revolutionary nature of PCR lies in that it:

makes abundant what was once scarce — the genetic material required for experimentation. Not only is this genetic material abundant, it is no longer embedded in a living system. Cloning had made scare genetic material abundant, but its obligatory use of living organisms as the medium of reproduction was also its limitation. PCR took a major step away from that dependency.[45]

Or as Mullis himself explains, with a bit more flourish, in an article in *Scientific American*:

(*Continued*)

(Continued)

Beginning with a single molecule of the genetic material DNA, the PCR can generate 100 billion similar molecules in an afternoon. The reaction is easy to execute. It requires no more than a test tube, a few simple reagents and a source of heat. The DNA sample that one wishes to copy can be pure, or it can be a minute part of an extremely complex mixture of biological materials. The DNA may come from a hospital tissue specimen, from a single human hair, from a drop of dried blood at the scene of a crime, from the tissues of a mummified brain or from a 40,000-year-old woolly mammoth frozen in a glacier.[46]

Mullis's experiments to make PCR work in practice were not entirely convincing, and getting it to do so reliably was a team effort with various Cetus scientists involved. One of the biggest difficulties in making PCR efficient was that most DNA polymerase, including the one initially employed, is unable to withstand the high temperatures needed to separate DNA strands during each PCR cycle. Consequently, polymerase needed to be added each time. Mullis had proposed that a thermostable polymerase be used. Consequently, Cetus settled on a DNA polymerase from a thermophilic (heat loving) microorganism discovered earlier in the Yellowstone National Park, famous of course for its geysers, *Thermus aquaticus*. The task of purifying this chemical ('taq polymerase') was carried out in-house but not by Mullis. Once achieved, PCR had become sufficiently refined to be an extremely power research tool, and a commercial product as well.

The self-consciously eccentric and individualistic Kary Mullis plays the part of the inventor hero with great aplomb. And like so many past inventors of renown like Charles Goodyear of rubber fame,[47] electrical engineer Nikola Tesla and plant breeder Luther Burbank[48] to name just three, he never did receive his financial due, or so he believes.[49] Then again, a share of a Nobel Prize doubtless made him feel a whole lot better. In his account of the invention Mullis regarded it as a true flash of inspiration. He used the word 'eureka' three times and said that he exclaimed 'Dear Thor!' on realising at that moment he 'had solved the most annoying problems in chemistry with a single lightning bolt'.[50]

Nonetheless, Mullis's PCR story did not convince everybody. The importance of Mullis's role, and the size of the creative leap that PCR represents, have both been questioned. The doubters included colleagues at Cetus who claimed he didn't really make it work (that is, in patent-speak, reduce it to practice). They also comprised some highly authoritative

(Continued)

people. Perhaps the most prominent doubter was the late Arthur Kornberg, a Nobel prizewinner who was first to isolate a DNA polymerase, and who testified to a court that Mullis's 'invention' had been anticipated by earlier researchers including himself. In 1991, the court upheld the patents as did the Patent and Trademark Office after a re-examination.[51] Whether or not PCR was all that original, Mullis, whether alone or with his colleagues at Cetus, had done enough as far as the jury was concerned. The patent system is not about originality as such, nor is it about genius; it is about being first to disclose something that has a practical, preferably commercial, application. The key patents protecting PCR were sold for the princely sum of $300,000,000. And Mullis got his Nobel Prize.

Cohen and Boyer worked at universities, Cohen at Stanford University and Boyer at University of California at San Francisco. The rDNA technique, which enables foreign genes to be inserted into micro-organisms and passed on to others through cell division, was patented by Stanford and licensed widely, earning over $200 million in royalties between 1975 and 1997, when the patent expired.[52] These were shared between the two universities and the inventors. A few years later, the era of commercial biotechnology got underway. This was largely due to its wide dissemination, and also to the fact that, following the *Diamond v. Chakrabarty* United States Supreme Court decision, this invention among others in the field was definitely patentable making this emergent sector attractive for investors.[53] One wonders how long the revolution might have been delayed had Stanford opted to grant exclusive rather than non-exclusive licenses. There would certainly have been the investment. But as a key research tool, the sector as a whole was dependent on it in those early years, and effective attempts to prevent others using it could have been as damaging as James Watt's patents were said to have been to progress during the age of steam.[54]

Genentech was one of the first companies started up to exploit the new biotechnological applications coming out of the universities, and quickly became a leader. It was founded in 1976 by a venture capitalist called Robert Swanson, with the aforementioned Herbert Boyer acting as an independent consultant. Genentech, whose name is short for 'genetic engineering technology', and is now owned by Hoffman LaRoche, was responsible for the first biotechnology-based health product to reach the market, which was genetically engineered human insulin, in 1982.

This product was developed by Genentech in collaboration with Eli Lilly, which as we know has had an interest in insulin going back to the 1920s. Lilly manufactured and marketed this 'new' insulin with cash and royalties from sales going to Genentech.[55] At that time, the insulin on the market was extracted from ground-up pig and cow pancreases and could cause allergic reactions in some diabetes sufferers. Claims that human insulin is better for diabetes sufferers despite its higher price have been widely accepted. According to Michael Sargant of the National Institute for Medical Research in London:

> Once genetically engineered insulin was established as an exact physiological equivalent of natural human insulin, some long-standing clinical problems could be overcome. Variants of insulin could be made in which certain amino acids were changed by redesigning the template — an unattainable goal with animal insulin. More effective control of blood sugar levels could be obtained using genetically engineered insulin modified either to be fast-acting or able to make a long-lasting response.[56]

But others are sceptical, pointing out that human insulin also produces harmful side-effects. Recent reports do suggest that it may be lethal for some users.[57] James Le Fanu also argues that its production is unnecessary because animal insulin is just as effective and was being produced in adequate quantities until 'Eli Lilly decided to "phase out" its production of animal-based insulin so it was less readily available'.[58]

During the 1980s Genentech followed up insulin with two more genetically engineered human proteins sold as pharmaceutical products. These were human growth hormone, which was approved in 1985 and marketed as Protropin, and tissue plasminogen activator (tPA), a 'clot-buster' drug for heart attack patients approved in 1987 and sold as Activase. Amgen followed in Genentech's footsteps two years later with

Epogen (erythropoietin), a hormone used to treat anaemia caused by kidney failure. Healthy kidneys produce erythopoietin to promote oxygen-carrying red blood cell formation.[59] Amgen, the most successful of all the new biotechnology firms established at this time, is now one of the world's biggest drug companies.

Genetic engineering became increasingly sophisticated with genes being transferred not just to microorganisms but also to plant and animal cells including mammalian ones. For example, patented methods were discovered to insert genes into cultivated plants.[60] In 1983, Richard Axel, Saul Silverstein and Michael Wigler were granted a broad patent covering methods and products concerning the transfer of genes into cultured mammalian cells. One of the important aspects of the invention is that their methods did not require the use of viral vectors for introducing the genes to the cells.[61] The patent and some follow on patents relating to the same technology were assigned to Columbia University. Non-exclusive licensing by Columbia of these patents generated nearly $800 million for the university.[62] A few years later, a cancer-causing gene was inserted into a mouse, resulting in the controversial Harvard oncomouse that was patented in 1988: the first granted patent that claimed a whole animal. Genetically modified mammal cells have since become the primary production systems for monocolonal antibodies, which are now major pharmaceutical products that generate huge profits for some companies.

Monoclonal antibodies and the emergence of 'living' medicines

One of the most exciting scientific breakthroughs of the 1970s — to the biomedical scientific community if not to the general public — was hybridoma technology developed by Georges Köhler and Cesar Milstein and announced in an issue of *Nature* in 1975. This can be seen as an update of serum therapy as discovered many decades earlier by Behring, Ehlich and others.[63] Like most but not all basic scientific achievements — PCR being a rare exception — this was not, and arguably could not have been, achieved in an industry laboratory but in a public institution: the Medical Research Council's Laboratory of Molecular Biology at Cambridge

(*Continued*)

(*Continued*)

University, the same institution where Watson and Crick made their famous discovery.

Hybridoma cells result from the fusion of a type of cancer cell known as a myeloma with an antibody-producing cell: a B lymphocyte. Hybridoma cell cultures are capable of mass-producing antibodies of a highly specific type, which are called monoclonal antibodies.[64] The MRC's culture was still not particularly pro-patent, and the NRDC did not see anything patentable in the discovery.[65] They were almost certainly incorrect about that. Thus it fell into the public domain, an outcome that later gave rise to some heavy criticism. There were high hopes that the technology would provide, without any great delay, a range of extremely powerful 'magic bullets' in both diagnostics and therapeutics. As it turned out, while several diagnostic tests were commercialised in the following years, it took two decades of expensive setbacks and disappointments before monoclonal antibody (MAb) drugs became available. It was the second, ReoPro (abciximab), a cardiovascular medicine marketed by Centocor and Eli Lilly, approved by the FDA and the European Committee on Proprietary Medicinal Products in December 1994, which proved to the doubters that MAbs did have immense commercial potential. Idec Pharmaceuticals' Rituxan (rituximab), which was approved in 1997 and is used to treat non-Hodgkin's lymphoma and rheumatoid arthritis, was the first MAb cancer treatment. It generated sales of $152 million in its first year alone, and is now marketed by Biogen-Idec and Genentech in the USA, and by Roche in Europe.[66] By 2000, it was reported that 'about a quarter of all biotech drugs in development are MAb, and around 30 products are in use or being investigated'.[67] Currently six of the best selling drugs in the world are monoclonal antibodies.[68] More significantly perhaps, especially given the first one was not introduced onto the pharmaceuticals market until 1986, MAb treatments reportedly take the second (AbbVie's Humira/adalimumab), fourth (Johnson & Johnson's Remicade/infliximab), sixth (Biogen and Genentech's Rituxan/rituximab), seventh (Amgen's Enbrel/etanercept), eighth (Genentech's Herceptin/trastuzumab), and ninth places (Genentech's Avastin/bevacizumab) in the world's top ten all-time best-selling medicines.[69]

(*Continued*)

MAbs are very large complex chemicals and can only be made in eukaryotic cells, not bacteria. Typically, Chinese hamster ovary (CHO) cells are selected as ideal host cell cultures for producing the antibodies.[70] The processes used to make them are immensely challenging. CHO cells take a long time to create and prepare for production, and yields are quite low. This has massive market and regulatory implications as we will see.

Another new technique developed during this period was animal cloning based on nuclear transfer; that is to say the insertion of an adult cell nucleus into an egg cell that has had its nucleus removed. In 1996, the now world famous sheep called Dolly was cloned by Ian Wilmut and Keith Campbell at Roslin Institute in Scotland from a cell taken from a mature sheep's udder. It was not the first cloned animal but the first to be cloned from an adult mammal.[71]

Biotechnology in the United States

The USA pioneered commercial biotechnology and continues to be the world leader by some considerable distance. Why is this? There is no single explanation, but the private sector has undoubtedly benefited enormously from basic research by universities, hospitals and the government, which has been a massive investor in biomedical research over several decades. And, since the early 1990s, the US government has adopted a more competitive attitude towards research it sponsors. Increasingly, government biomedical research funding there is aimed at strengthening the competitive positions of the national pharmaceutical and health biotechnology sectors, reducing healthcare costs (not very successfully one might add), and at securing higher returns on public research investment.[72] From 1994 to 1998, the federal government was spending at least $20 billion a year on biotechnology research, about double the expenditure in all the European Union member countries combined, and of course these figure have risen since then.

Private finance is also much easier to secure in the USA than else-where. Academics and businessmen wishing to found start-up biotech-nology firms can tap into venture capital funds that exist on a scale unmatched in any other country. And thanks to an early wave of opti-mism that new products would soon reach the market, many such firms secured extraordinarily large cash injections through public offerings enabling them to invest heavily in research. So although there are plenty of these businesses in Europe, they tend to be smaller, employ fewer sci-entists, and their market capitalisation is far lower.

As it turned out much of the initial optimism was misplaced. During the 1980s only 10 biologic drugs were approved for sale by the FDA, of which just three were developed and marketed by the new biotechnology firms. The others were licensed to established pharmaceutical compa-nies.[73] From the late 1980s, it became more difficult for many of these dedicated biotechnology firms to attract further investments, and few of them succeeded in generating enough new products to join the ranks of the large science-based transnational corporations. Clearly returns from the low-hanging fruits represented by the first wave of biologic medicines, has diminished.

In consequence, several biotechnology firms were taken over by their larger rivals, though others found ways to avoid this fate. Patenting has undoubtedly helped some small firms to maintain their independence. According to one commentator, 'outright acquisitions of the new bio-technology firms were effectively blocked by the extensive cross-licensing agreements among different partners'.[74] On the other hand, the owner-ship of a key patent or a large portfolio of patents may serve as a signal to a larger company that the biotechnology firm would make a good pur-chase. To some of the latter companies (or at least their investors), being bought by a bigger company is a mark of success rather than failure.

Those biotechnology firms that kept their independence did so by entering into strategic alliances with other ones as well as the bigger, longer-established firms, and by forming extensive research, development and marketing networks containing both small and large established firms, and government and university research institutions — often across national boundaries. Such alliances and networks held the promise of happily marrying the basic research expertise of the dedicated biotechnology firms and universities with the drug development experience and marketing strength of the pharmaceutical and chemical companies and of course their much deeper pockets. To give one example of the success (and perhaps the sheer necessity) of such collaborating, the aforementioned anti-cancer MAb drug Rituxan involved a worldwide partnership of companies including Idec, Genentech, Hoffman LaRoche and Zenyaku Kogyo Co.[75]

Biotechnology in Europe and Japan

Innovation in commercial biotechnology outside the USA has taken place almost exclusively in Europe and Japan, although this is starting to change with emerging hotbeds of innovation in South Korea and China where research investment commitments are substantial and local scientific capacity is now on a par with the first mover nations like the US, Britain, Germany and France. As with the US case, industry in those countries has enjoyed the benefit of ground-breaking research carried out in universities and public sector research agencies. However, while the US system has been relatively effective at turning new discoveries made by public sector and university researchers into commercial products, Europe and Japan have been less successful in putting together the downstream linkages from fundraising for basic research all the way to commercialisation. The most successful countries in commercial biotechnology are the UK, Germany and France. The first two countries have a relatively large number of dedicated biotechnology firms, many of which are university spin-offs, but in France and the rest of continental Europe, the existing large science-based pharmaceutical and chemical firms have from the start been responsible for virtually all the private-sector biotechnology research and development. Like their US counterparts, they tended to be quite cautious about biotechnology and were thus rather slow to set up in-house biotech research and development programmes. In Japan, early investment in biotechnology came from a wide range of industries and not just pharmaceutical and chemical firms. These include manufacturers of beer, foods and even watches.[76]

Since the 1980s, the European Community countries and Japan have been preoccupied with catching up with the USA. Both the European

Commission and the national governments have sought to stimulate biotechnology research and development through industrial policy and more business-friendly product and intellectual property regulation. The Japanese government has likewise acted to encourage commercial biotechnology and enhance international competitiveness.[77] It remains to be seen whether Europe or Japan can catch up with the USA, whose lead is considerable.

Most government funding and commercial activity during those early decades of biotechnology were in the area of health. The majority of the biotechnology firms (that is, dedicated biotechnology firms and other firms that do biotechnology) in the USA and Europe were engaged in human and animal health. The types of product being developed included biopharmaceuticals such as genetically engineered therapeutic proteins and vaccines. Other common types of product were diagnostic kits and testing services for diseases linked to genetic defects. Health biotechnology was used not only to develop new types of drug but also to enhance the efficiency of the drug discovery process. In fact, this became the main objective of health biotechnology research. According to one commentator,

> Partly…due to the high costs of production, using genetic engineering to make human proteins is currently seen to be a minor use in pharmaceuticals. The major use of genetic engineering is to improve the efficiency of the drug discovery process, in combination with a better understanding of the workings of the body. Combining that knowledge implies that pharmaceuticals can be more directly designed to do certain things.[78]

Agricultural biotechnology became the second most important biotechnology field in the USA and Europe, followed by industrial biotechnology. However, healthcare products tended to be more commercially attractive, as they still do, because they have potentially much higher returns, and because demand tends to be far less cyclical. The biotechnology and genomics revolutions created completely new commercial opportunities, and spawned four types of business. These were (i) the technology providers that manufactured the DNA sequencing machines and other equipment (for example, Applied Biosystems and Amersham Biosciences);

(ii) the information providers (such as Incyte and Celera) that collected and organised sequencing information; (iii) the research firms, consisting mainly of the dedicated biotechnology firms that generally did the upstream research but lacked the resources or the ambition to do the downstream product development and marketing; and (iv) the health, agricultural and industrial biotechnology firms. These included the larger vertically integrated dedicated biotechnology firms (for example, Amgen and Genentech) and much longer established businesses, which were mostly pharmaceutical, chemical and life science corporations. Businesses do not necessarily fall into a single category and stay there indefinitely. The information providers, for example, struggled to make money out of information that could be acquired for free elsewhere thanks to the Human Genome Project, and had to diversify to survive.

From genetics to genomics

Crucial as Watson's and Crick's great 1953 breakthrough was, assisted (with little in the way of gratitude at the time) by their seeing Rosalind Franklin's now famous photograph 51 image, it was more of a beginning than an end. At least as important was the discovery in the following decade of how DNA instructs cells to assemble amino acids, which form the building blocks of proteins. In brief, each gene contains the instructions for the synthesis of one or more proteins. Just as proteins consist of chains of amino acids, each gene may be sub-divided into units called codons that comprise three nucleotides and 'code for' (by way of a closely related chemical called ribonucleic acid (RNA)) the preparation of a particular amino acid. These amino acids are then combined in a specified way to form the required protein (that is, the one 'expressed' by the gene).

The fact that DNA rather than proteins was now known to bear the genetic coding did not make the study of proteins less important or new discoveries about them any less revolutionary. Also in the early 1950s, Linus Pauling had successfully worked out the basic rules determining the structures of proteins. This is important because the specificity of different types of protein and the processes by which they form cannot be inferred from their chemical composition alone, but requires one also to understand the three-dimensional form that they assume. This achievement was hugely important:

> Pauling's discovery ... inverted the hierarchy of science. For seventy-five years, researchers had been baffled about whether proteins conformed to discrete shapes and whether those shapes determined their activity. Pauling not only answered with a resounding yes, but detailed all the major motifs by which they were formed... In structure lay function, and what a molecule did determined its importance.[79]

What do we know about DNA now? As molecules go it is enormous. It can be broken up along its length into an almost infinite number of smaller pieces of varying sizes. It can also be pulled across-ways into two separate strands like an unzipped zipper. Sections of DNA can be assembled artificially in a lab. Among the three billion nucleotide bases on each strand are those which form genes. As such, these bases are essential in molecular processes leading to the production of proteins specified according to the order and identity of the nucleotide bases involved. DNA has four such bases: adenine ('A'), cytosine ('C'), guanine ('G'), and tyrosine ('T').

In brief, the coding regions of each gene specify one or more proteins for the cell to synthesise. Proteins comprise an ordered assembly of amino acids of which there are 20 in all. Each of these protein building blocks is added according to a three-part combination of the four nucleotide bases which for DNA are A, C, G and T, and for RNA — which is chemically similar to DNA but much more active in this three billion year-old manufacturing process — are A, C, G and U (for uracil). These three-base long DNA and RNA parts are called codons. If bases can be analogised to letters, codons are the words and as such are the smallest units of meaning in this whole process. Simple arithmetic shows that 64 types of codon are possible: AAA, AAC, ACA, CAA ... and so on. One codon signals the start of the process. This is AUG in eukaryotic cells, which codes for an amino acid called methionine, always the first 'brick' in the under-construction protein. Large proteins may contain vast numbers of amino acids. Others, of which there are three, serve to terminate the process: UAA, UAG and UGA.

Since the Human Genome Project was completed (see below), scientists have been working to identify all of the 20–25,000 or so genes and match them with their associated proteins, that is, the ones 'expressed' by each of the genes. Note here that more than one type of protein can be expressed by a gene as a result of a phenomenon called alternative splicing. Human and animal bodies have more proteins than genes. For a number of reasons, this endeavour is of huge importance for human health and therapeutics. In brief, mutations, in which 'misplaced' bases affect protein production, can have harmful effects that can at one extreme prove fatal, or else may increase susceptibility to certain health problems. Some mutations are inherited, others arise due to the attritional effects of a life well (or badly) lived, or to such insults as exposure to genotoxins ranging from the sun's ultraviolet rays to other natural and industrial chemicals such as heavy metals and some agrochemicals. Unsurprisingly mutations tend to accumulate as one ages, hence the increased risks of cancer as one gets older. Some diseases are caused by single gene defects. Others are directly associated with more than one defective gene. Many diseases are linked to a combination of genetic and environmental factors. Susceptibilities and risk factors identifiable in the human genome are worth knowing about — especially if you can do something in advance to reduce them through lifestyle changes among other possible actions. This is why it is important to understand the human genome in all its variability. Human genetic diversity is narrow compared to most other animals. We are a young species and there has not been sufficient time for isolated human populations to evolve separately. But individual and group variations exist and identifying and analysing those sequences associated with sickness and health can be very useful for example in developing diagnostic and predictive testing services, and in designing better tailored treatment regimes. In addition, linking genes to specific proteins is essential for the production of human protein drugs, such as insulin and monoclonal antibodies in cloned microbes and cultured cells such as those Chinese hamster ovary cells. This is something we ought to be doing better than we are. Africa is where *Homo sapiens* has lived longest and is thus a source of much of the world's genetic diversity, and yet DNA sequencing of Africans has largely been overlooked. As a recent article in the *Financial Times* stated:

Without including the genetic data of Africans, precision medicine, gene editing and other scientific advances risk becoming the province of the white and wealthy. Many genetic tests are already better at predicting breast cancer and type-1 diabetes in patients of European descent than clinical methods, because the tests are based on them.[80]

Thankfully, African scientists are stepping up their engagement in genomic research. But the failure up to now to study and incorporate such a rich source of potentially health-relevant data into genetic studies in which the majority of participants are of European descent is a wider problem for healthcare globally. This unfortunate bias is a major limitation on identifying and enhancing understanding of the full set of associations in existence between genetics and disease.[81]

Genomics refers to the mapping, sequencing and analysis of the full set of genes (that is, the genome) of different organisms or species. Nowadays many species — microbial, plant and animal — have been fully sequenced, but sequencing the human genome has understandably been seen as the most important one and became a massive international endeavour attracting huge funding from governments and foundations, even before we had the technology to be able to do it at any great speed.

The Human Genome Project was launched in 1990 as an international public consortium with the objective of sequencing every one of the three billion nucleotide pairs within the 23 chromosome pairs found in human cells,[82] and publicly disclosing the data for the benefit of science. Given that genes take up only about 3–5 percent of the genome, this was a much more ambitious task than just decoding the then estimated 100,000 or so genes, which in itself would have been a huge undertaking. The organisers expected the work to be completed by 2005.

Initially, two techniques were adopted for the mapping part of the work: physical mapping and gene mapping. Physical mapping involves breaking DNA into multiple fragments using bacterial enzymes called restriction enzymes, inserting them into bacteria or yeast cells, and then matching the overlapping pieces. Gene mapping dates back to the early twentieth century, but had become much more sophisticated in the early 1980s. Around that time, David Botstein at MIT and Ronald Davis at Stanford University, among others, proposed the idea of locating genes along the chromosomes by first randomly seeking out DNA sections which commonly vary between different individuals. These sections are known as markers, and the more of them that can be found the better. By studying families whose members frequently share distinctive traits such as faulty gene-related diseases, scientists can compare incidences of the markers with incidences of the traits. If the two tend to coincide, the responsible gene is likely to be nearby (though still not necessarily all that easy to find). The method considerably aided the search for gene variants (called 'alleles') causing, or increasing susceptibility to, dangerous diseases such as Huntington's chorea, cystic fibrosis and breast cancer. Robert Cook-Deegan describes Botstein and Davis' technique as 'the conceptual engine that drove human genetics from the era of the horse-drawn carriage into the age of the automobile'.[83] The actual sequencing, though, was based on methods pioneered by Frederick Sanger at Cambridge, who used it to sequence a virus in 1977. Interestingly, Craig Venter used similarly automotive and equally hyperbolic language to Cook-Deegan, but applied it instead to describe Sanger's great achievement: 'Sanger's methods had been as critical for genetics as the invention of the wheel or the first steam-powered cars in the seventeenth and eighteenth centuries had been for the automobile industry'.[84] Over time, the process was rapidly accelerated, thanks mainly to the introduction of increasingly fast sequencing machines.

In spite of being an international project, the USA made an extremely large contribution in terms of funding and the actual sequencing work. Britain made the second biggest overall contribution, ahead of France, Japan, Germany and China, which all participated. The Wellcome Trust, a British medical foundation, was one of the biggest single funders of the Project (though well behind the US government) providing £210 million by February 2001, and the Sanger Centre (now the Wellcome Sanger Institute) near Cambridge sequenced a total of eight chromosomes.[85] In fact, the Sanger Centre was the only non-American among the five institutions responsible for 85 percent of the sequencing achieved by October 2000.[86]

From the start, scientists debated priorities, concerned as they were to complete their work as quickly and cheaply as possible. Some felt it would be better to focus first on finding the genes and leave the whole genome sequencing for later. Others disagreed. Although many scientists went on to seek out, map and sequence genes, the whole genome strategy carried the day. As for methods, the first controversy[87] took place in 1991. A scientist at the National Institutes of Health called Craig Venter, eager to sequence and map protein coding regions of the genome, adopted a short-cut method of identifying genes using so-called expressed sequence tags (ESTs). The EST method takes advantage of the established principle that messenger RNA can be converted back to DNA using an enzyme called reverse transcriptase. Messenger RNA ('mRNA' for short) is the chemical that relays the genetic code from the nucleus to the site in the cell (the ribosome) where it is translated for the assembly of the protein-forming amino acids. The result of applying reverse transcriptase is a substance called complementary DNA (often shortened to 'cDNA'). Essentially, cDNA has the same sequence as the gene but without the non-coding nucleotide regions: the introns. By sequencing the ends of these pieces of cDNA, one obtains partially encoded gene fragments called ESTs. When stretches of RNA are extracted from specialised cells, such as brain cells, the ESTs derived from them can help to identify genes that are useful in the functioning of that particular cell or the organ of which it forms a part. Of course, the EST short-cut strategy does not provide the full gene sequence. Neither can an EST in itself provide enough information to indicate the function of the related gene. For these reasons, the strategy immediately attracted criticism from some quarters.

But what was even more controversial than the method itself was that in 1991 and 1992, the NIH filed patent applications claiming rights over thousands of ESTs. This move was condemned not only by other agencies involved in the Project but also by the Human Genome Organization, which had been set up by scientists to coordinate the project internationally. Even representatives of the biotechnology sector condemned the move. James Watson famously described NIH's actions as 'sheer lunacy' and resigned from his position at the NIH, where he was head of the Office of Human Genome Research and in this position the de facto leader of the international Project. The Medical Research Council decided in its wisdom to respond by also filing similar patent applications. In 1994, the NIH withdrew its appeal against the Patent and Trademark Office's initial rejection of its applications and agreed, as did the MRC, to no longer patent gene fragments having no known function.[88]

By 1998, the Human Genome Project had made considerable progress, although only 3–5 percent of the genome had actually been sequenced. This does not sound impressive, but the expectation from the start was that sequencing would accelerate quite rapidly in the final years. In May of that year a rival was to appear in the form of a new company called Celera Genomics that was headed by Craig Venter, who had since left the NIH. Celera was set up by a company called Perkin-Elmer which also owned Applied Biosystems, the leading producer of automated DNA sequencing machines. Armed with an initial investment of $75 million from Perkin-Elmer and an array of these machines, Celera got to work. The approach adopted was the so-called 'whole-genome shotgun strategy', which would entail breaking the human genome into tens of millions of fragments, sequencing the pieces about 10 times over (a plan that was subsequently scaled down by nearly half) and then reassembling them.

On 26 June 2000, at the White House in the presence of President Clinton, Craig Venter and Francis Collins, director of the NIH's National Human Genome Research Institute and coordinator of the public project, temporarily put aside their differences to announce jointly that they had ordered most of the full genome sequence. This was really just a public relations stunt, since the public project had only sequenced 90 percent of the genome and was just a 'rough draft'. And as Celera's 'first assembly' was only available to subscribers, Venter's claim to have a more complete version was not something that could be publicly verified.

In February 2001, the International Human Genome Sequencing Consortium that was implementing the public project and Celera both announced they had compiled almost complete human genetic sequences by publishing detailed reports of their work in *Nature*[89] and in *Science*.[90] The two reports came up with considerably reduced estimates of the total number of human genes as compared with the commonly cited figure of around 100,000.[91] The Consortium's estimated number was 30,000–40,000. Celera's was 26,000–38,000. An important implication of the reduced figure is that, since there are many more proteins than there are genes and not all genes code for proteins, many of those that do must be able somehow to generate (or help to generate) more than one protein. Another interesting finding was that a substantial proportion of the genome was of viral origin.

Despite being controversial at the time, Venter's and Celera's entry into the race was probably a good thing both for science and for the public domain however people might have felt at the time. First, the competition forced both entrants to commit themselves to rapid sequencing. A major consequence is that the public project completed its work earlier than it would otherwise have done, and the scientific community had not just one but two versions of the human genome sequence to choose from. Second, fears that Celera would adopt an aggressive privatisation strategy increased the public consortium's determination to make all its sequence data available as soon as it was generated. Indeed, doing this made Celera's original business model based on the provision of genetic data completely unworkable. However, there is evidence that Celera's intellectual property management strategy, which was largely contract-based rather than patent-dependent, was actually a hindrance to scientific research and product development.[92]

Apart from being a huge feat in itself, the mapping and sequencing of the human genome is certain to be a tremendously useful source of information for biomedical scientists for years to come, and of course for industry. At quite an early stage, data provided by the public consortium helped in the identification of about 30 diseases linked to faulty genes.[93] And knowing more about human genes and proteins should substantially increase the number of drug targets for drug discovery research.

All that said, the lack of early commercial and therapeutic spinoffs of the Human Genome Project was disappointing to many. One should not have been too surprised by this delay in the much hoped-for development of new health products. Human bodies at the molecular level are of course complex enough. Just knowing the order of the three billion nucleotide couplings cannot possibly be immediately translatable into medical solutions. Turning genetic code into medically-relevant information is difficult for many reasons not least of which is the almost baroque complexity of the human genome, defying simplistic views that genes code very specifically and exclusively for this or that protein, and the rest of the genome other than the protein-coding regions (that is, the genes) is mere 'junk' that is unworthy of study.[94] And this is even before you start to look into individual human variation. As mentioned before, a very necessary area for follow on work would be to identify, not the sameness of individual genomes, but their variability, hence the need, for example, of the HapMap Project described in the next chapter. This follow-on work has cost vast amounts of money and generated staggering amounts of data out of which bioinformaticians and others strive to glean patterns, connections and insights that can contribute to better healthcare. But we have a long way to go until we have discovered everything there is to know.

Ontologically, the main feature about DNA making it unique is that it has a dual nature being both a physical object and containing, or even itself being, information. Accordingly, it fits neatly within a wider perspective on life: that life itself is an information system. The idea that biological molecules and molecular processes can be defined in informational terms is hardly new. As we saw earlier, when Ernest Starling coined the word 'hormones' in 1905, he immediately referred to them as 'chemical messengers'.[95] From this, many are inclined to take the next step, which is to understand cells and organisms as highly sophisticated information-processing systems which are capable of being harnessed, reconstructed and improved for our benefit, the genome being the instruction manual. In reality, DNA sequences cannot be characterised as a how-to guide with instructions for making proteins correctly (or incorrectly in the case of mutant versions) as if they are a recipe, car repair manual, or flat-pack furniture assembly leaflet. If only things were that simple.

In reality, biology is not information technology, and there is no programmer — only natural selection. Life is far too complicated to be reducible in this sense, or in any other. As two firm critics of information talk in biology explain, just as planets do not 'compute their orbits around the sun' but just blindly go round elliptically according to the laws of physics, cells cannot 'compute' in any kind of intentional way.[96] Furthermore, complicated as genomes are, their informational value is limited. They simply cannot explain everything about such phenomena as growth and development. While a direct relationship can clearly be made between a codon (as we saw above, a three-base sequence) and a specific amino acid, that is about as far as one can go in treating DNA sequences as *pure* information, and even then that tells the cell little about what protein to assemble and how to do it properly so it folds in the right way.

There is in fact some considerable conceptual distance between a lengthy sequence of bases and a correctly folded protein; even more between those base 'letters' and a whole functional, or dysfunctional, cell or organism. The sheer complexity, subtlety, context-dependence and informational-incompleteness of DNA requires us to cast a sceptical eye on the view that genes may be treated as instructional texts using four letters and 64 words comprising all the necessary information for the cell or organism to use. It may be reasonable to say that cellular machinery 'reads off' the DNA 'code', but this does not make the genome an instruction manual for the cell; nor does disease causation become merely a search for typographical errors. It is far more complicated than that. That said, genomic variability between groups of people and individuals is well worth studying and, as we will see, there has been a great deal of research done in this area.

New cell therapies

The era of small molecule drugs is certainly not over. And yet as we have seen the market share captured by biologics has grown markedly in recent years. Another highly promising development is the new gene and cell therapies. Perhaps the most prominent are treatments comprising the use of human stem cells that are transformed into therapeutic cells to replace those that people normally have in their bodies but are not being produced, leading to sickness. Humans possess about 200 different kinds of cell. Since all except red blood cells contain in their nuclei each person's entire genome without variation, it follows that the kind they are depends on which genes are activated and which are 'switched off'. All cells in the body are descended from undifferentiated cells that first appear in the fertilised egg once cell division has started. These are stem cells, so called because it is from them that all other cell types branch out. When a fertilised human egg (zygote) starts to divide, each cell has the potential to develop into an entire human being with placenta. This cellular capability, called totipotency, exists for the first three divisions.

Once eight cells have become 16 this potential diminishes somewhat. These then pluripotent cells can develop into all cell types but no placenta or umbilical cord can form. This means that developing into a fully-fledged individual human from the separate growth of a single cell is no longer possible but in all respects these cells can still be converted into any somatic human cell. This makes them scientifically useful, and medically too for such purposes as regenerative treatments, drug testing and for basic research into human development, both normal and abnormal. For scientists, the property of pluripotency is what the philosopher's stone was to alchemists — something that converts the most basic and universal units of human life into precious cellular gold and silver.

After five days, the zygote has graduated to a blastocyst which looks under a microscope rather like an open clam, the 'shell' being the outer cell mass, and the 'fish' the inner cell mass. By that time the latter is a rich source of pluripotent cells that can be cultured in a laboratory. Although scientific definitions of 'embryo' vary to some extent, zygotes, blastocysts and morulas (those in the stage between the two) are all generally considered to be embryos in different states of development.[97] So, by most definitions a blastocyst is an embryo but it has not yet implanted in the womb, and neither are the cells differentiated. Differentiation takes place from about 14 days, from when splitting into twins becomes impossible. Of course, it takes longer still for the embryo to have any consciousness or feeling. Obviously, despite their genetic similarities, twins are completely different people. It follows from this obvious fact, and the total absence of a brain and nervous system, that the early-stage embryo is not yet a human being and arguably is not one for some time afterwards. Worldwide, 14 days tends to serve as the limit beyond which interventionist research becomes illegal. However, following reports of scientists keeping embryos alive *in vitro* for almost that length of time, some have argued for a reconsideration with a view to possibly extending the allowed term so as to learn more about human development.[98]

It is important to understand that 'Embryonic Stem Cells' (ES cells) are *in vitro* cell cultures (cell lines) from a single source — they are derived from embryos rather than being embryonic cells themselves. Accordingly, they are not cells existing in blastocysts but laboratory 'products' kept in artificial conditions to keep on dividing without differentiating for as long as possible so that cells can continue to be 'harvested' over time for experimentation and use. They are of course descended from the original cells obtained from the inner cell mass of a blastocyst but they are not the same ones due to the continuous process of division and subdivision. The embryo itself is destroyed in the process of extraction. What is controversial about all this is not just that embryos are destroyed but that they are being used at all for purposes that may be of medical benefit to patients but at the expense of foreclosing the potential that the destroyed embryo had while alive to develop into one (or more) people. It is others who will derive any advantage from their use. While it is possible to snip out a single cell from an early-stage embryo for examination without affecting its integrity, this is not yet a viable approach to producing an ES cell line.

Health benefits in terms of regenerative medicine and other fields of healthcare are largely for the future. However, some treatments have been used with success. Thus, the *New Scientist* reported on 25 May 2013 as follows:

> A man blinded by the degeneration of his retinal cells has had his sight restored in one eye after receiving a stem cell treatment. Human embryonic stem cells were turned into retinal pigment epithelial cells and then transplanted into his retina, as part of a trial by Advanced Cell Technology in Marlborough, Massachusetts.

Different countries adopt a range of positions on how far they support and the ways they regulate the development and use of ES cells. The European Commission funds stem cell research but it must be legal in the country where it is to be done. It is in fact illegal in Poland and Lithuania. Where legal it must also use leftover embryos from IVF. The reason is that these would ultimately be destroyed anyway. Currently, the UK, Belgium and Sweden allow creation of new embryos for research, whereas in Germany to do so is a criminal offence. Much research takes place in the United States where the first methods of deriving stem cell lines from human embryos were invented. However, the 1996 Dickey-Wicker Amendment bans federal funding for 'research in which a human embryo or embryos are destroyed'.

Government-funded research must use existing cell lines. Accordingly, the National Institutes of Health Guidelines for Human Stem Cell Research, 2009, permits funding as long as research 'utilizes cells from lines: (1) created by *in vitro* fertilization for reproductive purposes, (2) no longer needed for that purpose, and (3) voluntarily donated by the individuals who owned them.'

There are adult stem cells too. For example, haematopoietic stem cells in our bone marrow can differentiate into the various blood cells but not into other types of cell. These have been used medically for some time now for patients with certain bone marrow and immune system disorders that can be treated by the transplantation of these cells. But adult stem cells are a lot less versatile, forming at most a limited number of related cell types.

The science is moving rapidly and it gets harder to speak of inevitabilities and impossibilities. Scientists mostly in Japan have found out how to reprogram adult cells into pluripotent stem cells. These are known as Induced Pluripotent Stem cells (iPS cells). Compared to ES cells, use of these has both advantages and disadvantages. Because they may be derived from the cells of a patient-donor they may counter the problem of 'foreign' cell rejection and enhance personalised health care. They also do not require destruction of embryos, which may allay some of the ethical concerns. On the other hand, they may be less stable and effective than ES cells. There are also possible dangers in the use of retroviruses to deliver the genetic factors that induce the pluripotency, with the possibility of causing tumours. Other methods are in development and research is ongoing to find the safest and most effective one.[99] A new safer method was announced in January 2014 but was subsequently retracted. The first patient trials using cells derived from two patients receiving treatment took place in Japan in 2014, but they were discontinued a year later.

There has also been some success in deriving stem cells from cloned human embryos, which may possibly resolve some ethical concerns too. In 2014, scientific teams in South Korea and United States used the 'Dolly technique' to derive ES cells lines from skin cells donated by two men,[100] and to transform ES cells into insulin-producing cells using cells donated by a diabetic woman.[101] Of course, the fact that the embryos' genomes are identical to the adult donors' still makes them embryos no more nor less than if they were not cloned. Moreover, the enucleated eggs still had to come from somewhere.

In cancer especially, there is a great interest in immunotherapy as an alternative to the conventional approach of identifying a cytotoxin that is as specific as possible. The latter has of course led to successful treatments. Immunotherapy seeks to utilise and — ideally — improve the defensive abilities inherent to the body's immune system. The two are not necessarily in opposition. MAbs can be used as an immunotherapy, helping the immune system target cancer cells by attaching to them, or targeting the immune system itself by inhibiting proteins in the body that stop attacks on cancer cells ('checkpoint inhibitors'). As we will see below, ADCs are hybrids representing something of a halfway house between the two.

One highly promising approach is so-called Chimeric Antigen Receptor cell therapy, typically abbreviated to CAR-T. It has proven highly effective for some people. Here, T cells are taken from patients' blood and genetically engineered *ex vivo* in order to express the right antigen receptor specific to the type of blood cancer affecting the patient. They are then multiplied and returned to the patient's body. As an individualised treatment, it is complex, staggeringly expensive, may have potentially serious side-effects, and it only works so far for a limited number of blood cancers. The treatment is available only at certified health centres. Solid tumours are not yet treatable using this technology. Only two have been approved so far: Novartis's Kymriah (tisagenlecleucel) and Kite Pharma's Yescarta (axicabtagene ciloleucel). Kite is a specialised cancer immunotherapy company founded only in 2009 that was acquired by Gilead in October 2017, the same month that the FDA approved Yescarta. But it is likely that there will be more to come.

Personalisation, Digital Medicine and Precision Drugs

Modern-day healthcare is becoming increasingly information intensive including at the personal level. The intervention of data and informatics in medicine, including pharmaceuticals and diagnostic and predictive tests, is often referred to as digital medicine.[102] The genomic data made available by the Human Genome Project gave this trend a great deal of impetus as did the more recent emergence of big data analytics alongside unprecedented computing power including artificial intelligence, enabling the generation of useful health-relevant information out of vast genomic and other datasets. But as was explained earlier, genomic data alone is far from being enough. However, digitally recorded and annotated genetic and other molecular information acquired from large numbers of people, especially when combined with other information (lifestyle, family, personal electronic health history records etc.), can provide not only a massive volume of health related data for analysis, but also diversity in kinds of information we can derive, from responsiveness to drugs, to likelihood of contracting particular diseases, and ways to prevent or reduce risk of certain diseases later in life.

It is not just healthcare in the broad sense that is moving onto computer screens; medicine is becoming digital as much as it is chemical, especially when healthcase nowadays focuses so much on disease prediction, diagnosis, prognosis, and monitoring of sickness, health and treatment effects and side-effects, and of course with personalisation. The role of the drug is still quite central to a great deal of patient care. But prescribing a drug with a generalised instruction as to how much to take and when, except for minor ailments like colds, is becoming insufficient. According to one article on the subject, 'the patient is an enormous repository of information that needs to be harvested as a partnership not only in clinical care but in discovery... The ability to stratify the phenotypic expression of wellness and disease will ultimately lead to better validation of human therapeutic targets for drug discovery.'[103]

As any evolutionary biologist will tell you, inherited individual variability is essential for natural selection to work and drive evolution. Individual molecular-level variation is also highly relevant in the design and selection of precisely targeted medical interventions too, something we have come to appreciate more and more. Some variations that matter, such as rare mutations, may be possessed by just a few individuals; some by large groups of people.

It is well known that a powerful drug in a particular dosage can cure one person with minor or no side-effects, whereas the same dosage may not work on another person, cause harmful side-effects, or even endanger a patient's life. Being able to accurately predict how an individual will respond to a drug treatment and what the optimal mode of delivery should be for that person is very important, but it requires further research including the gathering of data big enough in volume and breadth of coverage to generate findings enabling precise and individualised treatment including the discovery of biomarkers.

Indeed, the word 'biomarker' is increasingly part of the discourse of modern medical research including personalised medicine, denoting 'a broad subcategory of medical signs — that is, objective indications of medical state observed from outside the patient — which can be measured accurately and reproducibly.'[104] It is a somewhat broad term. Traditional physiological biomarkers include blood pressure and pulse rate, but nowadays the most valuable ones to discover (and patent) are molecular including proteins, metabolites and gene sequences. They are hugely important as we move forward:

> Biomarkers and molecular individualized medicine are replacing the traditional 'one size fits all' medicine.... The essence of personalized oncology lies in the use of biomarkers.... Three different types of biomarkers are of particular importance: predictive, prognostic and early response ... Molecular diagnostics identify individual cancer patients who are more likely to respond positively to targeted chemotherapies. Molecular diagnostics include testing for genes, gene expression, proteins and metabolites.[105]

Precisely targeted treatments are based not just on significant genotypic characteristics of people but also on greater specificity as to the medical condition that the person has, or is at risk of having. One interesting aspect of our enhanced understanding of how cellular malfunctions lead to disease is that some disease categories are fragmenting so that out of what was once considered a single disease arise several or many diseases. (This is something we touched on in Chapter 3.) And out of one patient population sharing the same disease and being given the same treatment there may become several patient populations being treated for different, albeit closely related, diseases; or even patient sub-populations forming a larger population all having the same diseases but who need to be given either a completely different treatment, or a different dose or formulation of the same one. This latter observation leads us to two other forms of the complexification phenomenon we looked into earlier: first, the links between genomic variation and human health and disease;[106] and second, the differences between people having the same disease in terms of how they respond to the same treatment.

Lumping or splitting of people for the purposes of personalised treatment, not just medicines but dosage regimens for that drug, is matched by the lumping and splitting of diseases and categories of disease that we saw in Chapter 3. Instances of both exist. The latest version of the International Classification of Diseases brings together sexual health conditions that were previously classified separately.[107] But of the two, splitting seems to be more common, so the trend is to start off with some and progressively increase to more or many: patient type (which affect their treatment), medicines (for a disease that is narrowly defined, perhaps carved out of one previously more broadly applied), dosage regimens (such as 5 mg a day rather than 10 mg according to the individual), and diseases.

With regard to the latter, diseases of the blood, a catchall term a century ago, was split into leukaemia and lymphoma. As we saw in Chapter 3, nearly 40 leukaemias are now recognised as are over 50 lymphomas. So out of one disease, many can arise. Molecular analysis of variations in breast cancer tumours, for example, has revealed numerous sub-groups of the disease, and, as the authors of one key study claim, these findings 'provide a novel molecular stratification of the breast cancer population'.[108] The hope is that this will lead to more precise treatments to patients. According to Joe Gray and Brian Druker from the Oregon Health and Science University writing in the same issue of *Nature* as the above quote: 'the promise still remains that the precision with which breast cancers are diagnosed and managed will be improved by the identification of new drug targets and by the ability to assign cancers to molecular subtypes that are associated with effective treatments. This is being made possible only by the remarkable advances in measurement science and computational capability.'[109] There is also category re-lumping: diseases can be moved from one category where they are presently lumped to another one, such as stroke which is now a neurological disorder rather than one of the circulatory system, where it was previously placed.

If the scale of the business stakes is not already apparent, human molecular variability is very important to understand for another major commercial reason. Available medicines in many therapeutic areas are actually not very good even if they are very effective for some people. For every Glivec there are numerous products that do little for the majority of people who take them. According to a recent study not one of the ten bestselling drugs in the United States helps the majority of patients who are given them. In fact, they benefit only 'between 1 in 25 and 1 in 4 of the people who take them. For some drugs, such as statins — routinely used to lower cholesterol — as few as 1 in 50 may benefit.'[110] In a 2001 article on pharmacogenetics, the authors found efficacy rates of major medicines in several areas to be very low: a 25 percent efficacy rate in oncology, 30 percent in Alzheimer's, 47 percent for hepatitis C virus, and 48 percent in osteoporosis to give a few examples.[111] In addition, adverse drug reactions can cause deaths. Doubtless, some of these figures have improved in the years since then. For example, there are now medicines that can completely rid the body of the hepatitis C virus, and thereby cure the disease.

Is this a low-quality issue, or are there less negative ways to assess these apparently rather unspectacular treatments — in the sense of their disappointing efficacy rates? It may be fairer to say they are as good as they can be given the state of knowledge. If you do not know anything relevant about the individual patient that would enable the tailoring of the treatment to the person, you need to have a generalised treatment and dosage regimen that as such will not take individual molecular variability into account, and the likelihood is that responses will vary. Moreover, all medicines are 'for' an illness, obviously; but do we really know everything about the disease category for which the product is designated? A single disease may in fact be better subdivided into a series of related diseases each of which requires different therapeutic responses whether in the form of radically different drugs or alternative dosages or formulations of the same ones. If this is true, is the off-the-peg style of drug development now outmoded and ready for replacement by made-to-measure drugs? And if so, can drugs for the same disease still be cut from the same cloth or is it going to be a case of diverse treatment for different people having the same disease? As we will see in this chapter, the questions go beyond these rather simplistic ones. Note that I am not just talking about the science. How can firms make money from treatments that will be given to only some patients out of a much bigger population having a particular disease? And stratifying and personalising patients by drug responsiveness is not the end of it. It is no good giving the right sort of drug in the right amount to the right sort of patient if it is for the wrong version of the same disease. This is a serious issue in cancer which researchers over the years have been splitting into ever more cancers. Again, how can businesses make money from patients having a highly specific disease affecting very people that is part of a 'family' of diseases previously thought to be one single disease? The fact is that they can. Glivec (see below) bears this out amply. It may be possible too to make a great deal of money from turning a mediocre medicine prescribed for a large population of patients into an outstanding medicine for a selected few. In an article published several years ago in *Nature Biotechnology*, the author had this to say: 'personalized medicine is becoming a viable option, most notably in oncology, owing to its capacity to rescue drug candidates that would otherwise be doomed because they are of equivocal clinical utility.'[112] This is very true.

Personalised medicine is frequently held to be a very promising development that could dramatically enhance the health of millions of people. Under one definition, personalised medicine

> refers to the tailoring of medical treatment to the individual characteristics of each patient; to classify individuals into subpopulations that differ in their susceptibility to a particular disease or their response to a specific treatment so that preventive or therapeutic interventions can then be concentrated on those who will benefit, sparing expense and side effects for those who will not.[113]

There are those who doubt that the anticipated transformative effects of personalised medicine on healthcare will all come to pass, and that there is a certain amount of overhype.[114] And of course, not all of this turn to big data is convenient for industry. There is a genuine possibility, for example, that it can reveal links between a commercially successful drug and health risks for some people that would otherwise be very hard to detect. Nonetheless, the commercial benefits of finding biomarkers enabling a subset of patients to be selected whose response rates will be much better than the average and whose lives will not be endangered by a medicine, is fairly clear even when we consider that identifying such smaller patient groups shrinks the number of users of the medicine until new indications can be identified, and could result in withdrawal of the product from the market.

Before going further, it is important to place personalised medicine in context. Personalised medicine is in fact one aspect of the efforts currently being made by biomedical scientists and industry to enhance targeting of disease to achieve better health outcomes for more people. Personalised medicine deals with the tailoring of treatments in a way that responds to the variability of human beings, and to the fact that single diseases may really be families of sub-diseases. It implies individualisation of medical intervention but whereas it does involve the testing of people for certain biomarkers conveying diagnostic or therapy-related information, those biomarkers are typically ones shared with other people. Thus some prefer the term stratified medicine which makes it plainer that the focus is on those shared traits that are meaningful as far as medical intervention goes. All well and good, but attempts to stratify must be done with a certain amount of care, as BiDiL demonstrates (see box).

BiDiL: A racial drug?

The case of a medicine called BidiL, a combination of isosorbide dinitrate and hydralazine, is an intriguing and highly controversial one in this context, in which race, a sociological concept, is essentially used as a stratification marker.[115] In 1997, the FDA rejected a combination of hydralazine and isosorbite dinitrate, the subject matter of a US patent granted in 1989 as a general heart failure treatment. That might have been the end of the story: yet another medicine that failed to make the grade. What happened in the meantime? A few relevant clinical trials were undertaken, not just of the isosorbide dinitrate and hydralazine combination but also of two standard treatments: enalapril, a type of ACE inhibitor, and bucindolol, a beta blocker. These found that enalapril and bucindolol are medically efficient for 'white' patients but not for 'black' patients.[116] The authors of one report on these trials concluded by suggesting 'that the overall population

(*Continued*)

of black patients with heart failure may be underserved by current thera-peutic recommendations'[117] and that 'therapeutic recommendations may need to be tailored according to racial background'. A final trial was conducted exclusively on patients self-identifying as 'black' one group of whom were given the isosorbide dinitrate and hydralazine treatment with standard therapies (including ACE inhibitors), and the other given a placebo also with standard therapies. A report on this trial concluded thus: 'the addition of a fixed dose of isosorbide dinitrate plus hydralazine to standard therapy for heart failure including neurohormonal blockers is efficacious and increases survival among black patients with advanced heart failure.'[118] On this basis the medicine was approved by the FDA. This was even though trials had not demonstrated clinically that patient response rate to the combination product was affected by the ethnicity of the patient.

Let us turn to the follow-on US patent granted in 2002.[119] This was a methods of treatment patent rather than one on a product. Patenting the combined product was not possible because the chemical combination had been disclosed in the earlier patent granted 13 years earlier by one of the same inventors, and the two constituent substances were already known and in medical use. Looking first at the abstract, reference is made to African Americans. However, the patent specification and the claims make 75 references to 'black patients', with 'black' referring 'to a person of African descent or an African-American person'. Medically this all seems rather imprecise as a criterion for patient stratification. Indeed, researchers were unable to identify any reliable physiological or molecular biomarker. Despite this, FDA approval was given that would otherwise not have been granted for this product. The question arises of whether the aim of targeting black or African American people is purely commercial, and perhaps rather cynical, given that it lacks a proper scientific basis yet has justified, albeit rather shakily, the grant of a patent on something that seems not to be new in any genuine way. One might have expected marketing authorisation to have required further testing including to figure out how it interacts with the human body to produce a desirable effect on a specific biomarker-defined group of people but not on others.[120]

While digital medicine is clearly highly promising, and biodigital convergence seems to be an inevitable process, there is a tendency among some to overhype the information/data sciences as if traditional biology which highlights the 'thing-ness' of life and living processes is bound to be pushed to the sidelines. Yet reducing biology to digital information may not entirely be feasible. Organisms are far more complex than any human artefact, as are individual cells. Understanding and manipulating living processes such as cell metabolism are inherently empirical tasks, and they continue to require the input of conceptual systems and scientific approaches lying beyond the reach of today's digital technologies and analogies, such as biology, chemistry, clinical medicine, and physiology among other disciplines. In fact, no single discipline or conceptual system is sufficient by itself to make entire sense of cellular phenomena. As I suggested earlier in this chapter, the latter may be capable of being described in informational (or for that matter chemical) language — or even as being information itself — but only incompletely. It follows that juridical and regulatory authorities, who are already struggling to deal with biotechnology, should feel their way cautiously rather than embrace paradigms whose potentials and limits are not entirely clear thus far. Nonetheless, it remains the case that digital technologies are being applied in the life sciences and have been tremendously useful in, for example, enabling the sequencing, annotation, and even the synthesis of whole genomes.[121] The hype is not entirely unjustified either. But it would be a grave mistake to treat big data science and information and digital technologies as if they, and they alone, embody the future for medicine.

Precision medicine has emerged in the United States as an aspirational concept, alongside personalised medicine but is in my view different in terms of emphasis. The word 'precision' seems to imply the idea of the 'magic bullet', the smart drug that forcefully hits the right target head on and without collateral damage. Rational drug design is nothing new, Sir James Black's greatest achievements discussed earlier being classic examples. But precision medicine promises to make pinpoint accuracy in pharmaceutical design increasingly a routine achievement. This is extremely important for cancer where existing medicines, having to be toxic to the targeted cell but needing to avoid hitting the normal cells as well but often failing to do so, tend to have a very narrow therapeutic window. This makes treatment frequently a highly unpleasant experience and not always effective.

Glivec, a small-molecular medicine that likewise manifests high design of the purest gold, perhaps as much at least as any other, is a prime example of a precision medicine, and has a fascinating back-story bringing up interesting questions about credit, learning-trails, and drug company decisions on whether or not to market a product and at what price.

Making Glivec: An excursion or a long and winding road?

It is a common cliché that drug research and development is a linear one-way process in which one molecule in 10,000 will enter the market 10–15 years after its discovery, the discovery of the successful molecule marking the start of the trail, and the end being the placement of the approved drug on the market. This is in fact misleading nonsense. Every drug is different and each has its own story. The learning trails from the initial find (or set of initial finds) to a product or class of pharmaceutical products is frequently long and complex, especially long in the case of aspirin. Enormous lengths of time may elapse between the finding or rediscovery of some early and barely discernible clue, and the marketing of a pharmaceutical product whose therapeutic use may in fact be quite different. Trails have no obvious end, since one product leads to another. Trails may branch off in some very fruitful directions, possibly before any product has been developed, and also merge with others. Alternatively, one might suggest the complexity of research progress has more in common with trees having many spreading branches than with thoroughfares. Drug discovery and development processes clearly defy simple models. As we will see later, the Glivec learning trail — if we are to continue to use path-related metaphors — can apparently be traced to 1960. And yet, Peter Nowell, writing five decades after his famous discovery, extends the trail commonly assumed to begin with him and his co-discoverer further back to nineteenth century German pathologists and, among others, a biologist called Theodore Boveri, citing his work published in Germany in 1914.[122]

In 2003, then Novartis CEO Daniel Vasella published a book in praise of the great scientific and therapeutic achievement that is imatinib, or Glivec to give its trade name (as well as of his own company).[123] Undoubtedly it was an extraordinary attainment, historic even. Its

(Continued)

(Continued)

specificity and curative impact make it a major advance in cancer therapeutics. Arguably, it was the first anti-cancer weapon in the pharmaceutical armoury resembling the precision drugs envisaged by Paul Ehrlich over a century ago, to which the book's title clearly alludes.

But whose achievement was it really? Reading the front pages of the relevant patents helps us little. If we look at the original United States patent on Glivec,[124] only one person is named as inventor: Jürg Zimmermann of Ciba-Geigy, the company that merged with Sandoz to form Novartis in 1996. When we turn to the later US patent on the crystalline form held in India to be unpatentable, Zimmermann is joined by two Novartis colleagues, Bertrand Sutter and Hans Michael Bürger.[125]

Detailed published accounts of Glivec's discovery and development exemplify the lengthy, highly complex and collaborative nature of successful product conceptualisation, discovery and development in research intensive business sectors. Two people loom especially large in accounts, albeit not so much in Vasella's, neither of whom is named as inventor on the patents: Nicholas Lydon, who worked on Glivec for Ciba-Geigy in the 1980s and 90s and has become something of an international celebrity of pharmaceutical science for his crucial contribution; and the even more renowned Brian Druker, who did not work for the company. I once took up the issue of who invented Glivec with a senior member of Novartis's patent team, and to him the inventor was Zimmermann. Fair enough: his name is on the patents. However, he had not even heard of Lydon and Druker. This is despite the fact that both Lydon and Druker, but not Zimmermann, were esteemed enough to be awarded prestigious international prizes for Glivec from the Japan Prize Foundation (also with Janet Rowley), the Lasker Foundation (with Charles Sawyers, one of Druker's collaborators), and the Warren Alpert Foundation (with Baltimore, Matter and Witte).

The fact of Novartis's possession of Glivec is a matter for law, specifically patents and trademarks. In many countries this possession is pretty watertight. But *owning* a drug product is a separate matter from the question of whether the owner-company was the sole actor in bringing the drug into existence. The Glivec case exemplifies this point; at least it does if we think of it as something more than a molecule that just happened to have been synthesised in a company lab and then found to work. Vasella's statement in

(*Continued*)

his book, whose purpose clearly includes promoting his company, that 'when people dispute who should get credit for the discovery of a drug, nothing good can emerge'[126] seems right: the dispute between those credited with insulin was undoubtedly unfortunate, for example. But the fact he gives so much of the credit to Novartis and its scientists suggests it is also quite a convenient position to take in this case. Scathingly, a reviewer in the prestigious *Journal of the American Medical Association* dismissed the book as 'essentially a puff piece for Novartis'.[127]

Novartis's scientists *were* essential and the company invested a substantial sum of money in the research and development that made Glivec possible. But chronic myeloid leukaemia patients would never have received a product called Glivec if they had had to rely solely on Novartis and its highly competent teams of scientists. For the general public, and no doubt for many journalists and news reporters, the patent holding company and the named inventors are the ones that made the invention and this in turn implies some moral authority on the part of the firm in question. For the company it is obviously convenient for people to make such assumptions.

Credit is a devilishly tricky matter to be objective about. Effort, dedication, inspiration, vision, ambition, intuition, counter-intuition, advanced technical knowledge in one or more discipline, skill, serendipity, networking abilities, and sheer bloody-mindedness are all extremely relevant factors. Read together, the various accounts of the Glivec story bring together a large cast of players and numerous locations most of which are very distant from the Swiss city of Basel where Novartis is headquartered.[128] The cast expands as do the geographical locations in those accounts which take a longer and wider view that embraces the initial conceptualisation of chronic myeloid leukaemia as a disease ripe for targeting with a small molecule.[129] That is to say, those stories that treat Glivec, not merely as a chemical made in a laboratory, but as the highest point to date in a long and winding historical tale; one that begins in 1960 with a foundational discovery by two United States-based scientists of a chromosomal defect which they suggested at the time had a 'causal relationship' with 'chronic granulocytic leukemia'.[130] The impactful nature of the discovery turned out to be far greater than one might have assumed from the modest length of their article reporting it, of three paragraphs taking up less than half a page. According

(*Continued*)

(Continued)

to a well-known leukaemia specialist called Emil Freireich, 'It's three hundred words and it revolutionized everything'. Before we had Glivec, but essential to its existence, Nowell and Hungerford's discovery was followed by a series of insights from universities in several countries that built on this initial finding. Most appeared long before there was ever a Glivec but they were nonetheless essential to its eventual existence.

Here is a timeline of all the significant achievements and events.

1960 — Peter Nowell and David Hungerford identify chromosomal defect that becomes known as the 'Philadelphia chromosome' after its place of discovery, and in their article postulate a 'causal relationship between the chromosome abnormality observed and chronic granulocytic leukemia'.

1973 — Janet Rowley identifies specific location of the chromosomal translocation comprising a fusion of genes normally on separate chromosomes.

1982 — Scientists in Netherlands isolate the abl gene, which codes for the Abelson (ABL) protein.

1984 — The same team isolates the Breakpoint Cluster Region (bcr) gene which fuses with abl in individuals possessing the Philadelphia chromosome.

Mid 1980s — Alex Matter and Nicholas Lydon at Ciba-Geigy start work on kinase inhibitors.

1986 — Matter and Lydon find skeletal chemical structure that binds to protein kinases and controls function. Zimmermann makes multiple variants and Buchdunger tests *in vitro* for toxicity and solubility. Enhanced specificity achieved.

Late 1980s — Lydon meets Brian Druker and they attempt to set up collaboration between Ciba-Geigy and Dana-Farber Cancer Institute in USA to conduct tests on patients. Initially unsuccessful.

1987 — David Baltimore proves the chromosomal defect causes CML; with Owen Witte discovers that abl-brc codes for a kinase enzyme and that it is causing unregulated cell divisions.

1990 — George Daley (in Baltimore's lab) proves bcr-abl can cause CML by itself.

(*Continued*)

Early 1990s — Lydon successfully tests on kinases.

1993 — Lydon informs Druker of highly specific molecule find. Arrangement made between Ciba-Geigy and Oregon Health Science University (where Druker now works).

1996 — Druker publishes promising test results in *Nature Medicine*. Druker and Lydon two main authors with Zimmermann and Buchdunger added as co-authors.

1998 — Novartis send Druker enough Glivec to test on 100 patients.

2001 (May 10) — US Food and Drug Administration approves Glivec. Subsequently priced at $2,000 to $2,400 per month.

2003 — Novartis announces Glivec reached $1 billion in annual sales.

2013 — In a decision that attracted media attention around the world, the Indian Supreme Court dismisses appeal against rejection of patent on beta crystalline form of imatinib.

Read individually, the Glivec stories differ quite widely in terms of which actors are the stars, who played major supporting roles, who may be described as bit part players, and of who were basically extras. Which are most complete and accurate depends in large part on whether you think Glivec is the culmination of a long and winding road, or a brief excursion that starts at Ciba-Geigy. But either way, the credit largely lies outside the laboratories of Ciba-Geigy and its successor company Novartis. But it also depends on what you think Glivec is. Glivec the synthetic small molecule, a pyrimidine derivative generically known as imatinib, is one thing. If Zimmermann was the first and only person to make this molecule he is rightly the inventor of it as long as we are unconcerned about *scientific* credit and merely need to identify one or a few individuals closely associated with its first manufacture.

Let us now consider Glivec as being much more than this or that pyramidine derivative in this or that structural form. Glivec broad, as opposed to Glivec narrow, is a pharmaceutical product of a type known as a tyrosine kinase inhibitor and is extraordinarily effective in the treatment of chronic myeloid leukaemia, as with all cancers, a highly complex disease.[131] Potentially, an almost infinite variety of different molecules can be made in the laboratory. But to identify a class of chemicals to be made for a specific

(*Continued*)

(*Continued*)

purpose, analyse them, select a few for testing, test them in various ways, select the best one, optimise it, and finally get it approved for sale requires the contribution of many more people, especially if we include those involved in the basic science, and not just the applied work.

One way to look fairly at credit is to ask the question: which people were the most essential, the *sine qua nons* as it were: those without whom there would have been no Glivec? The importance of the individual who came up with the actual chemical doing the trick cannot be underestimated. But the inventor named on the patent can also be seen in such cases as the one who added the finishing touches, inching the idea forward over the novelty, inventive step and industrial applicability thresholds. Accordingly it is immaterial whether this person's effort or intellectual input was proportionately significant as compared to anybody else's. This may not necessarily be seen as unfair. Zimmermann did spend more than two years in developing the right molecule and then preparing it in a form that could be taken orally. Designing the last piece of the jigsaw was no quick and easy task.[132]

Was there one single individual who was most essential to Glivec? Competing claims can reasonably be made for Lydon, and for Alex Matter who led Ciba-Geigy's programme on kinase inhibitors from the start. But if it is possible at all to single out one irreplaceable person without whom there would have been neither an invention nor a pharmaceutical product called Glivec, then it would probably be a man who worked a hemisphere away and for a different employer: Brian Druker, initially working at the Dana-Farber Cancer Institute and then at the Oregon Health Sciences University. Neither is a corporation.

Druker was not just an outstanding scientist who happened to be the lead author of the *Nature Medicine* article which announced Glivec to the world under the name of CPG57148.[133] He was a keen collaborator across institutions, and he was driven by an intense determination to find a treatment for this disease *and* to make this treatment available to as many patients as possible. This commitment to do all that was necessary to cure leukaemia patients led him to collaborate with Lydon and Ciba-Geigy in order to harness the company's biochemical capacity in the field of kinase inhibitors to his search for a molecule that he could help prove specifically to block the action of a single aberrant enzyme common to the cells of sufferers of this particular cancer. His role did not end when the molecule was discovered and, largely under his direction, shown to work. He then had to

(*Continued*)

persuade Novartis, as Ciba-Geigy became, to invest in developing the drug and then selling it. It took two years for Novartis to relent to pressure from Druker and also from patients to provide the drug for more extensive testing. In Jessica Wapner's definitive account of Glivec,[134] and in an interview of Druker with author and biomedical scientist Siddhartha Mukherjee,[135] one can only be deeply impressed by his incredibly persistent efforts to persuade a reluctant Novartis, concerned about the small number of patients and therefore the lack of a market for the drug, into producing enough for clinical trials. Ironically, the specificity of Glivec which made it such an outstanding drug was not at first seen as being in its favour as a commercial product, from the perspective of Novartis: it kept the patient base small.

In the event, Novartis went ahead with Glivec, which turned out to be to its considerable advantage. On 10 May 2001, in unusually quick time, the US Food and Drug Administration approved Glivec. Approvals elsewhere followed. On 31 January of that year, in the US Novartis was granted orphan drug status under the 1983 Orphan Drugs Act.[136] The legislation is supposed to incentivise private sector investment in treatment for rare diseases, and while it seems to have been quite successful, evidently Novartis was not encouraged by it without Druker's influence. Novartis set a universal price of $2,400 per patient per month. Even with patient assistance for lower income people, which enabled some to get it for free, the drug proved to be highly profitable, besides which such programmes, beneficial as they obviously are to some patients at least, are an excellent way to discourage generic market entry where there are no patents. By 2003, annual sales had reached $1 billion per annum and revenues have risen considerably since then. Brian Druker's name may not be on any of the patents. But it would be hard to name any other individual to whom leukaemia patients should be more grateful. True to his convictions, Druker was one of more than 100 physicians who published an article in *Blood* criticising the high prices of drugs for cancer, especially chronic myeloid leukaemia.[137]

An exciting development of MAbs is the emerging technology of antibody-drug conjugates (ADCs) which arguably almost perfectly embody Ehrlich's dream.[138] With ADCs, the MAb finds the target and the cytotoxin attached to it is the payload. The toxin is supposed to overcome therapeutic window narrowness inherent to most anti-cancer treatment due to its precise targeting, which of course means also that its cytotoxicity can be made very high indeed. Fewer than 10 such medicines have been approved so far, of which perhaps the best known is the highly effective but eye-wateringly expensive Trastuzumab emtansine (T-DM1), marketed by Genentech and Roche as Kadcyla for HER2-positive metastatic breast cancer. The MAb involved is trastuzumab, which is an existing (and already highly expensive) product under its trade name of Herceptin. Truly impressive as these medicines are, undesirable side-effects are reported, so they are still not yet the drugs of perfection that we really need. That said, given the diversity in individual human responses to ingested chemical entities occasioned by genotypic and phenotypic differences between each and every one of us, it is hard to know when a true universal magic bullet of a medicine will ever come to exist.

Summing up, biomedical science innovation is multifaceted and diverse in terms of what is being done, who is doing it and where, and it is constantly evolving. Despite early biotech achievements like genetically engineered human insulin, the dominance of large molecule biologics, especially the very high molecular-weight monoclonal antibodies, has been a long time coming, much slower than was anticipated after their initial discovery; the reasons involving a combination of technical, financial, and regulatory factors. But nowadays they have a very large market presence (Table 8.3). That said, though, authorising price reducing

Table 8.3. Top-ten pharmaceuticals by global sales in 2018

Product	Type of medicine	Company	Sales (US$ billions)
1. Humira	MAb	AbbVie	19.9
2. Revlimid	small molecule	Celgene	9.7
3. Keytruda	MAb	Merck	7.2
4. Herceptin	MAb	Roche	7.1
5. Avastin	MAb	Roche	7.0
6. Rituxan	MAb	Roche	6.9
7. Opdivo	MAb	Bristol-Myers Squibb	6.7
8. Eliquis	small molecule	Bristol-Myers Squibb	6.4
9. Prevnar 13	Vaccine	Pfizer	5.8
10. Stelara	MAb	Johnson & Johnson	5.2

substitutes in most countries took an unjustifiably long time even when you consider the technical challenges to regulating in this area, and the approval requirements do have dysfunctional consequences unduly inhibiting competition and the introduction of better versions.

It is arguable that, as long as disease processes are not well understood and researchers must depend on serendipity, even the prepared mind must eventually contend with the law of diminishing returns.[139] Arguably, the antibiotics era took low-cost serendipitous drug discovery as far as it could go. Low hanging, they were the fruit that randomness could quite easily harvest. But afterwards, little else was in easy reach. And, while rational drug design has had some major successes, such as the ACE inhibitors, beta-blockers and cimetidine, and more recently with some of the new cancer drugs, its promise is far from being fully realized even now. Time lags between new scientific discoveries and their practical applications can be long ones. So perhaps the rest of the century's long transition period from randomness and hope, to precision and better prediction as to what can and cannot work, is more of a scientific issue, than it is a business or legal one. Nonetheless, to know what is going on and what might be done, we need to take all three into consideration.

Notes

1 Carlson (2011).
2 Bray (2009); Wohlsen (2014).
3 Ghosh (2020), 1.
4 *Ibid.*
5 Sideri (2020).
6 Deshaies (2020), 329.
7 Stockwell (2011), 8–9.
8 https://www.biospace.com/article/top-20-pharma-companies-by-market-cap-in-q1-2019/, visited 31/12/2019.
9 Mund (1969).
10 CIPA (1998).
11 Taylor and Silberston (1973), 365.
12 Hunt (2002), 3.
13 Le Fanu (1999), 247.

14 Quirke, (2013), 151.
15 For early discussion on this very issue on the United States, and in light of the 1962 Kefauver Harris Amendement, see Steele (1969).
16 See Stockwell (2011).
17 Scannell *et al.* (2012). The rest of this subsection draws on this article.
18 Wieseler and Kaiser (2019).
19 Fojo, Mailankody and Lo (2014).
20 Silverman and Lee (1974), 327.
21 *Ibid.*, 328.
22 Yi (2011), 456.
23 Quoted in Bud (1993), 27.
24 OTA (1989).
25 Kornberg (1995), 3.
26 Kornberg *op. cit.*, 4.
27 Rabinow (1996), 20.
28 Dawkins (2004), 558–62.
29 In this context it may be worth noting the definition of invention provided by the German Federal Supreme Court in the well-known Red Dove case, as mentioned in Chapter 2, and as reported in *International Review of Industrial Property and Copyright Law (IIC)* (1970), 1: 136, 138.
30 Albeit perhaps less than is commonly supposed.
31 Dahm (2005).
32 Among the most comprehensive historical accounts of the rise of molecular biology and the achievements of its practitioners are: de Chadarevian (2002); Cobb (2015); Judson (1996); Kay (1993, 2000); Morange (1998).
33 Kay (1993) *op. cit.*, 4–6.
34 Morange *op cit.* 1–2.
35 Schrödinger (1944).
36 Avery, MacLeod and McCarty (1944).
37 Morange *op cit.*, 36.
38 Based on similar table in Acharya (1999) with modifications.
39 On the huge controversy regarding the production of the HeLa cell line and its subsequent biomedical use, see Skloot (2010).
40 For a definitive history of the discovery of the DNA structure, see Olby (1974).
41 Watson and Crick (1953).
42 Yi (2008), 589.
43 Hughes (2001a), 549.

44 On PCR and its range of applications, see Mullis, Febré and Gibbs (1994).

45 Rabinow (1996), 1.

46 Mullis (1990).

47 Slack (2002).

48 Bugos and Kevles (1992).

49 His employers, Cetus Corporation paid him $10,000.

50 Mullis — Nobel Lecture.

51 *See* Fore *et al* (2006). The two patents were: US Patent no. 4,683,195 ('Process for amplifying, detecting and/or cloning nucleic acid sequences'), issued on 28 July 1987; and US Patent no. 4,683,202 ('Process for amplifying nucleic acid sequences'), issued on 28 July 1987. Mullis was named as sole inventor on the '202 patent, while four Cetus colleagues were added to Mullis's name as inventors on the '195 patent.

52 The initial patent application was filed in 1974, but was overridden by subsequent applications. The definitive patent (number 4,237,224) was filed in 1979 and awarded in 1980 following the Supreme Court decision in Diamond v. Chakrabarty. The title of the patent was 'Process for producing biologically functional molecular chimeras'. *See* McKelvey (1996), xix. Recombinant DNA aroused considerable scientific and political debate during the early years. For well documented accounts of the controversy, see Frederickson (2001) and Lear (1978).

53 For a discussion on the commercial significance of the patent, see Hughes (2001a), 571–2.

54 For views pro and contra this possibility, see Boldrin and Levine (2004) and Selgin and Turner (2006).

55 Wright (1986), 336. For an entertaining account of the race to clone insulin, see Hall (1987).

56 Sargant (2003), 246.

57 Picard (2002).

58 Le Fanu (1999), 289.

59 Sargant (2003), 256.

60 Dutfield and Suthersanen *op cit.*, 295–430; Kranakis (2020).

61 Fox (1983).

62 Rasmussen (2014), 188–9.

63 Marks (2012).

64 Kohler and Milstein (1975).

65 Milstein (2000), 360.

66 Robbins-Roth (2000), 56.

67 Breedveld (2000), 735.

68 Marks (2015) *op cit.*, 218.

69 Brumley (2017), The 15 All-Time Best-Selling Prescription Drugs. Kiplinger — Kiplinger.com, visited 21/9/2020.

70 The first product to be manufactured this way was Genentech's tissue plasminogen activator, Activase, in 1987. It has been suggested that microbial eukaryotes such as fungi are also suitable and may prove to be superior to CHO cells for some biologics in terms of production costs, expression yields, and quality. Emalfarb (2018). Algae are also considered promising candidates. Dahl (2018).

71 See Wilmut, Campbell and Tudge (2000); also, Dewar (2004).

72 Kornberg (1995), 11–3.

73 Powell (1999), 50.

74 Harrison (1997), 67.

75 Drug and Market Development (1998), 264.

76 Bud (1993) *op. cit.*, 198.

77 *See* Fransman and Tanaka (1999), 202–55; Howells and Neary (1995), 212–20.

78 McKelvey (1996), xxi.

79 Werth (1994), 203.

80 Munshi (2020); also, *Nature* (editorial) (2020).

81 *Nature Genetics* (editorial) (2019).

82 Males have 24 chromosomes that are different from each other, while females have 23. This is because in addition to the 22 pairs we all inherit, males also have an X and a Y chromosome while females have two Xs but no Ys.

83 Cook-Deegan (1994), 29–30.

84 Venter (2007), 198.

85 Cookson (2001).

86 Regalado (2001). The 'big five' were (in descending order): the MIT/Whitehead Institute Center for Genome Research; the Sanger Centre; Washington University Genome Sequencing Center; the US Department of Energy Joint Genome Institute; and Baylor College of Medicine Human Genome Sequencing Center.

87 Of course, the HGP was itself controversial. Many scientists felt the money allocated to it could have been used better on other endeavours with more practical outcomes.

88 Coghlan (1994).

89 See International Human Genome Sequencing Consortium (2001).

90 See Venter *et al.* (2001).

91 Some estimates ran as high as 300,000. In fact, two companies, Incyte and Human Genome Sciences, 'had both claimed to have isolated and patented more than 200,000 genes'. *See* Venter (2007), 322.

92 Williams (2013).

93 International Human Genome Sequencing Consortium (2001), 911.

94 Arguably, the human genome is far longer than it needs to be, and laden with error, repetition and redundancy. In describing this feature, one author refers to its design as 'baroque' and involving 'gratuitous genomic complexity'. Avise (2010). However, one may also infer that there is a tremendous amount of hidden meaning in the human genome that we are completely ignorant of, and which we need to know.

95 Starling (1905), 340.

96 Griffiths and Stotz (2007), 395.

97 Findlay *et al.*, (2007).

98 Hyun, Wilkerson and Johnston (2016).

99 Schlaeger *et al.* (2015).

100 Chung *et al.* (2014).

101 Yamada *et al.* (2014).

102 Elenco, Underwood and Zohar (2015).

103 Ibid.

104 Strimbu and Tavel (2010).

105 Kalia (2013).

106 Manolio *et al.* (2019).

107 The Lancet (editorial) (2019).

108 Curtis *et al.* (2012), 346.

109 Gray and Druker (2012), 329.

110 Schork (2015).

111 Spear, Heath-Chiozzi and Huff (2001), 202.

112 Allison *op cit.*

113 President's Council of Advisors on Science and Technology (2008), quoted in Kalia (2013).

114 Joyner and Paneth (2015).

115 Maglo *et al.* (2014).

116 Exner *et al.* (2001).

117 *Ibid.*

118 Taylor *et al.* (2004).

119 United States Patent no. 6,465,463: ('Methods of treating and preventing congestive heart failure with hydralazine compounds and isosorbide dinitrate or isosorbide mononitrate'). Date: October 15, 2002.

120   For in-depth critiques of the uses of race and other non-scientific categories to stratify patients for the purposes of medical treatment: Ghosh (2012); Kahn (2012).

121   Gibson *et al.* (inc. HO Smith and JC Venter) (2010).

122   Nowell (2007).

123   Vasella (2003).

124   United States Patent no. 5,521,184: ('Pyramidine derivatives and processes for the preparation thereof'). Date: May 28, 1996.

125   United States Patent no. 6,894,051: ('Crystal modification of a n-phenyl-2-pyramidineamine derivative, processes for its manufacture and its use'). Date: May 17, 2005.

126   Vasella *op cit.*, 188.

127   Relman (2003).

128   Brody (2007), 13–18; Keating and Cambrosio (2012); Mukherjee *op. cit.*; Nathan (2007); Vasella *op. cit.*

129   Wapner (2014).

130   Nowell and Hungerford (1960).

131   This narrow-broad distinction is analogous to Radick and MacLeod's IP narrow versus IP broad conceptualisation of the different ways that ownership interests in inventive work may be categorised and expressed, whether in legal, non-legal senses or perhaps a combination of both. Radick and MacLeod (2013).

132   Buchdunger and Zimmermann (undated).

133   Druker *et al.* (1996).

134   Wapner *op cit.*

135   Mukherjee *op. cit.*, 436.

136   Cohen, Moses and Pazdur (2002).

137   Experts in Chronic Myeloid Leukemia (2013).

138   Dan *et al.* (2018).

139   Le Fanu (1999), 237.

Chapter 9
Intellectual Property in Biomedicine

Introduction

Before the 1980s, governments and even courts were often ambivalent if not sceptical that patents were necessary for healthcare innovation in the public interest. In addition, there was a deep-seated sentiment among many scientists that patenting was not the done thing. Such mixed opinion was about as true for many developed countries as it was in the newly-independent nations, for whom suspicion as to the benefits of patents was to be expected. As we have seen, many European countries did not allow medicines to be patented for most of the twentieth century; even the UK prohibited them from 1919 to 1949. Many court judgements in the United States, where medicines were always patentable, implied an underlying doubt as to the public interest benefits of having strong patent protection in any field of technology.

This began to change from the late 1970s. We will not go into all the factors likely to have been at play behind this shift. But biotechnology as an emerging field of immense promise and the fact that the United States had a lead in this emerging area encouraged a more favourable disposition in government there. The same may be said for the country's growing anxiety about its post-war economic and technological dominance which was being challenged as never before. If other countries are catching up, many politicians and large corporations felt, it can only be because they are copying us. Europe similarly became eager to keep up with the competition, and the idea that to do so required a similarly pro-patent stance for the encouragement of innovation was an attractive one to some of the governments and to the European Community. The latter took up the cause internationally, alongside the United States and Japan which had by then joined the elite nations by way of the 1986–1994 Uruguay Round of trade negotiations. These talks culminated in the establishment of the World Trade Organization (WTO) and its intellectual property agreement (the TRIPS Agreement), at regional level by adopting a legal instrument that became EU law in 1998. Later on the European Union, as did the United States, sought to export their newly implemented intellectual property standards by means of bilateral and plurilateral trade agreements. Little thought was given to the fact that WTO rules forbid trade regulatory discrimination against foreigners. So overseas firms from emerging nations have the same rights to file patents in the US and Europe as do domestic ones. This was probably due to the supposition that these emerging economies were, and would for a long time remain, imitators with limited capabilities to create independently. To be fair pharmaceuticals is a field in which emerging nation catch-up has been relatively slow. Companies in the United States and Europe, and to a less extent Japan, continue to be highly dominant.

The first part of the chapter deals with how patent law currently deals with biomedicine. In the main, patent law is very friendly to pharmaceutical companies seeking to secure patent protection covering newly discovered features, methods and uses of existing medicines. But it is a mixed picture. One reason is the sheer complexity of today's patent laws especially in the countries where most of the corporate research takes place. Another is the fact that biomedicine, the biomedical infrastructure, and healthcare policy not only implicate a range of commercial, non-commercial and state entities and stakeholders whose interests are not necessarily in close alignment (to put it mildly!), and that there are massive social welfare implications. And as Parthasarathy[1] and Drahos[2] have separately shown us, patent granting offices have their own missions, cultures and ideologies, as do courts and those who draft legislation and who review and vote for relevant statutory instruments. We will also delve into the evolution of patent law of the past decades. The second part covers developments relating specifically to the biotechnology era which of course was not exclusively about biomedicine but had transformative effects on a number of scientific and industrial fields. The third part takes us away from patents, looking into a relatively new development, which is the increased use of non-traditional trademarks to protect the colour and shape of medicines. The fourth considers data protection, or data exclusivity, which as I suggested earlier is a *quasi*-intellectual property right and which bridges the domains of intellectual property law and pharmaceutical regulation. Finally, we will look into the ways that companies have been able to use the patent system together with other intellectual property rights, especially trademarks, for market advantage.

Beyond Product, Process and Use: What Drug Companies Actually Claim and What Patent Law Permits

Determining whether a product is new or not for the purpose of granting or refusing a patent would appear to be a fairly straightforward calculation. But this is far from being the case with medicines. Apart from the fact that the concept of novelty in patent law is in large part a matter of description, specialised knowledge and public availability as opposed to whether the invention had no prior existence in any absolute sense, chemistry and biology both present complications other types of invention do not necessarily share. The aforementioned coffee lid with a useful slide to unlock mechanism aiding the retention of heat and reducing the risk of the drinker getting scalded while dashing to catch the train is novel if no such device on a coffee lid was known to exist before. On the other hand, much invention in the biomedical sphere involves some kind of mimicry of nature. The patent system can apply novelty in a way that renders much incremental modification 'old'. Alternatively, it may be more accommodating towards protecting minor tweaks to what is out there already. By being strict, the system might demand some additional novelty requirement so that a small or trivial variation is disqualified because it is essentially the same thing as the disclosed or prior art chemical it most closely relates to. This is done in India (see below). If more tweak-friendly, the system will more readily accommodate variation on a theme: similar but different *is* different. Take two substances A and B. There is some difference of significance between them notwithstanding that they vary by as little as one being merely purer than the other but otherwise identical, or as one being a racemic mixture comprising both left- and right-handed versions (enantiomers) of the molecule, and the other being one or other of the enantiomers. Either way, A and B can be patented as separate inventions in Europe and in the United States. Accordingly, slightly different things are treated as being something else entirely if some new difference of therapeutic or other significance is disclosed (whether or not it is proven). Cumulative modifications to existing medicaments such as enantiomers, combinations, and minor variants of existing products may well be deemed patentable. This is exactly what the non-generic pharmaceutical corporations and their intellectual property lawyers and attorneys want. And it is what they normally get. But not necessarily in developing countries.

Generally, the system *has* become relaxed about novelty with respect to pharmaceuticals and this of course suits industry (albeit not the generics producers). Purified versions of existing substances can be patented on either side of the North Atlantic and in other jurisdictions too. There are old precedents for this as we saw in Chapter 6, including adrenaline[3] and insulin. The door may also be open to the patenting of naturally-occurring drug metabolites which are basically 'made' by the human body (see below).

There is of course a difference between the active pharmaceutical ingredient (API) and the drug product. A tablet contains a mixture of the API and other non-active chemicals called excipients which may perform certain functions such as protecting the API on its journey through the body, controlling its rate of absorption, or enabling more convenient modes of delivery. A huge cocktail of chemicals may be involved in production. Take remdesivir, a drug very much in the news as this book was about to go to press: 'even by the exacting standards of pharmaceuticals, remdesivir is tricky to produce — the months-long process involves 70 raw materials, reagents, and catalysts.'[4] It may be possible for the same API to be administered in liquid rather than solid form, or to be made to be chewable so it does not have to be swallowed whole. New dosage forms, such as a pill with a known API having a new coating offering some sort of advantage, genuinely therapeutic or otherwise, are patentable — like all other inventions for up to 20 years.

European patent law is generally accommodating towards the pharmaceutical industry, arguably excessively so. As we have seen, the industry is highly organised and spends large sums of money on promoting its interests. There are, however, certain exclusions in terms of methods claims. These date back to a time when, arguably, for the industry they were less objectionable in terms of business strategy. As we shall see, though, these can largely be circumvented by claiming new or additional uses. There are no such statutory exceptions in the United States. European Patent Convention (EPC) Article 53(c) excludes:

> (c) methods for treatment of the human or animal body by surgery or therapy and diagnostic methods practised on the human or animal

body; this provision shall not apply to products, in particular substances or compositions, for use in any of these methods.

This is somewhat similar to the allowable exclusions of 'diagnostic, therapeutic and surgical methods for the treatment of humans or animals' in the TRIPS Agreement, which unsurprisingly borrows language from both European and United States' intellectual property laws. The methods of treatment exclusions require some explanation in terms of their meaning, purpose and scope of application. In terms of its rationale, Article 53(c) of the EPC seeks to immunise physicians, surgeons and veterinarians from patent infringement suits. As such it is grounded in ethics and public health concerns, an interpretation affirmed in a series of European Patent Office (EPO) cases.[5] Boundaries need to be set, and the methods of treatment exclusion, conveniently for industry, does not extend to drugs or equipment that may be under patent. As far as therapy goes, a line of EPO appeal board decisions has distinguished between methods for treatment intended to benefit the health of patients in a range of possible ways which fall within these exclusions, from treatments that are cosmetic in nature that fall outside. Cosmetic treatments are quite broad. For example, EPO cases have found methods for treatment relating to weight control, baldness and hair removal, snoring and contraception to be cosmetic. Also falling outside the exclusion are treatments intended to kill humanely the recipient of the substance, for example euthanasia treatments for pets — but not for humans which is deemed immoral and thus not patentable.[6]

With respect to surgery, the EPO has struggled to be consistent. But surgery is now deemed to constitute physical intervention on the body involving the application of professional medical skill and which entails substantial health risk to the subject person or animal.[7] Sterckx and Cockbain helpfully sum up the situation by suggesting that 'interventions such as massage, tattooing, tanning, shaving, ear-piercing, blood-drawing, and routine injecting or catheterisation will not classify as excluded methods of surgery', whereas 'bone-setting, castration, embryo implantation and cosmetic surgery involving anaesthetics seem likely to be included.'[8]

Diagnosis of necessity involves at least two steps including data gathering or comparison followed by the act of diagnosis itself. These are all primarily mental, thus non-technical, acts that are outside of normal practice done on the body. But if diagnosis is inherently non-technical, diagnoses consist of 'methods for performing mental acts' and are therefore not inventions under EPC Article 52(2)(c). This would render the exclusion unnecessary. However, Enlarged Board of Appeal decision in G-1/04 identified technical steps: those implying 'an interaction with the human or animal body, necessitating the presence of the latter.'[9] Arguably, this is a questionable *ex post facto* justification for the existence of a redundant provision.

The European Patent Convention allows known chemicals to be patented for previously unknown uses in the above-mentioned unpatentable methods. Providing for this (under Article 54(4)) is really a special exemption to the novelty provision which reflects the fact that much pharmaceutical discovery concerns extant substances, not just ones brought into existence by pharmaceutical chemists and designed with a specific application in mind. As we will see, this is not the only relaxation of the novelty criterion provided in the EPC in favour of the pharmaceutical industry.

The question arose of what to do about discoveries of new medical uses of substances that were already being used as medicines for something else; that is, second medical uses. Given the genuine possibility of drugs turning out to be useful for treating diseases other than the ones they were initially indicated for, and increasing commercial desire to expand the supply of patients for existing medicines, the industry obviously had an interest in the patent system protecting second medical indications (NB: 'indication' in European patent law practice is more general in meaning and not confined to a specific disease or medical condition). Given that this is not product protection being sought, since of course there is no novelty there, the obstacle was the wording of Article 53(c). The solution arrived at in favour of those desiring to acquire patents was devised by the Swiss Patent Office and became commonly known in consequence as the 'Swiss-type claim'. Accordingly, a second medical indication could side-step the methods exclusions under Article 53(c) as long as the following claim language was adopted: 'Use of a substance or composition X for the manufacture of a medicament for therapeutic application Z'. However, as from 2011, such claims are no longer accepted for new patent applications. This came after a decision of the Enlarged Board to end Swiss form claims on the grounds that they cast serious doubt — rather damningly when one stops to think about it — on whether they fulfil novelty and inventiveness requirements (see below). Instead, a more straightforward claim is to be made: 'Product X for use in the treatment of Z'. This is a consequence of a clause added to the revised 2000 version of the EPC which renders Swiss form claims unnecessary anyway. Article 54(5) now states that the novelty requirement:

> shall also not exclude the patentability of any substance or composition referred to in paragraph 4 for any specific use in any method referred to in Article 53(c), provided that such use is not comprised in the state of the art.

That second and follow-on use claims may be under patent after the initial patent on the drug itself has expired gives rise to the following rather curious scenario: a generic version of a drug can enter the market, subject to regulatory approval, for the original indication. But if marketed for the second use, its manufacture and sale would be patent infringing. This potentially raises difficulties for national health providers, physicians and pharmacists, especially in jurisdictions in which doctors are encouraged to write prescriptions using international nonproprietary names (i.e. official generic names) and where indications may not necessarily be entered on the prescription note. It also means that generic drug-makers must be careful about the indications they mention on the label, making sure not to include ones that are under patent protection. Given the undesirability of exposing physicians and pharmacists to patent infringement suits for just doing their jobs, and here one might reflect also on the purposes of the commonly provided 'pharmacy exemption' written into the patent laws of several countries (see below), this is serious cause for concern. Admittedly, there is little evidence that the pharmaceutical industry in Europe at least has much appetite for suing doctors or pharmacists. But pharmacists generally do not know what the medicine on a prescription is to be used for unless the patient is present to be asked and is happy to answer. One may question why they should be expected to. As mentioned, physicians may be expected to prescribe the cheaper generic version. Furthermore, they are normally permitted to prescribe medicines for known off-label uses and this is generally assumed to be in the public interest where there is reliable evidence to justify it.

There are two other important issues. One relates to the patent incentive to invent such as it really exists, the other concerns competition. The first is part of a wider debate about whether the availability of 20-year legal monopolies for incremental inventions is a good thing if we would prefer to see breakthrough inventions that entail high risk and greater investment. It may be unfair to place all of the blame for the industry's conservatism on the patent system but clearly it does not seem to be helping. According to a recent article '… the human genome encodes more than 500 protein kinases, of which hundreds have been shown to have genetic links with human diseases. Yet around 65% of the 20,000 kinase papers published in 2009 focused on the 50 proteins that were the "hottest" in the early 1990s. Similarly, 75% of the research activity on nuclear hormone receptors in 2009 focused on the 6 receptors — out of the 48 encoded in the genome — that were most studied in the mid 1990s.'[10] As regards natural products we have a similar situation and this is reflected in the patent system: '… human innovative activity involving biodiversity in the patent system focuses on approximately 4% of taxonomically described species and between 0.8–1% of predicted global species… We conclude that the narrow focus of human innovative activity and ownership of genetic resources is unlikely to be in the long term interest of humanity.'[11]

Whereas many second use claims are targeted towards diseases and other health problems that were not previously indicated, there are further types of claim that may be allowed in some jurisdictions where the disease is actually *the same* as before. This is where the earlier discussion on personalised medicine becomes particularly relevant. Following the EISAI decision, claims may be allowed on further uses and methods for optimised or personalised dosage regimes, that is, for a specific schedule of doses such as take one 200 mg. tablet every six hours. This rather generous interpretation of European patent law concerning second and further use claims was reaffirmed by the TBA in *Genentech/Method of administration of IFG-1* T1020/03, [2006]. As an aside, it is important to differentiate between the terms 'formulation' when applied to a specific drug mixture in whatever type it is prepared for delivery, and a 'dosage form'. The latter tends to refer to the physical form of the drug. Dosage forms include tablets, capsules, injectable solutions, ointments or powders to give some examples. However, the term is also used to apply to the chemical composition of the drug. Thus, there is a certain overlap in the usage of the two terms, which can be a little confusing. As we will see below, new formulations such as different mixtures containing known APIs that might offer certain advantages to patients are patentable. Examples of such patient benefits include its enabling a more convenient dosage regimen (e.g. a-one-a-day version of a drug previously to be taken every four hours), or a reduction in side-effects. Dosage forms presented as novel and unobvious routes of administration for known drugs can also be patented.[12]

In 2008, the British Court of Appeal made an important ruling on a medical product called finasteride, which had first been patented in 1978 as a treatment for enlarged prostate. A decade later, the same company, Merck filed a patent application on the same product but for its use to treat male baldness at a daily dosage of over 5 mg. using the Swiss form of claim. In 1996 a new patent relating to the same product was granted to Merck claiming its use 'for the preparation of a medicament for oral administration useful for the treatment of androgenic alopecia [male baldness] in a person and wherein the dosage amount is about 0.05 to 1.0 mg'. The Court, taking relevant EPO decisions into account reversed its earlier revocation, finding the new dosage regime to be novel: 'A claim to a pill containing a 1mg dose of finasteride would be a claim to a new thing. No-one had made or proposed such a thing, so why should it not be novel?' It was deemed non-obvious because there was deemed a low expectation of success.[13] Ironically, it was shortly after that the EPO decided in Decision No. G02/08 — Dosage regime/ABBOT RESPIRATORY that use of Swiss-type claims should cease in light of the new language inserted into the EPC from 2000. This decision clarified two important points as follows:

1. Where it is already known to use a medicament to treat an illness, Article 54(5) EPC does not exclude that this medicament be patented for *use in a different treatment* by therapy of the *same illness*.

2.   Such patenting is also not excluded where *a dosage regime is the only feature claimed* which is not comprised in the state of the art. [emphasis added]

Is it possible to claim uses or methods relating to a patient population identified by a shared biomarker that forms part of a wider population of patients having the same disease *and who may already have received the medicine?*[14] Surely, if the drug has already been prescribed for that disease including to those members of the smaller population, there is no novelty. This is a tricky issue, but the EPO has allowed patents for uses targeted to clearly defined sub-populations. In T1399/04 (Combination therapy HCV/SCHERING), the TBA stated that prior public use is not necessarily novelty-destroying. Moreover, defining a group of patients where there is overlap with a population already receiving the same drug for the same purpose *can* lead to a patentable invention. As stated by the Board:

> If the use of a compound was known in the treatment or diagnosis of a disease of a particular group of subjects, the treatment or diagnosis of the same disease with the same compound could nevertheless represent a novel therapeutic or diagnostic application, provided that it is carried out on a new group of subjects which is distinguished from the former by its *physiological or pathological* status.

With these second and futher use claims, generic companies can supply the drug for one or some indications but not for all of them. This makes it harder to challenge the market power of the first entrant. If one believes in full patent rights for new medical uses that is fair enough. If one is more sceptical that this lengthy term of protection is justified for such minor, albeit not necessarily therapeutically trival, discoveries, it follows that the public may not be getting the full benefits it should from a truly competitive market in medicines. Every patent is for 20 years subject to payment of renewal fees. In addition, aggressive assertion of patent rights may have a chilling effect on generic market entry.

Generally speaking, if it is patentable in the United States, it is likely to be patentable in Europe and vice versa. However there are some differences in terms of eligible subject matter and in legal reasoning. It would be fair to say that the situation in the United States regarding eligibility is confusing and in a state of flux. The Supreme Court has missed a number of opportunities to provide legal clarity. One particularly interesting example is the 2012 *Mayo v. Prometheus* decision of the Supreme Court[15] which again concerned personalised medicine. The two patents at issue involved use of thiopurine drugs for treating auto-immune diseases. They claimed methods to calibrate dosage of known drugs for an individual patient to achieve optimal therapeutic efficacy. This was done by measuring the amount of a drug metabolite present in the patient such that the dosage could be adjusted accordingly. This is important because different patients metabolise the drug at different rates. Thus at a given dosage, one patient may have a relatively large amount of the metabolite in the body which if too high may cause harmful side-effects. Another patient may produce so little of the metabolite from the dosage administered as to be therapeutically ineffective. So clearly the disclosed methods offered a therapeutic advantage for patients. But did that make them patentable?

The USPTO had found the patents to comprise eligible subject matter on the grounds that administering the drug providing the metabolite was a transformative step that made the whole process patent-eligible. The Court of Appeals for the Federal Circuit reversed a lower court judgement and found the patents to claim eligible subject matter in which physical 'transformation', a word that European patent law and jurisprudence has little use for, was present in the first two steps of the process. This rendered as insignificant the third and last step being deemed a 'mental step': taken as a whole, the methods were patentable.

The Supreme Court reversed this, stating its view that the patents described a general method to apply a law of nature, with administration of the drug adding nothing inventive to the state of the art. While it seems reasonable to conclude that there was nothing especially inventive about the patents, arguably all inventions apply natural laws to something practically useful — assuming we accept that 'law of nature' has any clear meaning. To be fair, the Court did accept this point, but it still found that transforming a law of nature into a patentable invention requires more than merely applying the law, and the patents were thus held to claim ineligible subject matter by failing to achieve this.

Another patent-relevant aspect of personalisation is the preparation of medicines comprising certain active ingredients for specific patients. Using the patented ingredient to make a medicinal product is an infringing activity. However, it is not only physicians and surgeons that we do not like to see getting sued for patent infringement. The same applies to pharmacists preparing treatments for individual patients. In about 40 countries there is an express pharmacy exception.[16] For example, in the United Kingdom, an act that would otherwise infringe, is permitted if 'it consists of the extemporaneous preparation in a pharmacy of a medicine for an individual in accordance with a prescription given by a registered medical or dental practitioner or consists of dealing with a medicine so prepared.'[17]

Another defence to infringement that is probably better known, is the so-called Bolar exemption (or Bolar provision as it is sometimes called), which we looked at in Chapter 3.

Let us return to a point, and to a series of questions, first raised in Chapter 3 about variability among things that, it might be supposed, are for all practical intents and purposes, identical. Is a form or variant of a chemical the same thing as that chemical? Or is it something else entirely? What about drugs? While you ponder this last question, bear in mind that a pill is not just a package comprising multiple numbers of the specified active ingredient, but a collection of those plus various additional chemicals, formulated to enhance the effectiveness of the drug product after it has entered the body. Paradoxically, it is both a pure substance and a mixture.

Consider one potentially significant type of variability in the pharmaceutical context: stereoisomerism. Two or more compounds may consist of the same elements in the same atomic proportions but differ in shape. The basic chemical formula is the same but each variant may interact with the human body in different ways that give rise to different effects. Isomers that are mirror images of each other are called enantiomers. A racemate is a chemical that has two forms, each a mirror image of the other. Racemic mixtures tend to comprise both in equal measure, and many pharmaceutical products are such mixtures. Technically speaking, a racemate is a molecule of a certain type: it is chiral, meaning it comes in two opposite forms: left-handed and right-handed. Whether they are in the left-handed half of the mixture or in the right-handed one they do not differ in their atomic constituents. In terms of their relationship to the mixture and to their counterpart in the other half of the combination, they are referred to in chemistry-speak as enantiomers. Each may also be referred to as an optical isomer. It is possible that both enantiomers have the same therapeutic effect. But there may also be huge and crucial differences in the medical impacts of a different enantiomer. To make matters more complicated, it is possible for the human body to convert a supposedly safe and effective enantiomer taken as a drug into a potentially harmful racemic mixture in the body. In recent decades, separating enantiomers has become easier. Needless to say, the ability to carry out such a separation can provide genuine benefits for patients. It is much easier, as of course it should be, to acquire regulatory approval for an enantiomer than for a genuinely new chemical entity. Moreover, enantiomers are patentable. This might all appear to be reasonable, but the possibilities for 'gaming' the regulatory and patent systems are very much present. Chiral switching, that is, moving from the racemic mixture to an enantiomer, and filing a patent on the latter, is frequently attempted as the original patent covering the racemic mixture progresses through its 20-year life cycle. Such 'evergreening' efforts are nothing new, but are not necessarily successful, at least without the availability of effective trademark strategy. Benzedrine, the first medicinal amphetamine product, as a racemic mixture was patented in 1924. Facing competition, and the impending expiry of that patent, the company (Smith, Kline & French) separated the left-handed form from the right one and patented the method of doing so. Although efforts to separately patent both forms failed, the company, finding the right-handed isomer (dextroamphatamine) to have more pleasing effects on people than the left-handed one, successfully marketed the former under the brand-name of Dexedrine. The 'dex' prefix comes from the Greek word for right: δεξια.[18]

Stereoisomerism is not the only type of variability that can be managed for commercial advantage. Prodrugs are chemically inactive drugs that are converted in the human body into the active ingredient by the action of enzymes. There are numerous reasons why prodrug forms can provide benefits, such as by enhancing in-body transportation or reducing toxicity effects. However, the actual metabolised product which causes the therapeutic effect can itself lead to an improved patient experience if delivered in that form instead. For example, the antihistamine prodrug terfenadine, marketed as Seldane, has cardio-toxic effects on some people. The metabolite, fexofenadine, subsequently marketed as Allegra (among various other names), is not. Metabolites of previously patented prodrugs can be patented too, as were both these two products. However, the situation is far from certain for companies. In the United Kingdom, the House of Lords revoked the patent on fexofenadine as the earlier patent on terfenadine had rendered it no longer novel even though the metabolite product had not been explicitly disclosed in the earlier patent.[19] But this did not necessarily make it impossible to patent a metabolite given the facts of the case were specific to the patents at issue. Indeed, in a 2003 United States Court of Appeals for the Federal Circuit case, Judge Rader found a metabolite to be inherently anticipated (that is, not novel), but he went on to clarify that 'With proper claiming, patent protection is available for metabolites of known drugs'.[20] He suggested different ways to evade anticipation including claiming an isolated and purified form of the metabolite or on a method of administering it to a patient.

Follow-on patents of these kinds that claim meaningful distinctions between similar things that in other contexts might be regarded as practically identical may promise benefits for patients. For example, whereas one patented minor molecular modification to a drug may make no difference to the average patient, another could lead to a much improved therapeutic effect on at least some patients. The former type would appear to be commercially valueless. If so, why file patents on it?

Notwithstanding possible benefits, patenting strategy here is clearly aimed to extend the market exclusivity of an existing drug or to support marketing aimed at switching patients to a supposedly upgraded version of a company's existing product. This is why they are controversial. Such incremental inventions may be regarded as examples of gaming the system by acquiring extended or new patent monopolies that are not justified by the minor level of inventive contribution or the possibly negligible added benefit to the public. Such practices are commonly referred to as secondary patenting,[21] or 'evergreening', a curious metaphor choice when one stops to think about it.[22] The industry of course sees them as perfectly justifiable. For critics, they reflect a flaw in the patent system, one with serious implications for access to medicines, and for the promotion of innovation. If you can get 20 years' added monopoly for a modest change that may not even be an improvement relating to a product which you already enjoy a dominant market position in, why invest in more expensive and risky radical innovation? So much for the traditional justifications for patents: that they reward inventors for bringing new things into the world that benefit society, and incentivise the development and dissemination of innovations that would otherwise never exist. We will look into this further below and again in the next chapter.

The phenomenon of tertiary patenting has recently emerged, albeit as yet without attracting much attention. Here, the patent covered 'product' is not a new chemical, whether radically new or a cosmetically modified version of an old one; nor is it even a chemical, at least not by itself. Rather, what is patented is a drug delivery device to be used in combination with an existing drug.[23] Such devices include such items as self-injector pens for drugs like insulin and epinephrine. Given that these can have their effective monopoly terms extended by means of patenting incremental variations that may or may not provide enhanced therapeutic value, tertiary patenting seems bound to start attracting controversy.

Even when the end of the monopoly on the existing branded drug can no longer be delayed any further, with good marketing it may be possible to shift patients from an about to become off-patent drug onto a new version marketed under a different name that is fundamentally the same thing and thus hardly better therapeutically if at all. If the original drug was successful and profitable while the patent was valid, such product switching could well generate a lot of money. We will consider more of the contemporary criticisms of patents in the next chapter.

Intellectual Property in Biotechnology

As business tools, patents can profoundly influence investment patterns and, in consequence, even the whole structure of a business sector. This is bound to be especially the case for a sector that is very heavily science-based and has been utterly dependent on patents right from the time of its inception. The last four decades have seen the establishment of a growing number of small science-based firms seeking to develop or take advantage of new biological technologies. Given the high costs and risks, and the lengthy time horizons entailed by developing new medicines, they tended to focus more on the discovery side than on development. Their ability to remain in business, raise funds and grow is heavily reliant on patents. As we will see, realisation of this dependency makes such firms very interested in patent regulation to the point in some cases of seeking to influence policy-making.

Key to the success of biotechnology company initial public offerings (IPOs) was the possession of patents protecting important technologies and promising products in the making. The *Diamond v. Chakrabarty* decision provided a tremendous fillip in this respect. In that 1980 decision, the US Supreme Court ruled by a narrow majority that an engineered oil-eating bacterium produced by Anand Chakrabarty, an employee of General Electric, could be classed as a 'composition of matter' or a 'manufacture', and therefore be treated as a patentable invention. Before the 1980s, the patent situation with respect to biotechnology processes and products was highly uncertain. While clearly non-biological process technologies such as recombinant DNA could be patented in the USA, the court-crafted (i.e. non-statutory) product of nature doctrine, which dates back to the nineteenth century, was assumed by the Patent and Trademark Office — and by most scientists — entirely to preclude the patenting of life forms and their structural and functional components.[24] In the absence of statutory language treating 'discoveries' as not being inventions, the meaning of the product of nature doctrine is that organisms or substances as they occur in nature cannot be considered as patent eligible subject matter.

Up to that time, the new biotechnology firms were yet to organize themselves into a single trade association to further their collective legal and regulatory interests.[25] However, the Chakrabarty decision — highly successful for industry — was achieved neither by a such a firm or even a pharmaceutical company, but by a firm traditionally involved in quite unrelated research activities, General Electric.[26]

Diamond v Chakrabarty: The patenting of living organisms

Prior to 1972 when General Electric filed its patent in 1972, of the four million US patents issued since 1790, only 70 had protected 'mixtures or compounds that included microorganisms in unmodified form'.[27] Only Pasteur's yeast culture product patent exclusively covered living organisms. The product of nature doctrine had since the 1880s apparently precluded the patenting of any further life forms. At least, that was the view of the United States Patent and Trademark Office (USPTO) when it rejected the application's claims directed to the microorganism itself. Within the emergent biotechnology sector it was likewise generally assumed that microorganisms could not be patented.

General Electric's patent lawyers had a different attitude, working as they did for a long-established industrial corporation whose use of the patent system goes back to its formation in the 1890s. So while the scientist involved, Anand Chakrabarty, doubted that his microorganism could be patented, the company lawyer assigned to the case, Leo MaLossi, saw no logical reason why it could not. 'To MaLossi, aware that by now scientists understood living matter, including bacteria to be chemicals, Chakrabarty's bugs were manufactures, new compositions of matter — and, hence, patentable'.[28]

On appeal at the Court of Customs and Patent Appeals, the patent rejection was overturned. In hindsight this was the most likely outcome. A few months earlier, Judge Rich of the Court had made the following statement when delivering the majority opinion at the conclusion of a similar case[29]: 'we think the fact that microorganisms, as distinguished from chemical compounds, are more akin to inanimate chemical compositions such as reactants, reagents, and catalysts than they are to horses and honeybees or raspberries and roses'. There is no question that this life as chemistry conceptualization inherent to MaLossi and Rich's arguments is a powerful one. Indeed, it is now implicitly recognised by other patent offices, including the European Patent Office.[30,31] By treating micro-organisms as natural chemical substances into which a useful new characteristic has been introduced and thereby rendered unnatural, they are assumed to be patentable in accordance with long-established practice with respect to chemical products that allows a natural chemical to be the basis for an invention as long as the

(*Continued*)

(Continued)

version claimed differs by being more purer, modified chemically, or by being mixed with something else that results in a different effect.

In 1980, the USPTO's appeal at the Supreme Court was rejected by five to four. According to the majority opinion, the US legislature (that is, Congress) 'recognized that the relevant distinction was not between living and inanimate things, but between products of nature, whether living or not, and human-made inventions'. And any novelty and utility concerns, if there were any, were addressed by the Court's statement that 'the patentee has produced a new bacterium with markedly different characteristics from any found in nature and one having the potential for significant utility.' In making this decision, the Court was not of course taking the view that all parts of the microorganism had been made by Chakrabarty. Rather, it was treating the microorganism as a natural compound that had been structurally modified and thus transformed into a new 'article of manufacture' or 'composition of matter' that was no longer natural. By treating the microorganism as a natural chemical substance into which a useful new characteristic had been introduced and thereby rendered unnatural, the court found it patentable in accordance with long-established practice with respect to chemical products.[32]

Interestingly, the Pharmaceutical Manufacturers Association in its amicus brief was keen to assert that if a line should be drawn, it should not be placed between the living and the non-living but between unicellular and multicellular life forms. It referred to the British Patent Act of 1977 and the European Patent Convention, both of which explicitly excluded plant varieties and animals but not microorganisms. Indeed, Chakrabarty's British patent application on the same invention had been granted without fanfare or controversy. This was of course strategic. The PMA would have preferred no subject matter restrictions, but the battle to further extend patent protection could wait for another day.

The majority dismissed arguments that wider societal values being at play, the patent application should be rejected. As the Peoples Business Commission, whose most prominent leader was a well known activist called Jeremy Rifkin, stated in a submission to the Court:

It is PBC's contention that such a proliferation of genetically-based technologies is not in the public interest for a host of reasons. PBC believes that the

(*Continued*)

ecological, evolutionary, ethical, philosophical, political and economic questions that surround that patenting of living organisms have been given insufficient consideration by the Congress, the country as a whole and the lower court in issuing its ruling in favor of such patents.

The Commission also invoked a slippery slope argument, that — contrary to the PMA but in fact as was proven to be correct, once a life form was held patentable, any life form would become patentable. The Court specifically addressed the first point but — perhaps understandably given the absence of any statutory instruction to take account of societal values especially morality — refused to admit that such matters are relevant:

The briefs present a gruesome parade of horribles. Scientists, among them Nobel laureates, are quoted suggesting that genetic research may pose a serious threat to the human race, or, at the very least, that the dangers are far too substantial to permit such research to proceed apace at this time. We are told that genetic research and related technological developments may spread pollution and disease, that it may result in a loss of genetic diversity, and that its practice may tend to depreciate the value of human life. These arguments are forcefully, even passionately, presented; they remind us that, at times, human ingenuity seems unable to control fully the forces it creates — that, with Hamlet, it is sometimes better ;'to bear those ills we have than fly to others that we know not of.'

…

What is more important is that we are without competence to entertain these arguments — either to brush them aside as fantasies generated by fear of the unknown, or to act on them. The choice we are urged to make is a matter of high policy for resolution within the legislative process after the kind of investigation, examination, and study that legislative bodies can provide and courts cannot. That process involves the balancing of competing values and interests, which in our democratic system is the business of elected representatives. Whatever their validity, the contentions now pressed on us should be addressed to the political branches of the Government, the Congress and the Executive, and not to the courts.

The decision in *Diamond v. Chakrabarty* was the first success in a campaign by industry to clarify (and later to change) patent rules in the biotechnology field in ways that suited their interests. General Electric did not pursue this affair because the invention in question had commercial promise, of which there was little — but because the company was seeking to ensure that the barrier to the patenting of microorganisms would henceforth be lifted. Not surprisingly Generic Electric attracted support from pro-patent interests with several amicus briefs filed by companies and organizations such as Genentech, the Pharmaceutical Manufacturers Association, and the American Patent Law Association. (In fact, most of the ten amicus briefs supported General Electric's position). Among the arguments made to the Court by Genentech and the PMA were that patents as compared to trade secrecy allowed for greater public accountability, and that allowing patents would encourage innovation and enhance the country's competitiveness in an emerging high technology field.[33] In other words, according to these groups, permitting the patenting of microorganisms is in the national and public interest. In propounding such a justification, they were claiming patent rights on public interest grounds rather than on the basis of desert. This was clearly a prudent strategy, but should be contrasted with the way some of these same interests sought to frame similar claims at the international level later in that decade.

In hindsight it is difficult to imagine any other outcome given the collective economic power of the interests which stood to gain and the forum in which the legal breakthrough was achieved. According to Cary Fowler, then an anti-biotech patenting activist,

> The GE-Chakrabarty case was a major tactical victory for the industry. Not only did it secure the protection it had long sought, but it did so through a new arena, the court system. The courts were neither fast not cheap, but they were faster and cheaper than the political process. They were also foreign territory to most advocacy groups.[34]

Despite some recent reversals — most famously the Myriad decision (see below), the United States has tended to be the boldest jurisdiction for subject-matter expansiveness. We will consider the reasons for this below. Continued attempts by organizations such as farm, animal welfare and church groups[35] and organizations like Jeremy Rifkin's Foundation on Economic Trends to roll back the tide had to face the organized opposition of industry and even universities that saw the licensing of biotech patenting as a potentially huge earner for them. Yale historian of science Daniel Kevles explains that in congressional hearings during the early 1990s, 'patent attorneys, biotech representatives, and several congressmen warned that restrictions or a moratorium on the patenting of life or its parts would put the US at a competitive disadvantage internationally and impede research on cures and therapies for disease'.[36] These alleged negative consequences were clearly very persuasive, and opponents stood little chance of success.

In 1993, the patent interests of the domestic biotechnology sector were further strengthened — one might say even privileged — with the passage of the Biotechnology Patent Act. The law was intended to prevent a situation in which foreign companies could import into the USA a product manufactured through known processes that being so could not be claimed in a domestic firm's patent covering elements of the product. The legislation was inspired by a 1991 court decision involving Amgen and a Japanese company called Chugai, relating to the production and importation of recombinant erythropoietin (EPO). The court determined that Amgen could not assert its patent to prevent Chugai from importing EPO produced in Japan through the recombinant DNA technology. This was because previous court decisions had determined that the scope of Amgen's patent covered only the complementary DNA[37] coding for EPO and host cells transformed by the EPO-expressing gene. It did not cover the recombinant EPO itself, or the process which had of course been patented earlier by Cohen and Boyer. Chugai was in the advantageous position of having licensed a patent owned by Genetics Institute that covered the rEPO itself.[38] This allowed it to produce the EPO using the cDNA patented by Amgen and the same technique *as long as* its production was carried out abroad with the EPO then exported to the USA.

For lawmakers, this experience pointed to the need to change the law to protect an emerging industrial sector considered vital to the future of the US economy. The legislation essentially dispensed with the normal patentability requirements in respect of processes as long they were being employed to manufacture something new. In part, the Act stated that 'a claimed process of making or using a medicine, manufacture, or composition of matter is not obvious under this section if — (1) the machine, manufacture, or composition of matter is novel ... and nonobvious ... (2) the claimed process is a biotechnological process ...'.[39]

As regards patentable subject matter, in a 1985 patent appeals case, the Patent and Trademark Office affirmed the patentability of plants, seeds and plant tissue cultures. In 1987, the PTO Board produced another ground-breaking ruling (in ex parte Allen) concerning a patent application on oysters. Although the patent was rejected, the ruling established that multicellular organisms were patentable. A year later the first ever animal patent was granted for 'a transgenic nonhuman mammal' containing an activated oncogene sequence. The patent is commonly referred to as the oncomouse patent, since it describes a mouse into which a gene has been introduced which induces increased susceptibility to cancer (see below).

Genentech raised considerable funds with its post-Chakrabarty IPO, announced two months after the Supreme Court decision, and with the Bayh Dole Act enacted later that year, other university researchers moved into this emerging sector or opted to launch new firms themselves. Another factor in enhancing the sense that patents were not just necessary but actually valuable as business assets was the 1982 establishment by Congress of the Court of the Appeals for the Federal Circuit (CAFC) to hear all patent appeal cases. The Court is widely acknowledged to have reversed the tendency of many appeals courts in the USA to be sceptical about the validity of patents.

None of this should be surprising given that 'a very large group of large high technology firms and trade associations in the telecommunications, computer and pharmaceutical industries was essentially responsible for the creation of the CAFC. The group believed that a court devoted to patent cases would better represent its interests'.[40] In addition to these developments, the US government was also one of the main actors in strengthening intellectual property protection worldwide in support of its science-based corporations (and copyright and trade mark industries).

During the early and mid-1980s, there was a wave of successful IPOs by biotechnology start-up companies following in Genentech's footsteps, the biggest being that of Cetus, where PCR was discovered, which raised $107 million, and which was actually founded before Genentech.[41] The founders of many of these companies hoped eventually to turn them into integrated pharmaceutical corporations. Only in a few cases have such ambitions been realised. The costs of doing research in this field are very high, and the risks of investing in companies several years at least from having any products to sell are considerable. Consequently, there has been a tendency at times to make exaggerated claims about new discoveries and products. For some critics, recombinant insulin is a good example.

Biotech Patenting in Europe

During the 1980s and 90s, Europe tended to follow these trends, albeit with some important differences. In 1988 the European Patent Office granted the first patent on a plant. The European oncomouse patent, about which much more will be said below, was also granted after initially being rejected. In the late 1980s, the European Commission decided to draft a directive on the legal protection of biotechnological inventions. The European Commission was motivated by concerns about the legal uncertainties which, it was felt, could be prejudicial to the future of biotechnology in Europe, and fears that some European countries might respond to mounting controversy by banning patents on living organisms and genes. However, it was only in 1998 that the *Directive on the Legal Protection of Biotechnological Inventions* was finally adopted.

Let us consider the Directive's language in relation to synthesized and isolated chemicals that are copies of, or are themselves, natural products. There is no reason to suppose that the drafters had read the old US Cochrane (see Chapter 5) or Parke Davis (Chapter 6) cases, disapproving of the former judgment and approving the latter. After all, why would they have bothered to read these ancient cases from the United States? And yet, upon reading certain provisions of the Directive, one can be forgiven for wondering whether they had. Thus Recital 20 of the Directive states in part:

> ... an invention based on an element isolated from the human body
> or otherwise produced by means of a technical process, which is

susceptible of industrial application, is not excluded from patentability, even where the structure of that element is identical to that of a natural element, given that the rights conferred by the patent do not extend to the human body and its elements in their natural environment.

Reference is made to the human body rather than, as in Cochrane, to a produced 'element' that is identical to a natural element existing in a plant. Nonetheless, the issue of whether a synthetic or isolated chemical can be patented despite its being identical to a naturally occurring substance is again answered but this time affirmatively.

Turning to the question of whether a substance isolated from the human body or other life form can form the basis of an invention capable of passing the novelty test, Article 3.2 states that 'biological material which is isolated from its natural environment or produced by means of a technical process may be the subject of an invention even if it previously occurred in nature.' No doubt Learned Hand would approve. Article 5.2 follows this up linking this general principle specifically to gene sequences and the human body: 'an element isolated from the human body or otherwise produced by means of a technical process, including the sequence or partial sequence of a gene, may constitute a patentable invention, even if the structure of that element is identical to that of a natural element'. As we will see below, as a result of this language, Europe is now more welcoming of DNA patent claims than is the United States.

Animal patenting

Aside from patenting a human being, the most radical subject-matter for a patent would appear to be an animal. Let us now turn to the first animal patent, the oncomouse. One of the reasons why the oncomouse case is interesting is that patent-granting offices and courts in three important jurisdictions have been called on to assess the patentability of the oncomouse but have failed to come up with the same conclusions. This not only raises the question of how far patent law should go but also how far the harmonisation of patent standards in biotechnology can go.

The oncomouse patent saga begins in June 1985, when Harvard University filed a patent application for 'transgenic non-human mammals', naming as inventors Philip Leder and Timothy A. Stewart. The patent was granted in April 1988. The primary claim covers the following:

> A transgenic non-human mammal all of whose germ cells and somatic cells contain a recombinant activated oncogene sequence introduced into said mammal, or an ancestor of said animal, at an embryonic stage.

Three things are interesting here. The first is the obvious fact that a living organism is being claimed as an invention. The second is that the patent describes the successful introduction of oncogenes into mice and yet it claims not only mice but all transgenic non-human mammals transformed through the same process. The third is that the scope of the patent includes not just animals with activated oncogenes, of which an increasing number are being discovered, but also their ancestors into which the oncogenes were initially introduced by the inventors. In other words, the patent owners have rights to all future generations of mice that inherit the oncogenes up to the expiry date of the patent.

The first interesting feature, that for the first time, an animal has been claimed as a patentable invention, raises the question of whether this is consistent with well-established patent doctrines. While no US courts were called on to answer this question, the decision of the Supreme Court in *Diamond v. Chakrabarty* suggests that the Court may have answered in the affirmative. Indeed, the ruling in ex parte Allen, mentioned above, relied in part on the Chakrabarty decision. One interesting thing to note here is an amicus on behalf of the Pharmaceutical Manufacturers Association before the United States Supreme Court as it deliberated on the Chakrabarty microbe was intent on challenging efforts by others to raise 'slippery-slope' concerns. Falsely, as subsequent events would prove, it dismissed the possibility that the issue of patenting higher life forms could be settled without congressional action. In consistency with Judge Rich's statement in Bergy, the amicus expressed that 'if a line must be drawn, it may easily be drawn between the mindless, soulless microorganism involved in Chakrabarty (as well as Bergy) and higher forms of life'.

As for the second feature of the US oncomouse patent, this appears to claim too much, since for all anybody knew, the use of the technique to transform other animals may prove to be far more difficult and may require unobvious modifications to the technique. This is a problem of excessive patent breadth that is not limited to the life sciences, but is nonetheless very important and will be considered further below.

Turning to the third feature, this situation is clearly problematic. One of the ways in which the patent system seeks to balance the interests of owners and the public is through the concept of exhaustion of rights (or the first sale doctrine in the United States). Once a patent-protected product is sold by the owner or the licensee, his or her rights over that product are usually exhausted, unless there is a contract of sale imposing conditions on buyers. When it comes to patents on life forms, the rights are not exhausted when the 'product' is sold but extend to the progeny whether or not the progeny is directly 'manufactured' by the 'inventors'. In this sense, we are making a concession to the patent owner in order to make the patent monopoly meaningful. It is not necessarily wrong to do this. After all, the public may benefit from the use of transgenic animals for such purposes as medical research (as with the oncomouse) or so-called pharming (the use of transgenic animals as producers of thera-peutic proteins for human health).

As far as patentability goes, the oncomouse was treated quite differ-ently in Europe. From an early time all life forms were not equal as far as patentability went, and that applied also to methods of producing or utilis-ing them. To some extent at least, this is what industry wanted. The 1963 *Strasbourg Convention on the Unification of Certain Points of Substantive Law on Patents for Invention*, from which the relevant parts of the European Patent Convention and TRIPS borrowed language, stated that 'parties were not required to grant patents in respect of ... (b) plant or animal varieties or essentially biological processes for the production of plants or animals; this provision does not apply to microbiological processes and the products thereof'. The singling out of microbiological processes and prod-ucts was made at the suggestion of AIPPI, an influential international association of intellectual property practitioners, which pointed out that microorganisms were commonly used in well-established industrial activi-ties such as brewing alcoholic beverages and baking bread.[42]

As far as animal patenting goes, the story begins, as in the United States, with the oncomouse. The European one, though, is long reaching a final conclusion only in 2004. During prosecution of the patent application, the Examining Division objected to the broad scope of the product claims, which extended to 'transgenic non-human eukaryotic animals' despite, as with the US patent, only disclosing the insertion of the oncogenes in mice. In response, the applicants narrowed the claims to 'non-human mammalian animals'.

Nonetheless, while the Canadian Patent Office rejected the product claims alone, the European Patent Office in July 1989 rejected the patent entirely on two grounds. The first was that in claiming animals that were new on the basis of the introduction of oncogenes, the patent was to all intents and purposes claiming animal 'varieties'. According to Article 53(b) of the European Patent Convention (EPC), animal varieties are not patentable.

The second was insufficiency of disclosure, which was not satisfied by the narrowed-down product claims. According to Article 83 of the EPC, 'the European patent application must disclose the invention in a manner sufficiently clear and complete for it to be carried out by a person skilled in the art'. The Examining Division's reasons for rejecting the patent on the grounds of insufficient disclosure were as follows:

> The claims as they presently stand refer to non-human mammalian animals, i.e. not only to mice or more generally to rodents but to any kind of mammals such as anthropoid apes or elephants, all of which have a highly different number of genes and differently developed immune systems.

The Examining Division added that:

> Mr Philip Leder, one of the inventors of the present case, declared . . . before the United States Patent and Trademark Office how surprising it was to obtain positive results on the mouse and reasons are given why he thought that he might have failed. This clearly shows that the success with the transgenic mouse cannot be reasonably extrapolated to all mammals.[43]

On appeal, the Technical Board of Appeal (TBA) decided in October 1990 that animals *per se* were not excluded from patentability under Article 53(b) EPC. It followed that since claims to genetically modified animals, mammals or any other taxonomic groups higher than that of species were not animal varieties, the oncomouse patent could not therefore be rejected on such grounds. In addition, the TBA pointed out that animals produced by microbiological processes would not fall under the exception anyway. It therefore requested that the Examining Division reconsider its interpretation. The TBA also denied that the disclosure was insufficient. Furthermore, in light of the many objections to the patent from animal welfare, religious and environmental organisations on the basis of Article 53(a) of the EPC, according to which patents 'in respect of inventions the publication or exploitation of which would be contrary to ordre public or morality'[44] would not be granted, the TBA came up with a so-called balancing test which it requested the EPO Examining Division to apply. According to the test, the examiners were required by the TBA to conduct 'a careful weighing up of the suffering of animals and possible risks to the environment on the one hand, and the invention's usefulness to mankind on the other'.[45] In October 1992, the grant of European Patent 169,672 was formally announced.

But the story did not end there. Further oppositions to the patent were filed during the 1990s and led in 2001 to the EPO's Opposition Division's response of restricting the product-related scope of the patent from 'non-human mammalian animals' to 'transgenic rodents'. In 2003, an interlocutory decision of the EPO's Opposition Division held the patent to be valid on the basis of the reduced scope but also affirmed that EPC rule 23d(d),[46] which requires that patents not be granted for 'processes for modifying the genetic identity of animals which are likely to cause them suffering without any substantial medical benefit to man or animal, and also animals resulting from such processes', is applicable for drawing the appropriate scope of a patent such as the oncomouse one.

In July 2004, the TBA was again required to assess the validity of the patent. The TBA's application of both the balancing test it had formulated in 1990 and rule 23d(d) resulted in a finding that the patent was valid but only on the basis of claims confined to 'transgenic mouse',[47] thereby vindicating the Examining Division's objections 15 years earlier to the patent's over-broad scope!

The differing treatment of the oncomouse patents in these three jurisdictions suggests that without a clear understanding of why we have patent systems in the first place and what they are meant to achieve, it may not be easy to argue conclusively that patenting life departs from the basic tenets of patent law and should not therefore be allowed. However, one clear point of divergence from conventional patent norms is that since living things have a tendency to reproduce by themselves, or at least with willing partners, in granting patents on life forms we are being very generous to the owners when we allow them to claim ancestors and progeny. But in our view, to know whether this is right or wrong we need to consider what we, that is to say, the public, gets out of the bargain.

DNA *as patentable subject matter*

The ease with which DNA claims slipped into patent claims belies the subsequent controversies about such 'things' being patented. DNA sequences started being claimed in the early 1980s. By the end of the century this number had increased enormously.

In January 2001, the US Patent and Trademark Office announced a new rule for DNA-related patent examinations. Patent applications disclosing DNA sequences had to provide convincing evidence that their utility is specific, substantial, and credible.[48] This effectively closed the door on EST claims,[49] and this was confirmed in a 2005 decision at the Court of Appeals for the Federal Circuit.[50] However, many more far-reaching proposals were rejected. This was an incremental reform albeit still very welcome.

Human gene patenting and the assertion of patent rights have continued to be intensely controversial. There are three types of human DNA claim: (i) isolated pieces of genomic DNA (gDNA) cut out of the bigger DNA molecule extracted from living cells; (ii) synthetic DNA the order of whose sequences are unchanged; (iii) synthetic DNA the order of whose sequences differ from the equivalent section of gDNA by the exclusion of inactive bases. This product is called complementary DNA, or cDNA for short.

Patents on genes linked to particular diseases tend to claim a range of applications including diagnostic and predictive tests. Some patent owners have been quite determined in enforcing their rights, including in one instance against patients that had collaborated in the discovery of the gene resulting in a lawsuit.[51] Often the validity of such patents is considered to be extremely questionable. Even non-commercial entities like public sector hospitals may be the target of companies demanding royalties or forcing them to close down. For example, it was reported that 'after the gene for the iron overload condition haemochromatosis was patented, 30 percent of labs surveyed stopped testing for the disease-causing gene variant, or developing such tests'.[52]

Perhaps the best known case with the most far-reaching implications concerns the patenting activity of the aforementioned Myriad Genetics relating to and covering two large genes (BRCA1 and BRCA2) linked to a certain proportion of breast cancer cases. But before looking into the discovery of the BRCA genes and the patent cases in which the eligibility of DNA claims was considered, it is useful briefly to discuss the contested nature of DNA, which certainly creates difficulties for courts. DNA is a chemical, but is it not something more than *just* a chemical. What does 'being something more' imply for patent disclosures, how patent claims are evaluated, and how courts should determine whether and to what extent it qualifies as protectable subject matter? None of this is at clear, as should be evident from our discussion on DNA in the previous chapter.

Nobody doubts that DNA is a chemical. But is it just a chemical, and if it is not, is it appropriate for the law treat to treat is a chemical no more nor less? Humans 'share' genes with every single living thing from bacteria to beetles and beavers. Most of our genome is identical to that of chimpanzees and gorillas. Individually, our differences are minuscule. And yet the role of DNA in heredity, our individual destiny and in our sense of identity — as persons, and members of family and humankind — already makes human DNA patenting a sensitive issue to many even before we get into debates on access and supply of DNA-based diagnostic tests subject to patent monopolies.[53] For many of those taking issue with the notion that DNA is like any other chemical for the purposes of intellectual property law, it is an emotive issue. Here 'Playing God' types of objection come to the fore as do ones proffered by opponents of unbridled capitalism and other social critics concerned that commodification of life has no apparent limits. Wherever one stands on the matter, DNA undeniably has unusual properties.

DNA is not just a thing but a hybrid. But the nature of this hybridity and the question of why it matters in terms of law are a little unclear because we seem unable fully to agree on what exactly information has to do with DNA, genes, and life in general, other than, well, quite a lot obviously. Nonetheless to regard DNA as having a dual chemical-informational nature is certainly a lot more helpful than treating it as stuff and nothing but stuff whose scientific investigation and commercial exploitation requires one first to have a physical sample in one's test tube. Gleaning knowledge and extracting commercial value does not always require direct contact with a single DNA molecule. Vast amounts of sequence data are stored on computers and all the advantages of big data in other fields of human endeavour including science and business are available here too.

If this discussion is useful at all it is because it helps us to understand that DNA is a chemical but of a very special kind. As we will see, there is a danger of the conceptual differences leading to practical difficulties. Patent law must do more than treat DNA exactly as if it is any other type of chemical, but the question is how should it? We will look first into the different types of DNA product claims in patents. After this we will consider some of the practical concerns that have arisen. Then we will see how different jurisdictions have dealt with patentability of 'new' subject matter and determined the appropriate scope of protection.

Patenting human DNA and its limits: the Myriad story

Myriad Genetics is a company known as much for its aggressive assertion of its gene patents as for the genetic testing services it provides. The company's IP acquisition and management activities form an essential part of any account of the evolution of patent law in the field of molecular biology, especially genetics. This is because the controversies motivated litigation and legal reforms that in a few cases actually affected the scope of patent

---

(Continued)

(*Continued*)

protection in the field of genomics. Some European countries' opting for purpose bound patent protect appears to be a response of sorts to concerns arising from Myriad's aggressive patent acquisition and assertion practices. Myriad's patents have been litigated in a few countries, but we will focus just on those few cases which have resulted in changes to the scope of protectable subject matter: the recent United States Supreme Court and Australian High Court cases. But first, we present some background.

The discoveries of the afore-mentioned BRCA genes were not made by Myriad alone — far from it. Mary-Claire King of University of California, Berkeley showed in 1990 that both breast and ovarian cancer could run in families, and that a variant of a gene located somewhere on chromosome 17, given the name BRCA1, substantially increased a woman's susceptibility to both cancers.[54] BRCA1 codes for a protein that is 'critical for DNA repair and transcription regulation; when the gene is inactivated through mutation and the protein is altered, it leads to abnormal cellular gene expression'.[55] In April 1995, King filed a US patent assigned to the Regents of the University of California on 'genetic markers for breast, ovarian, and prostatic cancer', which was granted in April 1997.[56] However, two companies, Myriad Genetics and OncorMed, patented the sequenced gene.[57] In Myriad's case it was actually a collective effort involving scientists from the University of Utah, the National Institutes of Health (NIH) and McGill University. Myriad filed its BRCA1-related US patents on 7 June 1995.[58] These claimed the whole gene sequence plus some harmful mutations.[59] OncorMed's first US patent on BRCA1 sequences was filed a few months later, on 12 February 1996.[60] The sequences claimed were very similar to those of Myriad.

Subsequently, another variant gene linked to breast cancer incidence, dubbed BRCA2, was also patented by Myriad even though the claimed invention drew heavily on publicly available sequence data and a considerable amount of public sector research. It is probably more accurate, and certainly fairer, to say that BRCA2 was discovered by an international team led by Mike Stratton at the Institute of Cancer Research (ICR), which had determined that the gene was located somewhere on chromosome 13. According to Stratton, on 23 November 1995, the Sanger Centre in Cambridge and Washington University's Genome Sequencing Center

(*Continued*)

jointly released onto the internet a sequence of 900,000 nucleotide bases containing the gene. Their intention in doing this was to accelerate the identification of the gene's precise location but without favouring any of the research groups involved in the race. The Cancer Research Campaign (CRC) filed two UK patents, the first on the very same day that the sequence was released on the internet in the same month, the second on 21 December. The applications claimed a 1,000 base pair stretch of cDNA but not the whole sequence of the gene. The idea of doing so was controversial but it was meant as a public-spirited gesture. In this case it was done to try and prevent Myriad from controlling both genes and also to ensure the test would be widely available on the National Health Service and that it would be marketed and carried out in an ethical manner respectful towards patients. It achieved this by licensing the patent to OncorMed with very strict pro public health stipulations.[61]

On December 22, the ICR-led consortium publicly announced the sequencing of BRCA2, that they had filed the above UK patents, and that an article would be coming out the following day in *Nature*.[62] However, Myriad, who had downloaded the internet data, and drawing on automated sequencing technological capacity that the public consortium could not match, had very quickly sequenced the whole gene. Myriad made its own announcement on the same day, and filed an initial US patent application one day before the second and most important of the UK patent applications.[63] As with BRCA1, it subsequently filed patents on BRCA2 elsewhere including at the European Patent Office.

Myriad, which was spun off the University of Utah and was receiving some funding from Eli Lilly and the NIH, was determined to assert its priority and monopolise diagnostic testing services in the United States for hereditary breast and ovarian cancer. It was successful on both counts. But the company's behaviour not only made it hugely unpopular, but also brought gene patenting itself into disrepute.

By 1996, four institutions in the US offered commercial testing services: Myriad, OncorMed, the Genetics and IVF Institute, and the University of Pennsylvania's Genetics Diagnostics Laboratory. These were all a bit different in terms of how they did the testing, the specific sequences being tested for, and the types of people they tested. Myriad claimed that its test called

(*Continued*)

(Continued)

'BRACAnalysis' was the so-called 'gold standard', but none of them was perfect, and Myriad's was very expensive, in part because it was done in-house at the company's headquarters in Salt Lake City. The company came to an arrangement with OncorMed, which had licensed King's and the CRC's patents, according to which Myriad took over the latter firm's patents. It then used its patent rights to have all of its rival testing programmes closed down. Having cornered the US market it sought aggressively to do the same thing in Canada and Europe. In Europe the only legal obstacle was the ICR patent and the fact that its aggressive commercial practices were running into opposition at various levels, from patient groups who believed Myriad was taking improper advantage of women's anxiety about their health,[64] to professional medical associations, genetics laboratories and other public health organisations and parliamentarians, who were in varying degrees shocked by the sheer ruthlessness of Myriad and were questioning the wisdom of allowing genes to be patented at all. The outrage was perhaps greatest in those countries, like the UK, Canada and France, which have largely state-provided healthcare systems with fairly tight budgets. In Europe, the French Institut Curie, whose own research in this area cast doubts as to the quality of Myriad's test, organised a campaign to have the company's European patents revoked. The Institut and its partners in this effort relied primarily on classic patentability grounds rather than resorting to moral arguments, and this strategy proved to be successful with Myriad's patents either being invalidated or having their claims drastically reduced.[65]

The Myriad patents in the United States were challenged in court by public interest groups and patients, initially successfully. The lower court threw out all of Myriad's 15 patent claims in seven patents relating to BRCA1 and BRCA2 on isolated DNA, cDNA, and methods of comparing and analysing.[66] On appeal, the court's decision regarding the product claims to isolated DNA and cDNA was reversed. After some toing and froing between the Court of Appeals for the Federal Circuit and the Supreme Court, the later made its final decision in 2013.[67] In answer to the question of whether human genes are patentable, Judge Thomas speaking for the Court declared that isolated DNA is ineligible under section 101 of the Patent Act. However, cDNA was eligible subject to fulfilment of the criteria. Interestingly, the Court took a utilitarian approach. Citing an earlier case, the Court stated that in deciding what is naturally occurring, a law of nature, or a product of nature,

(Continued)

one must take into account the purpose of patent law — as if patent law itself must form the source by which practical meanings for these difficult concepts are to be sought. That makes sense as long as the malleability of such terminology, as Justice Frankfurter recognised decades before, in that earlier case, is kept within some reasonable limits. Accordingly, the Court argued, the inventive capacity of people should not be restrained by patenting what should be freely available to all. Finding the location of something already in existence is not patent-eligible under section 101 however extensive the effort entailed. As for the nature of the DNA disclosed and claimed in the patents, the Court noted that it was not DNA as chemistry but as information. Therefore breaking chemical bonds to isolate DNA is not significant because the information is not altered by doing so. Claiming a separated fragment of code that is part of much long code, none of which you have written yourself is not inventive and would be harmful for innovation. Oddly, when it came to cDNA the fact of its being a chemical synthesised in the laboratory seems to make it a new thing. Clearly it is not new as information since the messenger RNA leaving the nucleus would only differ from it by the substitution of a U for a T but it was at least 'made' by human effort and this makes it a new artefact: it is 'an exons-only molecule, that is not naturally occurring.' As expressed by Thomas:

[The petitioners] argue that cDNA is not patent eligible because '[t]he nucleotide sequence of cDNA is dictated by nature, not by the lab technician.'… That may be so, but the lab technician unquestionably creates something new when cDNA is made. cDNA retains the naturally occurring exons of DNA, but it is distinct from the DNA from which it was derived. As a result, cDNA is not a 'product of nature' and is patent eligible under §101 …

What the Court did not consider was the patent status of synthetic single-strand DNA primers?[68] These are not isolated but are, like cDNA made in the lab. So they are human artefacts, not natural products. However, unlike cDNA the sequences are identical to the naturally-occurring ones. The Court of Appeals faced this question a year later and, treating such claims as chemical rather than informational, considered them to be patent ineligible:

[N]either naturally occurring compositions of matter, nor synthetically created compositions that are structurally identical to the naturally occurring

(Continued)

(Continued)

compositions, are patent eligible. … A DNA structure with a function similar to that found in nature can only be patent eligible as a composition of matter if it has a unique structure, different from anything found in nature… Primers do not have such a different structure and are patent ineligible.

Primers necessarily contain the identical sequence of the BRCA sequence directly opposite to the strand to which they are designed to bind. They are structurally identical to the ends of DNA strands found in nature.[69]

Since the case, in the United States, the availability of BRCA1 and 2 test options has reportedly improved whilst prices have fallen.[70] Nonetheless, the decision has highlighted the fact that Myriad (and other patent owners) have been enjoying legal monopolies they should not have been given, and this has had negative social impacts in terms of people being deprived of access to the test. Moreover, Myriad used its monopoly position to generate vast amounts of data acquired through its testing service which it has been refusing to disclose since 2004. It has been argued that it now has a moral obligation now to freely disclose it.[71]

The US may be part of a trend to roll back patent rights in this area to promote genuine innovation. Courts from Australia to Turkey (an EPC member) have followed the example of the United States in excluding isolated DNA from patentability. In Australia's case, Myriad was one of the parties in the litigation. Previously, courts in Australia in deciding on relevant inventions were guided by the 1959 NRDC case which was not about natural products *per se* but that considered the patentability of certain weed control measures in light of the language of the English Statute of Monopolies.[72] It is worth discussing this case in some detail before moving onto the Myriad litigation. Previously the patent examiner had rejected the weed control method claims on the basis of not being 'not directed to any manner of manufacture in that they are claims to the mere use of known substances — which use also does not result in any vendible product'. The court dismissed the value of seeking to draw a distinction between invention and discovery:

The truth is that the distinction between discovery and invention is not precise enough to be other than misleading in this area of discussion. There may indeed be a discovery without invention — either because the discovery is of some piece of abstract information without any suggestion of a practical application of it to a useful end, or because its application lies outside the realm of 'manufacture'. But where a person finds out that a useful result may be produced by doing something

(*Continued*)

which has not been done by that procedure before, his claim for a patent is not validly answered by telling him that although there was ingenuity in his discovery that the materials used in the process would produce the useful result no ingenuity was involved in showing how the discovery, once it had been made, might be applied. The fallacy lies in dividing up the process that he puts forward as his invention. It is the whole process that must be considered.

The Court affirmed the view that to be inherently patentable in line with a reasonable understanding of the statutory language there much be a product, and it must be a 'vendible product'. As such, to be patentable the claimed invention, whether a product, use or method, must 'consist[s] in an artificially created state of affairs', and it must be of economic significance, hence vendible. In 2014, the Federal Court of Australia cited this case favourably in support of an expansive interpretation of inherent patentability finding isolated DNA claims to be patentable.[73] However, the High Court of Australia reversed this decision finding unanimously all three isolated DNA claims in Myriad's just-previously expired Australian patent to be invalid.[74] It is worth noting that in doing so it took much more of an informational view of DNA than did the Federal Court, and it also took public policy matters into account in making its decision. According to three of the judges in their joint opinion:

Despite the formulation of the claimed invention as a class of product, its substance is information embodied in arrangements of nucleotides. The information is not 'made' by human action. It is discerned. That feature of the claims raises a question about how they fit within the concept of a 'manner of manufacture'. As appears from s 6 of the Statute of Monopolies, an invention is something which involves 'making'. It must reside in something. It may be a product. It may be a process. It may be an outcome which can be characterised, in the language of NRDC, as an 'artificially created state of affairs'. Whatever it is, it must be something brought about by human action.

As for public policy and the purposes of the patent system:

There is a real risk that the chilling effect of the claims, on the use of any isolation process in relation to the BRCA1 gene, would lead to the creation of an exorbitant and unwarranted de facto monopoly on all methods of isolating nucleic acids containing the sequences coding for the BRCA1 protein. The infringement of the formal monopoly would not be ascertainable until the mutations and polymorphisms were detected. Such a result would be at odds with the purposes of the patent system.

In response to arguments that full product patent protection of DNA sequences is undesirable, France and Germany have opted, in the case of human sequences, for so-called 'purpose-bound protection' according to which DNA can only be claimed in respect of a specified use. Let us suppose there is a gene that codes for proteins A, B and C. The company that finds the gene discovers only that it codes for A and patents it on that basis. In the United Kingdom and the United States, that company can control use of the gene for any application or function subsequently discovered while the patent remains in force. But in Germany and France, another company that discovers the gene's role in producing proteins B and C can independently patent the gene in relation to those functions (but only those functions). It appears that this limitation to full product patent rights was a response at least in part to popular concerns in Europe (including the European Parliament) about the behaviour of Myriad Genetics.

So what is the appropriate position to adopt: full product protection or purpose-bound protection? The only honest answer is the underwhelming one of 'it's difficult to say for sure'. Nonetheless, the purpose-bound approach makes much sense whether or not it makes much difference in actual practice.

One can argue on sound scientific grounds that treating genes as patentable inventions on the basis of a single disclosed function or discovery such as that it codes for a particular protein, or that it is associated with a disease, is a rather generous interpretation of the 'inventor's' relatively modest addition to the state of the art. This is not to say that such discoveries are necessarily easy or inexpensive to attain and undeserving of any reward. The point is that there may well be much more to be discovered about the gene of both scientific and commercial interest, and such future discoveries may well be a whole lot more important. This is not just academic. Gene patenting can be a life or death issue.[75]

However, just as it is difficult to prove that extending the coverage of the patent system to cover DNA sequences as protectable subject matter guarantees there will be more investment in public health-improving research and development than there would be otherwise, proving the opposite is just as difficult. The well-publicised patenting by Myriad

Genetics relating to and covering two genes (BRCA1 and BRCA2) linked to a certain proportion of breast cancer cases and the aggressive assertion of these patents by the company lend plausibility to the view that DNA patenting is bad for public health research (see box above).[76] Human Genome Sciences' patenting of the CC-chemokine receptor 5 (CCR5) gene that was subsequently discovered by other scientists to have a link to HIV human cell infection raises serious doubts about the wisdom of allowing genes to be patented when very little is known about them.[77] Nonetheless, the use of a limited number of examples such as these does not prove beyond doubt that DNA patenting is necessarily *per se* a bad thing. But while empirical studies have been published that find little evidence to support the view that there would be more and better public health-oriented research without DNA patenting,[78] one should not rely too much on such findings. It is very difficult to estimate the size of the 'chilling effect' of patents on such research, which anecdotal evidence suggests may be substantial. Furthermore, reliable empirical evidence exists to support the claim that the aggressive assertion of DNA patent rights is unduly restricting the availability of diagnostic tests for patients in hospitals and other public service institutions.[79] This is sometimes the case even when testing by others does not require access to information disclosed in a patent.[80]

Of course concerns about DNA patenting are not confined to their effects on research. To the extent that patents are legal monopolies that can in some cases create market monopolies, they are bound to affect the prices of health products protected by patents including in developing countries. While the relationship between DNA patents and the prices of drugs, vaccines, diagnostic kits and other health products in the developed and developing worlds is often a complex one, to the extent that patents restrict competition it seems implausible, as is sometimes claimed, that patents can have no effect on prices.

In a detailed newspaper article published in Canada, Abraham, Gold and Castle critiqued the role of patents in the field of human genetics that the US Myriad decision might have gone some way towards mitigating, albeit not yet in that country.[81] These authors point out that most gene patents focus on single gene defects linked to disease. Often they fail to take into account other genes, and the wider complexities involved in disease development. Thus patents tend to be awarded on the basis of discovery of a single gene. However, the real innovation lies not in discovery but 'interpretation of errors — mutations — in those genes and the analysis of their interaction with other genes ... gene testing today involves innovation in data interpretation, competition between ways of analyzing the data and constant questioning and review of results.' Despite this, the patent system allows owners to restrict access to data. This is because 'firms holding gene patents are motivated to keep data to themselves and ... not share their insights into the impact of particular errors on disease development. Unlocking those patents will enable new generation of firms that compete not on the basis of exclusive rights, but on the accuracy of their methods of analysis, their service to patients and doctors and the reliability and reproducibility of their results.' They conclude that 'patents on these methods, rather than on genes themselves, will spur innovation as competing groups will try to outdo each other, provided that all have access to same basic data.' This sounds plausible but even if entirely true, this does not preclude the possibility also of negative impacts of reducing patent scope, such as small firms developing tests whose business models depend on being able to acquire patents on subject matter the Supreme Court now — following *Myriad* and *Prometheus* — prevents applicants from protecting.[82] However, it has been suggested that patenting DNA sequences is becoming less interesting for business. Genetic data mining is where much of the commercial interest is moving to. One scholar has even gone so far as to suggest that restrictions in the United States on patents claiming isolated DNA may accelerate this shift towards data mining by making such genetic information freely available.[83]

Concerns from industry have led to private ordering whereby actors take the initiative to devise collective solutions to shared concerns, in this case shared among companies and the public sector. Institutions, including companies concerned about the potential for intellectual property over-privatization's deleterious consequences for science, business and public health can of course agree on procedures to publicly disclose their data if they have a shared desire to do so. If the amount of data they collectively produce constitutes a large proportion of all the data likely to be generated, this will make it more difficult for individual data-provider companies to operate patent-based business models where the learning curve is steep and the 'novelty' of many patentable inventions would be very short-lived anyway. Companies may well be interested in joining such a consortium if they see a commercial advantage in agreeing to treat raw data generation as being a 'precompetitive' activity and therefore are happy to share it without IP restrictions. As the Human Genome Project was coming to an end it became clearer than ever that much would be gained both scientifically and therapeutically from studying the genetic variability within the human species. One key unit of such variability was at the tiny level of the individual nucleotide base. Such variations shared by reasonably large numbers of people, and forming 90 percent of the genetic variability of our species, are called single nucleotide polymorphisms (SNPs). In 1999, a group of companies and research organisations together with the Wellcome Trust, then the world's largest medical charity, established the SNP Consortium. Its aim was to identify all of the common SNPs, of which there are now believed to be around 10 million, and map them onto the human genome. From the private sector, Glaxo Wellcome (as it was then called) took the initiative in starting such an endeavour but after meeting the Wellcome Trust and some other companies during 1998, it was decided that the ideal approach would be to establish a consortium. Funding came from the Trust and several large pharmaceutical company members, including Aventis (now Sanofi), Bayer, Bristol-Myers Squibb, Glaxo Wellcome and SmithKline Beecham (now merged as GSK), Pfizer, Roche, Searle (then part of Monsanto which is now Bayer), and Zeneca (now AstraZeneca). Non-pharmaceutical concerns IBM and Motorola were also part of the consortium. In 2001 their shared data on SNPs was publicly released.

A similar pooling of public data was undertaken by the International HapMap Consortium, which comprised an international group of funders, government agencies and universities from the United States, the UK, Canada, China, Japan, Nigeria, as well as the SNP Consortium plus two biotech firms, Illumina and ParAllele Bioscience.[84] It has turned out that many SNPs throughout the genome are inherited together as 'blocks'. A haplotype is the arrangement of SNPs on each of these blocks. Given that the number of haplotypes is far lower than the quantity of SNPs, generating such a map offered an extremely convenient short cut in studying human genetic variability. The HapMap Project, the first phase of which was completed in 2005,[85] and the final one in 2009, required users to agree to a license that undertook them not to reduce access to the data or to pass data on to non-licensees.[86]

Such collaborative approaches and licensing schemes are not a rejection of intellectual property rights *per se*. But they do emphasize and seek to encourage collaboration of the kind that aggressive assertion of patent and other intellectual property claims would certainly preclude. Indeed, intellectual property protection may be necessary for 'open source' collaborative models to work. The assertion of intellectual property rights is the best available sanction against those who acquire data and then seek legal protection covering elements of the received data and who may not be bound by any license. This has been the case in software development, where open source collaborative models and licensing were first tried out with great success.[87] In fact, the SNP Consortium's intellectual property procedures were for patent applications to be filed for any inventions arising, but not to pursue them in order to record their priority dates so as to block patenting by others.[88] Currently the Structural Genomics Consortium, a charitable international partnership of non-profit foundations corporations has a policy of sharing freely and filing no patents on its discoveries.

Stem cell patenting

Despite the lack of practical outcomes to date, there has been an immense amount of patent activity in the area of stem cell research. In 2014 it was reported in a survey of patent filings that globally there are 650 patent families on iPS cell production technologies, and over 1,300 relating to cell differentiation methods.[89] The United States is the source of more than half of these inventions, with Japan coming a very distant second.

The United States treats stem cell-related inventions no differently from other types with the restriction under Section 33 of the *America Invents Act, 2011* that 'no patent may issue on a claim directed to or encompassing a human organism.' Indeed, Brüstle's invention, which will be discussed below, was patented there as it was in Japan, Australia and Israel.

In Europe the situation is completely different.[90] The sources of law concerning the morality of biotechnological inventions are the European Patent Convention and its internal rules, and the EU Directive discussed above. We need to say more about the latter instrument here.

Recital 16 states in part that 'patent law must be applied so as to respect the fundamental principles safeguarding the dignity and integrity of the person'. This would appear to be inapplicable to stem-cell related inventions given that blastocysts are not yet persons having any dignity or integrity to safeguard. As we will see below, things are not as simple as that.

Article 6, which has been incorporated almost verbatim into the Implementing Regulations of the EPC (Rule 28), states as follows:

1. Inventions shall be considered unpatentable where their commercial exploitation would be contrary to ordre public or morality; however, exploitation shall not be deemed to be so contrary merely because it is prohibited by law or regulation.
2. On the basis of paragraph 1, the following, in particular, shall be considered unpatentable:

    (a)   processes for cloning human beings;
    (b)   processes for modifying the germ line genetic identity of human beings;
    (c)   uses of human embryos for industrial or commercial purposes;
    (d)   processes for modifying the genetic identity of animals which are likely to cause them suffering without any substantial medical benefit to man or animal, and also animals resulting from such processes.

It should first be noted that (a) to (c) are quite definite, absolute even. Commercially exploiting these processes and uses, which patents are assumed to promote or facilitate, is immoral or contrary to ordre public. Therefore there can be no patents on them. Whether there are societal benefits and how substantial they may be are not considerations to be applied. There are sound reasons to ban patents on (a) and (b) given that human reproductive cloning and germ line modification are illegal in most countries, as they should be. Such practices are unethical, highly risky, and raise profound concerns regarding whether or not we wish to live in a society in which babies can be designed and 'created' to order. Interested readers are referred to Aldous Huxley's dystopian novel *Brave New World*, an ever-increasing number of science fiction novels and movies, as well as some weighty bioethical writings expressing a diverse range of opinions as to the ability of humankind to use such technologies wisely if we are to use them at all. But what about (c) and (d)? (d) differs from the others in being utilitarian. It is also somewhat vague in practice given the lack of guidance regarding the level of medical benefits needed to attain substantiality, besides which they may be no more than future possibilities as opposed to present day certainties. What is it that is immoral here for which denying a patent is the right response? What really is the point of these exclusions? Is it that nobody should commercially exploit such inventions as if we are to leave the research to governments, public universities, and public domain-oriented scientists with no commercial agenda? Or is it that gaining legal monopolies over these processes and uses with monetary gain in mind is itself immoral? There is nothing in the text to say unequivocally that the inventions in themselves are immoral, just the base motives of those who might wish to patent them to make money.

In the 1990s, James Thomson of University of Wisconsin succeeded in isolating primate including human embryonic cells and generating sustainable purified cell lines. Subsequently, three US patents — all titled 'Primate embryonic stem cells' — were granted with Wisconsin Alumni Research Foundation as assignee: 5,843,780, 6,200,806 and 7,029,913. These patents have attracted controversy, including about their broad scope and the rather restrictive licensing practices employed by WARF especially in the early years.[91] But they have never been successfully challenged. The first patent has expired but the latter two remain in force. One could perhaps see this as a case of evergreening through secondary (and tertiary) patenting, but we will leave it to others to assess the extent to which the '806 and '913 patents disclose substantial technological advances over the '780 invention. As we saw earlier in this book, WARF's experience of effective patent management goes back to the early twentieth century.

In Europe things turned out very differently. When law, moral philosophy and bioethics meet in the same forum, religious dogma shouts to get a word in, and somehow a decision must be made, unimpeachable logic is probably too much to hope for. The welfare of future sick people standing to benefit from the research was not to be a concern, but that of the embryo whose actual or potential personhood made dignity a relevant consideration in its treatment by the authorities. Accordingly, WARF's efforts to patent Thomson's work ended in failure. In 2008, the EPO Enlarged Board of Appeal handed down a decision concerning WARF's patent application rejecting it on the basis of the immorality/contrary to ordre public exclusion and more specifically the language of Rule 28(c) incorporating the text of Article 6.2(c) of the EU Directive.[92] It was irrelevant that the method involving the embryo destruction was not claimed in the patent. At first glance, the decision appears entirely straightforward:

> Since ... the only teaching of how to perform the invention to make human embryonic stem cell cultures is the use (involving their destruction) of human embryos, this invention falls under the prohibition of Rule 28(c) (formerly 23d(c)) EPC.

Obviously there was an underlying industrial purpose to this necessarily embryo-destroying invention. Industrial application is a basic criterion and one wonders why anybody would file a patent on something lacking this capability. As for commercial purpose, one wonders why anybody files a patent if there is no commercial purpose behind the invention. It is perhaps noteworthy here that WARF had been actively licensing its patents in the US for a few years by this time. But of course the exception applied specifically not to purposes of the invention as a whole but to the embryo use. Destruction of something to extract useful parts is without a doubt a use of it so to escape the exception that part of the invention's performance would have to have not been for industrial or commercial purposes. Up to this point, the EBA's reasoning appears perfectly sound given the text of the exclusion and the original intent of the framers.

The EBA might have just let those facts speak for themselves and kept its decision as short as possible. But it did not do that, declaring that patenting the invention was not the source of the immorality, but the invention itself. That was perhaps implicit but by stating it expressly, it raised legitimate concerns about overreaching, that is, going well beyond the bounds of what a patent-granting organisation should have to take into account when deciding to grant or not. This is what the EBA went on to say:

> … it is not the fact of the patenting itself that is considered to be against ordre public or morality, but it is the performing of the invention, which includes a step (the use involving its destruction of a human embryo) that has to be considered to contravene those concepts.

If so, why is a patent-granting organisation the one to decide and why should its views carry any weight or have legal implications of any kind? As we saw, several European governments had already deemed the legality of practicing the invented techniques to be in the public interest. In this field, inventions are original bio-scientific achievements with potential for practical use. But in most countries non-IP regulations exist setting limits as to what scientists can do in their labs. What is the purpose of a patent office telling us that what they achieved is immoral when they are perfectly legal?

The Enlarged Board clarified that the decision was not a blanket prohibition on patenting in the stem cell field:

> … this decision is not concerned with the patentability in general of inventions relating to human stem cells or human stem cell cultures. It holds unpatentable inventions concerning products (here human stem cell cultures) which can only be obtained by the use involving their destruction of human embryos.

What if the invention starts and ends with the transformation of stem cells in laboratory cultures and their use in therapy, and not their isolation and derivation from embryos? Wouldn't the invention also be morally tainted in the sense that at some point in time there would have had to be actual use of embryos in order to produce the stem cell line? And if so, wouldn't this invention also fall under the exception? These questions were answered by the Court of Justice of the European Union in the Brüstle case.[93] Brüstle's German patent was one concerning 'isolated and purified neural precursor cells, processes for their production from embryonic stem cells and the use of neural precursor cells for the treatment of neural defects'. Whereas Thomson's inventions teach how to produce lines of undifferentiated stem cells, this invention takes matters much further, providing a means to differentiate those cells into ones with genuine applications in regenerative medicine, specifically treatment of neural defects. On its face, this appears to be a great leap forward towards actual therapy. To class this invention as immoral is troubling to say the least. The Court did not dispute that:

> In order to remedy such neural defects, it is necessary to transplant immature precursor cells, still capable of developing. In essence, that type of cell exists only during the brain's development phase. The use of cerebral tissue from human embryos raises significant ethical questions and means that it is not possible to meet the need for the precursor cells which are required to provide publicly available cell treatment

So the claimed invention resolves a serious ethical difficulty: that the only other possible source of the cells would be far more developed human embryos and in a more morally discomfiting context. Indeed, Brüstle's invention appears to preclude sourcing such cells from the brain tissue of aborted foetuses which one would expect the sort of people who object to the patent on moral ground to find even more offensive. And yet the Court, again, would have none of such considerations. His invention was still immoral:

> Article 6(2)(c) of the Directive excludes an invention from patentability where the technical teaching which is the subject-matter of the patent application requires the prior destruction of human embryos or their use as base material, whatever the stage at which that takes place and even if the description of the technical teaching claimed does not refer to the use of human embryos.

Further,

> ... an invention must be regarded as unpatentable, even if the claims of the patent do not concern the use of human embryos, where the

implementation of the invention requires the destruction of human embryos…. The fact that destruction may occur at a stage long before the implementation of the invention, as in the case of the production of embryonic stem cells from a lineage of stem cells the mere reproduction of which implied the destruction of human embryos is, in that regard, irrelevant.

Again, as long as embryos' destruction whenever it took place is indispensable to practicing the invention, there can be no patent, an approach that the EPO followed in a later decision of the TBA.[94] The CJEU overreached and to a greater extent than the EBA. But in doing so it shifted focus also to the patent and patent rights, not just to the invention. Whereas the EBA sought to claim that it is the invention that is immoral not the patent, for the CJEU the patent and the rights attached are 'connected with acts of an industrial or commercial nature' whether or not the invention is. In a sense, then, filing the patent application is an admission of 'guilt' — that the purposes of the research, including the use of the embryos, are industrial or commercial.

The Court took an extremely broad interpretation of 'embryo', bizarrely including unfertilised human eggs. It took the view that a broad and uniform definition was necessary not just to uphold human dignity but for the sake of the internal market. On the other hand the Court left it up to national courts to decide whether a pluripotent stem cell isolated from an embryo at the blastocyst stage is itself a 'human embryo'. In the present case, following this CJEU ruling the German Federal Supreme Court correctly concluded in the negative.[95]

It did not take long for the Court to correct the first error following a referral from the UK. Unfertilised human eggs can be engineered to begin cell division but the fact remains that these are incapable of developing beyond the blastocyst stage. Such embryos are called parthenotes. In 2014, the CJEU clarified as follows:

An organism which is incapable of developing into a human being does not constitute a human embryo within the meaning of the Biotech Directive.

Accordingly, uses of such an organism for industrial or commercial purposes may, as a rule, be patented.

This is a rather perplexing situation. It is true that the Directive's text had to accommodate some of the scepticism of many European Parliamentarians about patenting in this field and about biotechnology in general. Nonetheless, whereas the benefits of genetic modification in agriculture are arguably more contestable in light of concerns about the environment, human health, and corporate control over the food chain, the encouragement of biomedical research, especially done by public sector organisations, is surely an unambiguously good thing and something that we ought to encourage. Parthasarathy's comparative research on the US and European patent system, which considers laws, cases, legislative hearings among other sources, offers us an answer of sorts.

There are legal explanations for the different treatment of biotechnological inventions. In the United States, under the legislation and according to Patent Office practice, patents are subjected almost entirely to technical enquiries: are the disclosed inventions eligible subject matter? Or are they natural? Courts may take into account the United States Constitution, the intent of the legislators, as well as public policy matters such as whether a given invention if patented claims what should not be owned because to do so would hinder research or harm the public interest. But technical matters are very much to the fore: is it eligible, is it new, useful, unobvious, and something that is not natural or abstract? It is true that similar technical considerations are applied rigorously in Europe too. However, Parthasarathy's political framework of analysis reveals underlying issues that shape patent institutions somewhat differently and has made the United States generally — albeit not always — more welcoming to inventions in the field of biotechnology, at least up to the Myriad decision. Accordingly, her analysis 'reveals the often-overlooked differences in the structures, orientations, and ongoing political work of supposedly similar patent systems.'[96] These differences include divergencies with respect to what should be 'the roles and responsibilities of patent system institutions, different understandings of who should participate and how they should do so, and different perspectives on how life itself should be governed.'[97] A major consequence of all this is that 'what is treated as technical and legal in the United States, ... is seen as moral and social in the European patent system'.[98]

Parthasarathy is correct to say that European patent law exclusions of immoral inventions and those contrary to what the English, French, and

German official versions of the European Patent Convention all call *ordre public* have deep historical roots. However, their persistence in European patent law as the continent began work to harmonize from the late 1940s, initially through the good offices of the Council of Europe, surely also had much to do with the politics of early postwar Europe. Much of Europe was in ruins; poverty, ill health, and hunger were rife; and countries generally chose left of centre governments, or else moderate right of centre ones. Welfare state ideology was quite dominant and populations were not necessarily keen to hand overwhelming market power over to corporations trading in food and health products. Of course, politics has changed in Europe and so has patent law. In terms of political culture and ideology Europe has become more similar to the United States, but Parthasarthy's market making/market shaping dichotomy still largely holds; hence the persistence of the various patent law exclusions, including plant and animal varieties and immoral inventions, and the much higher levels of civil society engagement. What is less clear of course is why European patent law is currently more permissive about DNA and cloned animals. Perhaps it just proves that civil society organizations do not necessarily get their way. Meanwhile the success of the campaign in the United States to restrict patents on human DNA may suggest a surprising area of potential convergence in terms of civil society involvement.

Harking back to our earlier chapter on regulation, regulatory capture seems more possible in the United States than in Europe whose continent-wide patent system with biotechnological inventions coming under the jurisdiction of the Court of Justice of the European Union is more pluralistic in terms of the values that need to be taken account of. This is despite much industry lobbying that takes place in Brussels and elsewhere. Such values include not just that biotechnology is a good thing to be encouraged and that doing so is good for the economy, but also that biotechnological inventions must not be harmful to human dignity, animal welfare, and the environment, or contrary to prevalent societal norms as to what is wrongful behaviour. Moreover, the ideology of patents being good for America is a powerful one and encourages a view that patent rights should be respected and governments should not intervene unless they are associated with excessive market power of a dominant company exhibiting anticompetitive behaviour, or a corporate giant resulting from a merger or acquisitions of other firms deemed, on account of its large intellectual property rights portfolio to be too much of a monopolist. Consequently, the research and non-commercial exceptions have been construed very narrowly. Moreover, the government is deeply reluctant to compulsorily grant a license to a third-party applicant or to itself on a patent whose government-funded invention is not being manufactured or made available for public use.[99,100]

An unbalanced system?

As we have seen, various approaches have emerged to fine-tuning bio-medical research in ways that take account of human variability at the molecular level, and that enable a drug design methodology that 'homes in' on a target with greater accuracy. The patent system has generally been very supportive, among other ways by accommodating chemical, therapeutic and physiological variabilities to a very fine degree and by treating novelty as a legal fiction in some areas. If we accept that the incentives for investment in innovation provided by the patent system are genuine here as elsewhere in the biomedical field, there are good arguments to justify such expansive patentable subject matter practices. However, there are convincing counter-arguments suggesting some rein-ing in of the scope of patentability or of the legal extent of the rights conferred would almost certainly be desirable. Let us now consider two such arguments and offers some policy approaches for consideration.

One argument is based on the well-known fact that the research-based pharmaceutical industry is a master at strategic patenting practices that can be used to unjustifiably extend market exclusivity over essential medicines well beyond the life of the original patent. The greater the number of ways companies can file additional patents surrounding this or that product, the greater is the opportunity to adopt business practices that reduce competition for ever longer periods of time. Why do we privilege the industry this way? While we continue to do so these legal monopolies on minor tweaks of existing medicines and their therapeutic application, despite being unworthy of patent protection as compared to inventions in other fields where novelty is applied more strictly, unrea-sonably lock up products with extended periods of legal monopoly protection. Obviously this has negative effects on patients. Competition is essential for reducing prices but it is being held back.

There are ample grounds to give serious consideration to the potential advantages of a more rigorous and consistent application of the novelty criterion to render unpatentable new discoveries of the kinds discussed earlier. This would of course leave them legally unprotected, and this may not be ideal either. Surely, we would not wish to discourage all personalised medical research, nor other modest but meaningful improvements. Devising a limited exclusivity scheme that is narrower in scope and shorter in duration than what is normally available under the patent system is an approach that may be well worth considering.

The other argument is that the ease of patenting incremental inventions and the expanded market power which doing so allows may be discouraging more radical innovation which is riskier, costs more money and takes more time to achieve. And yet the patent system does not discriminate between minor inventions protectable thanks to legal fictions (such as Nexium — see below), and breakthrough inventions (like the original Glivec — see Chapter 8). This seems unfair and poor policy. Modifying the patent system so that the latter get more favourable treatment may help to shift research efforts towards such areas and channel corporate marketing expenditures aimed to present the similar as radically different into *actually* producing the radically different.

As we have seen, and leaving to one side the vexed question of how accommodating the patent system should be towards such claims as well as to DNA, isolated natural substances, modified compounds, new uses and formulations, and other types of apparent discoveries or seemingly incremental life-science 'inventions', the invention itself may well offer a genuine public benefit.

More specifically, this period is characterised by a change to a more marketing-based business model facilitated by patent law and drug regulation and a shift away from a heavy reliance on end-to-end in-house research and development covering discovery to approval and all points between, albeit often benefiting from taxpayer funded basic research, towards an expansion of value chain participants. These phenomena — of new regulation- and law-driven business model changes and outsourcing and networking helped turn the industry into one that was more profitable and more global than ever — the one we have today.

Whereas rigorous application of the novelty and inventive step criteria by patent offices and court decision may prevent the most egregious attempts to unfairly extend patent monopolies, India's patent law actually has an anti-evergreening provision. Accordingly, Article 3(d) of the Patents (Amendment) Act, 2005 states as follows.

The following are not inventions within the meaning of this Act, ...

(d) the mere discovery of a new form of a known substance which does not result in the enhancement of the known efficacy of that substance or the mere discovery of any new property or new use for a known substance or of the mere use of a known process, machine or apparatus unless such known process results in a new product or employs at least one new reactant.

Explanation. — For the purposes of this clause, salts, esters, ethers, polymorphs, metabolites, pure form, particle size, isomers, mixtures of isomers, complexes, combinations and other derivatives of known substance shall be considered to be the same substance, unless they differ significantly in properties with regard to efficacy.

This measure was the subject of a highly publicised Supreme Court case which decided on the patentability of a new form of the anti-cancer drug Glivec and found it not to be, interpreting 'efficacy' for a medicine of necessity to mean 'therapeutic efficacy'. Novartis failed to prove that the new form had an enhanced and significantly different efficacy as compared to the earlier version of Glivec.[101]

Anti-evergreening measures have been adopted elsewhere. Indonesia revised its patent law in July 2016 along the lines of India's Article 3(d), ruling out patents for discoveries of new uses of existing or known products and new forms showing no increased efficacy. In Brazil, an agency set up by the health ministry (ANVISA) scrutinises pharmaceutical patents explicitly to reduce secondary patent grants. However, a recent empirical study strongly suggests that India's and Brazil's anti-evergreening approaches have made little difference in filtering out the grant of secondary patents, although the reasons are not entirely clear.[102]

Elsewhere, with good marketing (and clever use of trademark law) it may be possible to shift patients from an about to become off-patent drug onto a new version marketed under a different name that is really no better. If the original drug was successful and profitable while the patent was valid, such product switching could well generate a lot of money. We will see this with Nexium (see below).

Non-traditional Trademarks and Product Differentiation

There is a whole political economy of sameness and difference and companies uses trademarks to manage the boundaries in ways that can render drug products as unstable things whose names may confuse one as to whether other products with different names are or are not the same *and* thus interchangeable (see also Chapter 3).

A medicine is a rather undistinguished-looking object. There are limits as to how to make a pill's appearance communicate information, desirability or distinction. Of course, there is a brand name and its useful properties are indicated on the label. But its appearance *by itself* tells you nothing about what it is or can do. Hence the need for companies to consider imaginatively how to brand these boring looking and inherently uninformative goods. As historian Antoine Lentacker puts it, 'since drugs both contain and conceal their special powers against disease, they cannot circulate unless supplemented by some set of signs, whether textual or visual, that informs consumers or prescribers of their effects on the body.'[103] Consequently companies make 'uncommon investments… in building credit, gaining recognition, or accumulating *symbolic capital*'[104] the latter being embodied in brands such that the names of drugs form 'the basic currency'[105] of this form of capital.

It is hardly surprising, then, that the industry has taken full advantage of the expansion of the subject matter of trademarks from words, phrases and figurative marks to the full range of visual and other perceptible aspects of products and the packaging they are dressed up in. The trend to extend trademark protection this way has proved to be useful for many pharmaceutical companies. Some examples show us, though, that trademarks are not necessarily there to *reduce* confusion, an essential function of trademark law, but on the contrary to *increase* it. Some scholars have been aware of this for quite some time, but it is becoming increasingly evident now.[106]

Tablet form, including visual appearance, and function are hardly separate considerations. Tablet design must take into account such factors as therapeutic efficacy, ease of swallowing, and practicality from a manufacturing perspective.[107] But with imagination the appearance of a medicine itself *can* be made to tell you what it is and is supposed to do, and what its origin is. The industry can be creative in its use of trademark law and the expansion to non-traditional marks can be very helpful in this regard. We will look into some illustrative examples below.

Pharmaceutical Test Data Exclusivity and Other Restrictions on Competition

Intellectual property rights exclude competition by preventing others from doing certain acts relating to what is protected. But there are other forms of exclusivity that are available which are not based on property. The best known one is pharmaceutical test data exclusivity which has become something akin to an intellectual property right. Initially this type of exclusivity was part of a legal settlement to encourage the growth of a generic drugs industry while helping ensure that originator companies were able to enjoy a fair return on the potentially massive investment in the production of clinical trials data for experimental medical products. This settlement was the US Hatch-Waxman Act discussed above which provided patent term extensions and test data exclusivity for Big Pharma, and an abbreviated approval process and the Bolar exemption for the benefit of generic firms.[108]

TRIPS Article 39 concerns undisclosed information, whose meaning is somewhat broader than that of trade secrets. Paragraph 3 provides for the protection of test data in respect of pharmaceutical and agricultural chemical products that utilise new chemical entities. It must be protected against 'unfair commercial use'. Disclosure of such data is prohibited but may be allowed if necessary to protect the public or if legal protection measures against unfair commercial use are already in place. In justifying such provisions, Article 39.1 refers to Article 10*bis* of the Paris Convention, according to which 'any act of competition contrary to honest practices in industrial or commercial matters constitutes an act of unfair competition'.

How countries may give effect to Article 39.3 did not immediately attract heated debate. This is because the vagueness of the TRIPS language appears to allow for broad interpretative freedom. Things changed with the emergence of bilateral and regional trade agreements having health related intellectual property rights provisions, accompanied by a greater understanding of the economic and social welfare stakes involved.[109] Typically these trade agreements require parties to introduce data exclusivity modelled on U.S. or European standards which provide extended periods of exclusivity — typically at least five years — to the originator of the data during which drug regulators may not use the data to determine whether to approve the marketing of purportedly equivalent products.[110] The provision in TRIPS can be interpreted as not prohibiting regulators from doing this but merely as preventing generic producers from being able to acquire the data through dishonest commercial practices.[111] Needless to say, the United States and the European Union, which provides much longer exclusivity periods than the US, have been very keen to promote the former interpretation, and they have been quite successful in doing so despite the lack of any global consensus as to what is the correct or most socially optimal way to give effect to Article 39.3.[112]

Market and regulatory issues with biologic drugs

Superficially, the fact that — as we saw in Chapter 8 — biologic drugs comprise very large molecules whereas traditional pharmaceuticals usually consist of small molecule active ingredients might well seem rather unimportant. Surely existing norms apply, and industry can take this particular 'revolution' in its stride just as it did with hormones, antibiotics and other classes of medicine that were novel when they came onto the market. On the contrary, implications for the pharmaceuticals market and for regulation have been transformative in their nature.

To accurately and consistently mass-produce these large molecule products with a minimum of variability between batches, avoiding contamination, and without so-called post-translational modifications such as glycosylation, which can potentially drastically change the behaviour of the protein when it enters the body, is technically difficult and expensive. The manufacturing process itself is absolutely critical to what comes out at the end, and an originator company will certainly not disclose all of the details in a patent specification. As compared to small molecule generics, proving equivalence with biosimilars is far more difficult. 'Developing a biopharmaceutical is incredibly challenging... The difficulty comes in ensuring that your biosimilar has the same protein and glycosylation profile as the originator drug, within specified limits. In this regard, the innovator company perhaps had the easy job — they made the drug and showed that it was safe and non-toxic.'[113] 'Development of a biosimilar has been estimated to take 7–8 years and to cost between $100–250 million; in contrast, a small-molecule generic takes just 3–5 years and costs $1–4'.[114] One interesting proposal for accelerating and enhancing price-reducing competition is to require that the original biologic's cell-line be deposited as a condition for marketing approval, and that after a fixed period this be made accessible for generic companies seeking to produce an alternative product.[115]

Given the tremendous technical difficulties and enormous cost of manufacturing biosimilars and of getting marketing approval, there is quite a small number on the market thus far; admittedly, the first biologics only became available in 1980s[116] and these products are quite unique. Regulators struggled for a long time to find a way to approve generic versions which can never be considered to be exact reproductions as is possible with the active ingredients of small molecule drugs. So-called biosimilars have now been approved in some countries. The European Medicines Agency has been publishing its regularly updated biosimilars guidelines since 2005. The United States was slow to start approving biosimilars. Politics was no doubt a factor in the delay: how to regulate has massive financial stakes. Despite passage of the Biologics Price Competition and Innovation (BPCI) Act, 2010, the first biosimilar was not approved in that country until 2015 when the FDA allowed Sandoz's product Zarxio, which is similar to the reference product Neupogen. It is important to note that under the legislation 'similar' is not the same as 'interchangeable', which requires further successful clinical studies. An interchangeable product may be substituted for the reference product even where the doctor prescribes the reference product.

The substantial added time, expense and risk as well as the regulatory entry barriers in respect of biosimilars as compared to small molecule generics makes it enormously difficult for any firm other than a large generics or research-based business to enter this growing market. Moreover, the possibility of developing enhanced versions ('biobetters') is one that the regulatory system does not encourage because of the likelihood that clinical trials would need to be undertaken prior to grant of marketing approval. To add insult to injury, there are likely to be vast numbers of patents to navigate. According to medical historian Lara Marks, 'in 1986 it was estimated that there were only 830 patents relating to the hybridoma technology. This number grew exponentially thereafter, making the field difficult and expensive to navigate for anyone wishing to enter the space.'

Integrated Intellectual Property Management Strategy: Examples

As we have seen, industry has experience of using patents and trademarks together to ensure and perpetuate market power, going back to its beginnings. But now non-traditional trademarks are available. This matters a great deal. Trademarks and trademark expansionism counter free competition beyond the lifetime of patents and can assist in the transfer of value to related products from the same company. Arguably, this extends the scope of legal/regulatory monopolies too far in the direction of originator companies' interests by encouraging opportunistic behaviours that are detrimental to the ability of consumers to make choices in their best interests, in doing so running counter to a fundamental justification of trademarks;[117] and that also unduly restrict healthy competition benefiting the public.

As for patents, we now see the legal fictionalisation of novelty in patent law sitting alongside the admittedly longer-established low imagination quotient imputed to the fictional person skilled in the art: the one whose task it is to judge, on behalf of patent examiners and judges, the disclosed invention's not being obvious. Consequently, the opportunities for strengthened and extended market control have never been more promising. These opportunities are explained as well as any other way by considering a succession of four blockbuster-status drugs dealing with gastric and digestive tract complaints, such as peptic (stomach and duodenal) ulcers, and acid reflux, all of which speak of hugely effective marketing and intellectual property management of products on which the companies concerned were hugely dependent for revenue. Three were world number one bestsellers. These are cimetidine (marketed as Tagamet), ranitidine (Zantac) and omeprazole (branded as Prilosec in the USA, or Losec everywhere else). A fourth, esomeprazole (Nexium), shows how managing the boundaries between associated products in apparently contradictory ways can be done despite not being in the public interest.

The first two, cimetidine and ranitidine are closely related functionally, being so-called histamine H2 receptor antagonists, of which cimetidine was the pioneer. Yet both were patentable. The other, Losec, was a close competitor but of a different type, known technically as a proton pump inhibitor after its mode of action. The story shows the pharmaceutical industry at its best — applying brilliant science to develop products of great benefit to patients — and also at its worst.

These drugs testified above all to the massive profits to be gained from marrying hard-nosed business strategy to good science. Concerning the latter, while most of the drugs discussed so far relied a great deal on serendipity and trial and error with very little actual design or even knowledge of how they worked, these drugs were quite different. Cimetidine was an early triumph of so-called rational drug design in which the drug was specifically tailored to perform a highly specific task in the human body, an idea originally envisioned by Paul Ehrlich with his famous 'magic bullets' for the finely targeted drugs he aimed to discover.[118] The research leading to cimetidine and its discovery has been recognised by the American Chemical Society and the Royal Chemistry Society as a momentous achievement. As the American Chemical Society expressed it on its webpage:

> The research program leading to cimetidine … represented a revolution in the way pharmaceuticals are developed. Traditionally, the development of a new drug would often depend on the fortuitous discovery of a plant or microbial extract that showed some of the required biological activity. Using that first extract as a lead, many similar compounds

would be made and tested for pharmacological effectiveness. In many cases, the researchers did not know how the drug worked, so finding an optimal compound was difficult. The development of cimetidine was radically different: it was one of the first drugs to be designed logically from first principles... Using a step by step analysis of structural and physical properties, the team made a series of histamine-based molecules, which were then tested for antagonist activity using carefully designed pharmacological assays. *Today, this approach of rational drug design underpins the discovery programs of many major pharmaceutical companies.* (Emphasis added.)

In brief, the problem facing a research team led by James Black working at Smith, Kline & French Research Institute in the UK during the 1960s and 70s was that of how to prevent the secretion of acid caused by histamines reacting with the stomach. Up to that time, ulceration caused by these secretions was difficult to prevent and surgery was often necessary. It was known that the antihistamines, which inhibited the effects of histamines elsewhere in the body, could not do so in the stomach.[119] This suggested that the histamines were blocking a different receptor in the stomach's parietal cells to the receptor type that they blocked in other parts of the body which the antihistamines targeted.[120] The known receptor type was referred to as H in a 1966 journal article that postulated the existence of the second type.[121] The task then became that of identifying a chemical — a competitive antagonist in the language of pharmacology — that would successfully compete with histamines for this second receptor (labelled H_2) and reduce acid production. In 1972 they came up with cimetidine, the first of an entirely new class of drugs, which became available to patients in 1976.

Unlike the practices of some companies, the researchers were allowed to publish their findings as they went.[122] No doubt, this alerted competitors to the possibilities, and as soon as 1978, Glaxo — standing on the proverbial shoulders of giants — had come up with a more powerful H_2 receptor antagonist with fewer side-effects. For several years, ranitidine was the world's top selling drug with cimetidine as number two, and made Glaxo one of the biggest pharmaceutical companies in the world. This product was much better known under the name Zantac. However, now that ranitidine is a generic drug and Glaxo no longer has a need for the name, 'Zantac' is no longer what it was. Now called Zantac 75 it does continue to be applied to ranitidine. But the use of Zantac is now associated also with a quite different medicine albeit targeted at the same health problems as the original Zantac product, i.e. digestive tract disorders. This second medicine is a product called Rapidol Express whose active ingredient is not ranitidine but an extract of brown algae which itself is marketed under the registered name of Phycodol. This time Zantac is not the name of the product (which is in fact classed as a medical device) but serves instead as an indicator of the product's origin. Thus it is marketed as 'Rapidol™ Express by Zantac™'.

The Swedish company Astra, later merged with Zeneca, adopted a different approach, focusing on the mechanism by which the parietal cells produce gastric acid. It discovered omeprazole in 1979, which by its original mode of action was another class of drugs entirely, one which also had its subsequent followers: the proton pump inhibitors.

The massive commercial success of these three drugs relied on patent protection. Cimetidine, for example, had made \$14 billion by 1994, the year its United States patent expired.[123] Also key was the fact that they were found to be effective against other gastric disorders than just peptic ulcers including heartburn and indigestion to name just two.

Cimetidine was unique not only in the way it was developed; it was the world's first blockbuster drug. Since it came on the market and was followed by others, companies have desperately sought such products. The anti-ulcerant drugs we looked out suggest they have sometimes done so by developing a revolutionary new class of drug as did both Smith Kline & French and Astra. However, we have also seen how they may market a similar product to an existing one that is either more effective or safer, or, and this might sound cynical, that can be marketed so well that people are persuaded that it is. Ranitidine was a genuine improvement but in other cases there are reasonable grounds for scepticism that the 'me too' is any better at all than the original.

Blockbuster drugs can only be blockbusters if they are patented and for only as long as the patents remain in force. The value of the patent system then becomes more apparent than ever as is the threat once the patents expire. Companies nowadays are obsessed with the problem of what to do once patents on blockbuster drugs expire, when generic products enter the market and the price normally drops quite dramatically. They can be very creative, and often quite devious, in their efforts to continue the effective monopoly period or else to ensure that patients continue to use their products on the basis of having better versions available. A good example is AstraZeneca's Nexium, a product that was both chemically and therapeutically virtually identical to Losec. What difference *is there* between the two, other than the name? It's a very good question!

When its highly successful anti-ulcer drug omeprazole (sold as Losec, or Prilosec) was coming to the end of its patent life, and attempts to evergreen its monopoly were thwarted, the company sought to switch users to esomeprazole, branded as Nexium, a product that was both chemically and therapeutically virtually identical to Losec, but was ten times more expensive than the former drug. They did this by deploying aggressive marketing tactics claiming that it was both newer and better. Admittedly, the fact that it comprises optically pure salts of omeprazole enabled it to pass the novelty test in the key jurisdictions. But novelty in this context is of course a legal fiction. Like more than half of the drugs currently on the market, the active ingredient of Losec is a racemic mixture: a 50–50 mix of molecules that are mirror images of each other. Nexium is the so-called (S) enantiomer of omeprazole, the one that is therapeutically active. Putting it another way, esomeprazole is one of two optically pure salts of omeprazole. Therefore esomeprazole was part of the contents of omeprazole. In other words it was contained in the API of Losec.

This effort cost hundreds of million dollars in marketing, but it was worth it. 'About 40 percent of Prilosec users made the switch to Nexium earning the drug over \$3 billion in 2003 and almost \$5 billion in 2004'.[124,125] So *was* Nexium any better than Losec to which it is chemically very closely related? It appears that the improvement was modest to say the least.[126] Apart from needing less of it to have the same therapeutic effect by dint of the fact that the other enantiomer is inactive, both Losec and Nexium are prodrugs. Prodrugs are those which are converted by the human body into the substance which is the real active ingredient. Both Losec and Nexium are converted into the same compound, sulfenic acid, which only has a single-handed form: it is achiral, not chiral. Therefore, whether omeprazole or esomeprazole are taken, an optically and pharmacologically identical API is formed *in vivo* which goes about its business in a way that does not depend on which of the two products it is derived from.

However, the story does not end there. Losec and Nexium are of course closely associated products. Chemically and therapeutically, the differences between the two are negligible. However, by giving them two very different names it became possible to mask this similarity to impressive commercial effect. And yet, in the United States at least, AstraZeneca chose to exploit the goodwill the company has built up in the purple colouring of Prilosec pills by making Nexium the same colour. This seems ironic. Differentiation has been accentuated by the choice of names, but has been blurred by the strategy of blending the appearance of the pills themselves.

One presumes that the company was convinced that the commercial advantages of transferring the goodwill outweighed the risk of the public assuming Nexium by its visual similarity to Losec as being nothing more than the latter by another name. But perhaps we should not be too surprised by this or see any contradiction. Empirical research suggests that people make assumptions about what their experience of a drug will be by its physical appearance including its shape and colour.[127] Doubtless, this merely confirms what AstraZeneca knew anyway, hence 'The Purple Pill®'. If just looking at it evokes a warm feeling in the gut, why squander that goodwill so expensively acquired with a different-looking pill?

In 2015, the company submitted a complaint to the US district court for Delaware alleging trademark infringement and other offences by an Indian drug company selling purple coloured generic esomeprazole without licenses to use the 'The Purple Pill' and any of the purple colouring trademarks covering 'preparations and substances for the treatment of gastrointestinal diseases'.[128] The court responded with a temporary injunction. At the very least this testifies to the extent of determination to protect its investments in associating AstraZeneca with purple-coloured capsules for treating certain digestive tract ailments and its commercial success in doing so.

On the face of it, the impacts of making DRL change the colour of its pills seem unlikely to have much effect on the public. Teva and Mylan also sell esomeprozole using other colours so there is competition and esomeprozole is not expensive. However, in what sense did DRL's purple colouring cause the consumer confusion which trademarks are supposed to prevent? As long as consumers have visual access to the packaging they will be aware that the source is DRL and not AstraZeneca, but that it is still esomeprazole. So there is little or no confusion as far as they are concerned from making the pills look the same. On the other hand, preventing other producers from using the same colour arguably causes confusion by the aforementioned blurring of the chemically equivalent and substitutable relationship between brand name and generic medication. This could matter a great deal in the market for medicines where there is little competition and the original market entrant has been able to keep prices high.

There are other ways to use non-traditional trademarks for commercial advantage, and not just as an adjunct to patents or to extend monopoly protection beyond patent terms. With Nexium, the colour marks were aimed at shifting goodwill to a replacement product. But they can also be used to turn one product into two non-competing ones to be sold in separate markets. 'Prozac, an antidepressant, was about to lose its patent protection. Its manufacturer, Eli Lilly, rebranded the active ingredient — fluoxetine — by producing pink and lavender pills (Prozac was green and white), naming it Sarafem, and marketing it for the treatment of premenstrual dysphoric disorder.'[129] The blue Viagra pill with its diamond shape is another excellent example.

It was suggested in Chapter 3 that Viagra's success was partially attributable to disease-mongering, and we already looked into this particular aspect of the Viagra story. However, other factors were obviously at play including very effective intellectual property management and marketing. The fact it was so successful belies the fact that the patent status of the active ingredient was challenged in some countries and found to be less than watertight. Viagra is an interesting case study also in showing how the nature of a medicine is not necessarily a simple factual matter requiring no ontological reflection. Indeed, a consideration of the essence of a medicine like Viagra implicates product regulation and trademark law in quite intriguing ways. Additionally, it illustrates how unforeseen side-effects can be turned into approved new indications and massive market opportunities, even in the face of effective legal challenges from competitors.

But first: what *is* Viagra? Viagra cannot be adequately defined by what it is made of, what it is for, or by what it does when the human body absorbs it. In fact, what Viagra is, and is not, is determined not just by the regulatory regimes controlling its use, but by the intellectual property rights used to protect it, the scope of these rights, and their boundaries with the rights, duties and freedoms of others, and with the public domain. What is the relationship between Viagra and intellectual property? And can we reduce Viagra to a fixed legal construct 'created' by intellectual property law? Answering both questions should tell us much about not just the market power intellectual property rights can underpin, but also about how in some way, what a thing is isn't necessarily for scientists to determine but IP lawyers.

Viagra, like medicines other than mixtures, is a highly specific product in pill form containing a single active ingredient and other substances called excipients whose typical functions are to protect it on its journey through the body, control the active ingredient's rate of absorption, and enhance palatability. Scientifically the active ingredient can be identified as either: (i) the tongue-twisting 1-[[3-(6,7-dihydro-1-methyl7-oxo-3-propyl-1H-pyrazolo[4,3-d]pyrimidin-5-yl)4-ethoxyphenyl]sulphonyl]-4-methylpiperazine, as (ii) the somewhat simpler $C_{22}H_{30}N_6O_4S$, or as (iii) sildenafil citrate, or its non-proprietary generic name of sildenafil. For obvious reasons we will settle for the latter name.

To say that Viagra *is* sildenafil citrate is surely a statement of fact. However, Pfizer stakes its ownership claims in far more subtle ways than that. This is why it is more accurate to say that Viagra *has* — rather than *is* — sildenafil citrate. Even then, this does not mean that only Viagra has sildenafil citrate. Pfizer's management of its intellectual property surrounding Viagra does not make things that simple. Indeed, the boundaries secured and guarded by the patent and trademark rights around 'Viagra' or, to be absolutely specific as to what it really is: '*a sildenafil-containing Erectile Dysfunction treatment called Viagra*', are much broader than the active ingredient alone, albeit not as broad as Pfizer, the company responsible, would have liked.

Sildenafil citrate was discovered with the aim of producing cardiovascular benefits to patients. More specifically it purposely disrupts a naturally occurring enzyme called phosphodiesterase type 5 (PDE5) in order to deal with disorders like hypertension and angina. As such it was intended as a better version of a failed and now largely forgotten drug candidate called zaprinast. The initial results from tests on patients started in 1991 were disappointing in part due to the chemical's short half-life in the body making its effects a little too temporary. However, a group of people given the substance described increased incidences of erections. It turned out that PDE5 inhibition enables the flow of blood into the penis by relaxing certain muscle in the erectile tissue.

Central to any marketing strategy in the pharmaceutical industry is to have a good name for the product, one which directs those purchasing drugs to that product and not to alternative ones. Without question, Viagra as a product name has been hugely successful. Registration of the word mark is of course the first step in protecting the name of your drug (or any other product). Being ready to guard the mark through enforcement actions and opposition to the registration of similar marks is essential. Doing so has ensured that there is no such thing as 'Natural Viagra', at least in law, notwithstanding attempts still made to use the term for herbal products of varying levels of dubiety. Here trademark and patent strategy supported each other, as they often do in this business. Until Pfizer informs us otherwise, Viagra *must* consist of sildenafil citrate, a substance patented in the early 1990s. (These patents have of course now mostly expired). As such, this remains a defining quality. On the other hand, when sildenafil citrate is prescribed for pulmonary arterial hypertension (PAH), it is not Viagra™ but Revatio™, the only difference other than name and appearance being that the therapeutic effect and the side effect are reversed. All Viagra is sildenafil citrate but not all sildenafil citrate in the form of a pill is Viagra. In this sense one can say that Pfizer is narrowing the boundaries of its monopoly to accommodate another one, so that it is sildenafil citrate *only* when indicated for erectile dysfunction. But in a sense it is even more specific than this. Pfizer has numerous trademarks relating to Viagra include ones covering the blue-coloured and diamond-shaped appearance of the tablet, and even a European design right. Thus in the minds of the consumer and indeed the general public Viagra is that 'little blue pill'. In this case the specificity of Viagra's look will prevent generic firms selling sildenafil — its non-proprietary name — from making their copies look like Pfizer's original product.

Pfizer, as one would expect, did its utmost to expand the scope of its monopoly on the product as much, and for as long, as possible. The challenge facing the company as for others is that after its initial discovery as a novel substance with a plausible medicinal use, it turned out to be much more effective for something else, in this case for the main reported side effect. Thankfully for the industry it is possible to file patent applications for new medical indications of substances that themselves lack novelty having been discovered earlier. Pfizer availed itself of this possibility as far as it was able. In this endeavour it was only partially successful. The tendency to file new medical use patents claiming a class of compounds, of which sildenafil citrate was one member, sharing the ability to inhibit the action of PDE5 helped to render these patents vulnerable to attack. The UK and European patents were revoked or successfully opposed primarily on grounds of obviousness. The Chinese State Intellectual Property Organization revoked the counterpart Chinese patent in 2004 for the same reasons. In 2012, the Canadian Supreme Court revoked the patent there for insufficient disclosure. The fate of the United States patent on the use of Viagra for ED, which remained in force until 2019 albeit with reduced scope, is particularly interesting.

As the first pharmaceutical product for treating erectile dysfunction, one might expect Pfizer being keen to associate its invention with PDE5 inhibition as a unique feature. In fact, Pfizer's attempt in the United States to do this failed. In February 2010, the Board of Patent Appeals and Interferences of the US Patent and Trademark Office decided on an appeal by Pfizer relating to a patent on Viagra. The claim at issue, which the examiner had rejected, was this:

> A method of treating erectile dysfunction in a male human, comprising orally administering to a male human in need of such treatment an effective amount of a selective cGMP PDEV inhibitor, or a pharmaceutically acceptable salt thereof, of [sic, or] a pharmaceutical composition containing either entity.

By its interpretation of the law, the Board set a reasonably high bar for anticipation (that is, novelty negation) by prior publication:

> A reference is anticipatory under § 102(b) when it (i) discloses each and every element of the claimed invention, either explicitly or inherently, and (ii) enables one of ordinary skill in the art to make the invention.

Four of the references held by the examiner to anticipate the claim disclosed use of Yin Yang Huo ('horny goat weed') in traditional medicine. These together were referred to by the Board as the 'Yin Yang Huo references'. For the Board, the key point at issue was whether or not these references 'describe oral administration of the selective PDEV inhibitor icariin *in an amount effective to treat ED* [erectile dysfunction]'.

In his rejection, the examiner had relied on expert testimony showing that Ying Yang Huo contains icariin and that this substance is effective as a selective cGMP PDEV inhibitor. The question then arose of whether or not the Yin Yang Huo oral preparations as used in traditional Chinese medicine as an aphrodisiac that were described in the publications effectively delivered icariin to the patients and therefore anticipated the claim. In fact of the four relevant publications, one of them (by Yin) did not mention icariin; evidently the preparation was not well known to this author by its chemical composition. In arguing its case, Pfizer observed that the Yin article's 'disclosed treatment comprises a mixture of Yin Yang Huo and Tu Si Zi, as well as yellow rice wine, genital massage, rest, bathing in a herbal mixture, and abstinence from intercourse and, therefore, does not establish that the treatment effect was due to Yin Yang Huo alone'. Accordingly, Pfizer's lawyers claimed, this was not enabling. The Board rejected this view, concluding that the disclosure was sufficient to enable the oral delivery of enough of the enzyme inhibitory substance to treat erectile dysfunction. Therefore, each of the four publications was held by the examiner to anticipate claim 24, and the Board upheld this rejection.

Is Viagra no more nor less than what Pfizer tells us it is, in accordance with the intellectual property rights that it owns? Of course, the market (and marketing) power lent by intellectual property rights over Viagra allows a large measure of control over how the product is represented to the public *as a medical entity*. However, what patents and trademarks could never do is enable Pfizer to control all of the narratives, stories, meanings and representations about Viagra in society including popular culture. Consumers, social commentators, and comedians, among others, have also had much to say about Viagra and Erectile Dysfunction. That is of course a measure of its success. Viagra, whatever it is and whatever it is for, has joined Aspirin, Valium, Prozac and of course 'the pill' as a cultural icon, one that for Pfizer has been extraordinarily profitable. Indeed, Viagra may well be the first billion dollar a year drug whose sales were so much attributable to direct-to-consumer publicity and attendant media hype underpinned by a creative mix of patents and trademarks.

In closing this chapter, it suffices to say that in the past few years there has been much controversy about the lifecycle management practices of drug companies. These include extending the market power of a given medicine beyond the lifetime of the first patent covering the active pharmaceutical ingredient ('evergreening'); or shifting that power over to a follow-on product that may or may not be much different from, or better than, the previous one ('producing line extensions'). Sometimes in the latter case it may entail withdrawing the initial brand-name product so as not to undermine the market for the second one whilst — in some cases — carrying over other protectable 'signs' like shape and colour to the newer product. Such practices are enabled by intellectual property protection as well as by regulations dealing with approval, naming and pricing that concern, or that otherwise impact, the medical products trade. Numerous reports from intergovernmental organisations[130] and non-governmental[131] ones concerning these practices and their impacts on pricing, access and competition have contributed to the debates. Current concerns about pharmaceutical pricing, access and competition issues have tended to focus largely if not exclusively on patents, though. I have sought to diverge just a little from the tendency to discuss each intellectual property right in isolation, most commonly the right under analysis being patents.[132,133] That this is so frequently done is not unjustified. But trademarks now need more than ever to be part of the discussion.

Patents and trademarks in fact can be seen in many ways as functioning together: to both secure *and maintain* market power. Arguably, and history suggests this is largely true, using both is fundamental to how actors in this industrial sector have always done their business. We need briefly also to mention copyright. In some jurisdictions copyright provides legal protection from reproduction of the information included in the box. This is despite the rather obvious lack of creative choices in explaining how many pills are to be taken each day.

Finally, from a policy perspective, patents, trademarks and other intellectual property rights (include *quasi*-ones providing market and other types of exclusivity) are part of something much bigger. As mentioned in Chapter 2, intellectual property law generally, as well as those elements provided specifically with the pharmaceutical industry in mind, sit within a regulatory complex *and* a national ecosystem of biomedical innovation underpinned by research expenditures from various sources. In consequence, whether one is analysising their impacts or going further by proposing reforms, we must take account of this interactive and evolving regulatory and institutional embeddedness, in which the different parts interact with each other and potentially impact on the whole. This takes us to the final part of the book.

Notes

1 Parthasarathy *op cit.*, 2017.
2 Drahos (2010).
3 Parke Davis and Co. v. H.K. Mulford and Co., 189 Fed. 95 (S.D.N.Y. 1911) affirmed, 196 Fed. 496 (2nd Cir. 1912).
4 Langreth (2020).
5 Most notably, see G-5/83 Second medical indication/EISAI [1985], G-1/04 Diagnostic methods [2006], G-1/07 Treatment by surgery/MEDI-PHYSICS, [2011].
6 T-866/01 Euthenasia composition/MICHIGAN STATE UNIVERSITY, 2005.
7 G-1/07 Treatment by surgery/MEDI-PHYSICS, [2011].
8 Sterckx and Cockbain (2012).
9 G-1/04 Diagnostic methods [2006].
10 Edwards *et al.* (2011). Nicholas Lydon himself confirmed to the present author (pers. comm. 29 Sept. 2014) that Big Pharma remains overly conservative in relation to research directions and commercial opportunities from drugs that would only benefit relatively small numbers of patients.

Lydon continues to research kinase inhibitors by way of much smaller companies.

11 Oldham, Hall and Forero (2013).

12 Gupta *et al.* (2010).

13 Actavis UK Ltd v Merck & Co Inc [2008] EWCA Civ 444.

14 Parker and Hall (2014).

15 *Mayo Collaborative Services v. Prometheus Laboratories, Inc.*, 566 U.S. (2012).

16 See WIPO Document SPC/20/5 (9 Oct. 2013)

17 UK Patents Act — Section 60 (Meaning of Infringement).

18 Rasmussen (2008), 115–6. I am grateful to Nic Rasmussen for alerting me to this interesting example.

19 *Merrell Dow Pharmaceuticals Inc. and Anor v. HN Norton & Co.Ltd.* [1995] UKHL 14.

20 *Schering v. Geneva Pharmaceutical*, 339 F.3d 1373 (FCCA, 2003).

21 Amin and Kesselheim (2012).

22 For a justified critique of the vague usage of the term, for which the present author may be guilty, see Lietzan (2020). This author first heard the term uttered by Yusuf Hamied, chairman of the Indian generic firm Cipla, at a conference in London sometime around 2000.

23 Beall and Kesselheim (2018).

24 Other non-statutory exclusions in the United States are laws of nature, abstract ideas, and natural phenomena.

25 The Biotechnology Industry Organization was not founded until 1993, when two smaller organizations agreed to merge.

26 Although the USPTO was responsible for the shift in forum, GE was aware that the Supreme Court was an ideal arena to achieve its aim.

27 Kevles (1994), 111.

28 *Ibid.*, 117.

29 In re Bergy — Application of Malcolm E. Bergy (1977) *United States Patent Quarterly* 195:344, 346.

30 'DNA is Not 'Life', but a Chemical Substance which Carries Genetic Information', *Howard Florey/Relaxin*, EPOR 1995, 541, 551.

31 Having made this point, though, ground-breaking as this case may have been in the United States, the fact is that Europe was hardly a follower. Five years earlier, the German Federal Supreme Court had affirmed the patentability of micro-organisms. Chakrabarty's invention was quietly patented in the United Kingdom.

32 See Bozicevic (1987), 422–3.

33   Kevles (1994), 129–30.

34   Fowler (1994), 150.

35   See Kell (1992).

36   Kevles (2001), 31.

37   Complementary DNA (cDNA) comprises sections of DNA but without the non protein-encoding sequences ('introns').

38   See Barton (1991), 44, 46.

39   Borson (1995), 485–6.

40   Silverman (1990), quoted in Macdonald (2001), 11.

41   Robbins-Roth (2000), 21.

42   Bent *et al.* (1987), 66–67.

43   Decision of the Examining Division dated 14 July 1989, OJEPO (1989) volume 12, pp 451–61.

44   In 2000, the contracting states agree to strike out the words 'publication or' from the Convention text, and this and other amendments agreed at the time have now entered into force.

45   Decision of Technical Board of Appeal 3.3.2 dated 3 October 1990. T 19/90 — 3.3.2 OJEPO 13, 476–91, 1990.

46   This is the updated version of the TBA's balancing test referred to earlier.

47   T 0315/03 — 3.3.8.

48   USPTO (2001).

49   Calvert (2004), 305.

50   Kintisch (2005).

51   Andrews and Nelkin (2001).

52   Kleiner (2002), 6.

53   Ghosh (2012).

54   Hall (1990).

55   Williams-Jones (2002), 127.

56   US Patent no. 5,622,829 ('Genetic markers for breast, ovarian, and prostatic cancer'), issued on 22 April 1997.

57   Patents on BRCA1 were granted to Myriad at the USPTO in 1999 and the EPO in 2001.

58   US Patent no. 5,707,999 ('Linked breast and ovarian cancer susceptibility gene'), issued on 20 January 1998; and US Patent no. 5,710,001 ('17q-linked breast and ovarian cancer susceptibility gene'), issued on 20 January 1998. In each case ownership of the patents was shared, with Canada's Centre de Recherche du Chul and Japan's Cancer Institute ('999), with the University of Utah and the US government ('001).

59   Williams-Jones, *op cit.*, 131.

60   US Patent no. 5,654,155 ('Consensus sequence of the human BRCA1 gene'), issued on 5 August 1997. This was superseded exactly one year later by the filing of Patent no. 5,750,400 ('Coding sequences of the human BRCA1 gene'), issued on 12 May 1998.

61   Notes from a presentation delivered by Prof. Mike Stratton ('Patenting of genes — a case study of BRCA2') at St Catharine's College, University of Oxford, 1 June 2000. On file with author. *See* Parthasarathy (2005); Williams-Jones, *op cit.*, 137.

62   Wooster *et al.* (1995).

63   US Patent no. 5,837,492 ('Chromosome 13-linked breast cancer susceptibility gene'), issued on 17 November 1998. The patent was jointly filed with Endo Recherche, HSC Research and Development and University of Pennsylvania.

64   'In the United States, where its patents are still valid [when the cited article was published in 2008], Myriad has launched wide-ranging direct mailing shots to women, urging them to ask their doctors for a diagnostic test. This sort of scaremongering plays on patients' understandable confusion about the effect of the genes: although the vast majority of women with the BRCA1 gene will develop breast cancer, most breast cancers are not caused by the gene. So urging women to undergo an expensive genetic test for the sake of peace of mind raises both false alarm and false hope: false alarm because the gene is comparatively rare, false hope because even if you test negative for the gene, you can still develop breast cancer.' *See* Dickenson (2008), 92.

65   For details of the challenges to Myriad's European patents relating to BRCA 1 and 2, as well as a pending counter-challenge by Myriad to CRC's main BRCA2 patent, see Rimmer (2008), 190–200. For a very fair and objective presentation and commentary on the Myriad BRCA controversy, see Gold and Carbone (2008).

66   Association for Molecular Pathology v. U.S. Patent and Trademark Office (S.D.N.Y., 2010).

67   AMP v. USPTO (569 U.S. 2013).

68   'Probes' and 'primers' are commonly used terms in genomics. A very useful explanation of the terms and of their uses in the laboratory is provided in University of Utah Research Foundation *et al.* v. Ambry Genetics (*D. Utah* 2014). The case is interesting in itself, representing a failure by Myriad to get a preliminary injunction to stop a company selling BRCA tests after the Supreme Court judgement.

69   *In re BRCA 1 — and BRCA2 — Based Heredity Cancer Test Patent Litigation* (Fed. Cir. 2014).

70   Clain *et al.* (2015).

71   Conley, Cook-Deegan and Lázaro-Muñoz (2014). For further discussion on the implications of the Myriad decision, see Levy (2013).

72   National Research Development Corporation v. Commissioner of Patents [1959] *HCA* 67; (1959) *CLR* 252.

73   D'Arcy v. Myriad Genetics Inc [2014] *FCAFC* 115.

74   D'Arcy v. Myriad Genetics Inc [2015] *HCA* 35.

75   See Montgomery (2001), 5; Anand (2001), 1, 11.

76   See Aldhous (1996); Brown and Kleiner (1994); Ernhofer (2003); Henley (2001); Krimsky (2003), 67–8; Meek (2000).

77   Jackson (2015); see also Nuffield Council on Bioethics (2002), 39–42. CCR5 may be an appropriate target for medicines to treat other health problems, including stroke and traumatic brain injury. Villanueva (2019).

78   National Academies of Science (2005); Howlett and Christie (2004).

79   Merz *et al.* (2002).

80   Meek, *op cit*

81   Abraham, Castle and Gold (2014).

82   Liddicoat, Liddell and Aboy (2019). Research on the United States concludes that human gene patenting has neither promoted or hindered follow-on innovation. Sampat and Williams (2019).

83   Ghosh (2020).

84   The International HapMap Consortium (2003).

85   Goldstein and Cavalleri (2005); International HapMap Consortium (2005).

86   For criticisms of the HapMap licensing policy, see Hope (2008), 308–9.

87   For an excellent and highly detailed discussion on the applicability of open source to biotechnology including reviews of several ongoing open source biotechnology initiatives, see Hope *op cit.*

88   Holden (2002).

89   Roberts *et al.* (2014).

90   For a detailed comparative study on treatment of stem cell-related patents in the U.S., Europe and China, see Jiang (2016).

91   Golden (2010).

92   *Wisconsin Alumni Research Foundation (WARF)*. EPO, Decision of the Enlarged Board of Appeal of 25 November 2008, G 0002/06.

93   C34/10. *Oliver Brüstle v. Greenpeace eV, judgment of 18 October 2011.*

94   T2221/10 — 3.3.08.

95   *Case X ZR 58/07, 2012.*

96   Parthasarathy (2017), 3.

97   *Ibid.,* 3.

98 *Ibid.*, 9.

99 35 USC 201 ('March-in rights').

100 This has not always been the case. For much of the twentieth century American courts had few qualms about using compulsory licensing in response to abuses by patentees including antitrust violations. The Federal Trade Commission has also issued compulsory licensees when regulating corporate mergers and acquisitions. In addition, government use measures have been invoked on occasions, usually for national defence purposes, but also to reduce drug prices and in pursuit of environment protection and economic development. It is rather ironic, then, that today the United States actively discourages other countries from resorting to compulsory licensing. Reichman and Hasenzahl (2002).

101 *Novartis v. Union of India*, Civil Appeal No. 2706–2716 of 2013 before the Supreme Court of India (2013). For commentaries on the case, see Thikkavarapu (2014); Thambisetty (2014).

102 Sampat and Shadlen (2015).

103 Lentacker (2016), 142.

104 Lentacker *op. cit.*, 142.

105 Lentacker *op. cit.*, 143.

106 See for example, Wickremasinghe and Bibile (1971). I am grateful to Thiru Balasubramaniam for drawing my attention to this article.

107 Calvin and Lapinsky (2019).

108 Buick (2019).

109 Shaikh (2016), 2–3.

110 UNCTAD-ICTSD (2005), 531.

111 *Ibid*, 531.

112 Michael (2016). For a definitive exploration of how different countries have implemented TRIPS Article 39.3, and of the anticipated market impacts, see Buick (2019).

113 Rudd (2016), 54.

114 Von Hertzen (2016), 70.

115 Diependaele (2018); Diependaele, Cockbain and Sterckx (2018), 776.

116 Smith Hughes (2011b); Rasmussen (2014); Hoffman and Furcht (2014).

117 Brennan *op cit*.

118 The basis of rational drug design has been referred to as 'one target: one drug (1T1D)'. This involves starting with a drug target, and then coming up with a molecule that binds to it in order to enhance or inhibit its function (Deshaies (2020), 329). Glivec is a classic example, but the ACE inhibitors were arguably the first drugs resulting from the approach.

119 Ash and Schild (1966).

120 *Ibid.*

121 *Ibid.*

122 Black *et al.* (1972).

123 Freudenheim (1994).

124 Manners (2006) 46.

125 In Europe, the company sought also to delay generic competition with Losec by means that the European Commission found in June 2005 to be an abuse of its dominant position. AstraZeneca was fined 60 million. *See* Lawrence and Treacy (2005)

126 Angell (2004), 79; Goozner (2004), 222; Law (2006), 76–8.

127 Wan *et al.* (2015).

128 In the United States District Court for the District of Delaware, AstraZenica v. Dr Reddy's Lab, Complaint for Trademark Infringement, Counterfeiting, False designation of origin, Dilution, False Advertising, Deceptive Trade Practices.

129 E Jackson (2013), 509.

130 European Commission (DG Competition) (2009); European Commission (2019); OECD (2018); United Nations Secretary-General's High-Level Panel on Access to Medicines (2016). The latter report does acknowledge the need for what I am suggesting here: 'The panel's deliberations focused on patent law, and understandably so. But trademarks and copyright can exert monopolistic effects in the market that rival those associated with patents and with a far greater duration. The Report is silent on these issues, but there is much work that should be done to tackle the combined effects of different of different IP rights and other non-IP factors on the cost, distribution accessibility of medicines and health technologies.'

131 I-MAK (2018a).

132 E.g. Amin and Kesselheim (2012); Dutfield (2017); Gurgula (2017); I-MAK (2018b).

133 Two book-length exceptions, both of which mainly cover the United States are Gabriel (2014) and Greene (2014). See also Brennan (2015).

Part 4

The Pharmaceutical Sector and the Public Interest

Chapter 10

Prescriptions for a Healthier Pharmaceutical Industry

The Current State of Play

From a superficial glance at the new medicines becoming available (Table 10.1), things seem to be looking up again. For newly approved medicines, 2019 was a bumper year by recent standards with 45 FDA approvals. Of these, 11 are for cancer, and there are numerous treatments for some very serious infectious and non-communicable diseases like liver fluke infection — which is especially prevalent in developing countries — and Parkinson's disease. There are two new medicines for sickle cell disease, which is most common among Africans where it tends to be neglected by governments despite its significant role in child mortality rates there,[1] and among people of African descent elsewhere in the world. Approvals are not just for strictly new entities, though. Triclabendazole, the active ingredient of Egaten (called Fasinex when used as a veterinary medicine), has been used as an anti-parasitic in animals for a long time.

Two other interesting takeaways from an analysis of these approvals are, first, that as is common nowadays, the companies concerned were not necessarily the originators of these products. AveXis, founded as late as 2015 to develop gene therapy products, was acquired by Novartis in 2018 who were attracted to the company by its innovative product Zolgensma, which is predicted to become a huge seller. The trend for Big Pharma to take on products discovered and developed by small specialist biotech firms, is an ongoing one. Second, BeiGene's Brukinsa is the first approval from a Chinese company, an early sign perhaps of long-term change in the geography of pharmaceutical research and development.

Table 10.1. FDA new drug approvals in 2019

Brand name	Prescribed for	Type	Company
1. Jeuveau	frown lines	small molecule	Evolus
2. Cablivi	acquired thrombotic thrombocytopenic purpura	nano-antibody	Sanofi
3. Egaten	liver fluke infection	small molecule	Novartis
4. Zulresso	postpartum depression	small molecule	Sage Therapeutics
5. Sunosi	sleepiness from obstructive sleep apnea	small molecule	Jazz
6. Mayzent	multiple sclerosis	small molecule	Novartis
7. Evenity	osteoporosis	MAb	Amgen
8. Balversa	bladder cancer	small molecule	Johnson & Johnson
9. Skyrizi	psoriasis	MAb	AbbVie
10. Vyndaqel	transthyretin-mediated amyloidosis cardiomyopathy	small molecule	Pfizer
11. Zolgensma	spinal muscular atrophy	gene therapy/biologic	Novartis
12. Piqray	HR+/HER2- breast cancer (PIK3CA mutation)	small molecule	Novartis
13. Polivy	diffuse large B-cell lymphoma	antibody drug conjugate (ADC)	Roche
14. Vyleesi	hypoactive sexual desire disorder	small molecule	AMAG
15. Xpovio	multiple myeloma	small molecule	Karyopharm
16. Revarbrio	complicated UTIs and abdominal infections	small molecule (3 APIs)	Merck
17. Nubeqa	prostate cancer	small molecule	Bayer
18. Turalio	tenosynovial giant cell tumour	small molecule	Daiichi Sankyo
19. Pretomanid (unbranded)	drug-resistant tuberculosis	small molecule	Global Alliance for TB Drug Development
20. Wakix	narcolepsy	small molecule	Harmony Biosciences
21. Rozlytrek	ROS1-positive non-small cell lung cancer and NTRK fusion-positive tumours	small molecule	Roche
22. Rinvoq	rheumatoid arthritis	small molecule	AbbVie
23. Inrebic	myelofibrosis	small molecule	Bristol-Myers Squibb (Celgene)

Table 10.1.   (*Continued*)

Brand name	Prescribed for	Type	Company
24. Xenleta	community-acquired bacterial pneumonia	small molecule	Nabriva Therapeutics
25. Nourianz	Parkinson's disease	small molecule	Kiowa Kyrin
26. Ibsrela	irritable bowel syndrome with constipation	small molecule	Ardelyx
27. Aklief	acne	small molecule	Galderma
28. Beovu	wet age-related macular degeneration	MAb	Novartis
29. Scenesse	erythropoietic protoporphyria	small molecule	Clinuvel
30. Reyvow	migraine	small molecule	Eli Lilly
31. Trikafta	cystic fibrosis	small molecule (3 APIs)	Vertex
32. Reblozyl	anaemia in patients with beta thalassemia	Recombinant fusion protein	Bristol-Myers Squibb (Celgene) and Acceleron
33. Brukinsa	mantle cell lymphoma	small molecule	BeiGene
34. Fetroja	urinary tract infections	small molecule	Shionogi
35. Adakveo	sickle cell disease	MAb	Novartis
36. Givlaari	acute hepatic porphyria	small molecule	Alnylam
37. Xcopri	partial-onset adult seizure	small molecule	SK Life Science
38. Oxbryta	sickle cell disease	small molecule	Global Blood Therapeutics
39. Vyondys 53	Duchenne muscular dystrophy	small molecule	Sarepta Therapeutics
40. Padcev	metastatic bladder cancer	antibody drug conjugate (ADC)	Seattle Genetics and Astellas
41. Ervebo	ebola	Vaccine	Merck
42. Caplyta	schizophrenia	small molecule	Galderma
43. Dayvigo	insomnia	small molecule	Eisai
44. Enhertu	HER2-positive breast cancer	antibody drug conjugate (ADC)	AstraZeneca/Daiichi Sankyo
45. Ubrelvy	migraine	small molecule	Allergan

This feels like progress, not decline. While small molecule drugs continue to predominate, there is a strong presence of antibody drugs with eight (of which three are ADCs), plus a gene therapy biology and a recombinant fusion protein. There is one vaccine, for ebola, which is obviously very welcome.

And it is not just the last few years. From the 1990s we have achieved genuine advances in what were, and admittedly remain, hard cases. We now have sophisticated treatments for cancer. Not all of these are cures but they are still highly valuable in terms of extending lives. We have effective medicines to treat AIDS and cure hepatitis C, and these are benefitting patients around the world.

Nonetheless, progress in complex diseases is mixed. Alzheimer's, for example, remains a major disappointment, and infectious diseases are neglected. The latter remains a concern despite the global problem of antimicrobial resistance, the very real threats of viral pandemics, and their frightening consequences becoming better understood. And achievements in basic research carried out in universities and other non-corporate laboratories and hospitals, are still very hard for industry to translate into pharmaceutical products that make a difference. As with MAbs, obstacles are scientific, financial and regulatory, though in what proportions, and how far they are of the industry's own making — such as the excessive dependence on intellectual property rights as well as their frequently aggressive assertion — remains a matter for considerable debate.

Assessing the health of the industry four sets of question arise as follows:

(1) To what extent are these new and recent medicines *independently* discovered and developed by industry without public sector or other scientific input and funding? In other words, is the industry self-sufficient and therefore deserving of all the credit when 'their' medicines come on the market, typically protected from competition thanks to state-granted exclusivities? And finally, does this matter?

(2) Are these the *right* medicines we need? If not, why do we get these particular treatments for these particular diseases? What are the therapeutic areas tending to be neglected? What factors drive decisions on which ones to develop and which ones not to?

(3) Are the medicines they market fully accessible to those who need them? And if not, what are the obstacles to optimal access? And is this the 'fault' of industry legitimately maximising profit, or is it a regularory problem that can be resolved?

(4) What is to be done? Are there ways to use law and regulation to shape decision-making in maximally socially optimal directions? Even if we know what needs to be done, *can* it be done?

The rest of this chapter — and of this book — addresses these questions, and offers alternative approaches to looking at how to reorientate the profit-driven innovation model.

From Examination to Diagnosis

How much is industry responsible for new medicines? And does it matter?

Critics, including the present author, have for long pointed out that industry is inclined to give itself too much credit for genuine therapeutic contributions that the public sector and taxpayers contributed a great deal towards scientifically and/or financially. Universities have been and continue to be important sources of pharmaceutical innovation. Along with foundations, hospital research laboratories and public sector research agencies, they have been responsible for discovering *and* funding many of the most innovative and welfare-enhancing drugs.

It is not hard to find examples of the public sector and, on occasions, non-profit private institutions including charitable organisations, playing critical roles in the development of many new medicines, which industry often downplays. This is certainly true of the new ebola vaccine, where 'Canadian government scientists drove the development of rVSV-ZEBOV,[2] from laboratory bench to a commercial grade product for use in clinical trials, while private sector partners failed to substantively advance development in the years leading up to the [2014–15] West African epidemic.'[3] Every new medicine has its own story, but this kind of thing is hardly uncommon.

This is not a recent controvery. In the 1970s, Duncan Reekie and Michael Weber reviewed several studies addressing this issue and found that every one showed beyond their reasonable doubt that industry was responsible for developing *and* discovering the vast majority of drugs introduced in the USA during the 1950s and 1960s.[4] But a more recent finding is that the NIH, whose research budget has now reached nearly $40 billion per annum, played a significant role in the development of all five best-selling drugs in 1995.[5] The results of an empirical study published in 2011 based on new drug approvals from 1988 to 2005 does nothing to counter this trend towards heavy dependence on the public sector, finding this especially the case for the most innovative (priority-review) medicines:

> Government funding has played an indirect role — for example, by funding basic underlying research that is built on in the drug discovery process — in almost half of the drugs approved and in almost two-thirds of priority-review drugs.[6]

Most recently, a study published in 2019 in *British Medical Journal* on the 248 new molecular entities approved in the United States from 2008 to 2017, showed a marked upward trend in the scale of public sector research contributions to new drugs discovered. Out of those 248 a quarter 'had documented late stage research contributions from a public supported research institution or spin-off company'.[7] Some public sector research and expenditure can take a discovery quite far up the value chain towards approval.

But is any of this a problem? Perhaps not necessarily. We may justly accuse the industry associations and their spokespeople of hypocrisy when they downplay the public sector contributions to their products by implying they are their achievements alone. But hypocrisy is not a hanging offence. Besides which, clinical trials are hugely expensive and time-consuming and we normally place the burden of getting these done and properly documented on the companies. This is without doubt a considerable investment whose positive outcomes are far from certain.

The United States is a country that partially socialises research and development costs on the basis that we cannot expect the pharmaceutical industry unaided to discover, develop and acquire approval for all of the biomedical solutions needed to optimise health to the satisfaction of a population comprising individuals of all ages, socio-economic circumstances, and health conditions. That is largely true for many other countries. To enable this industry to generate income streams to support continuous research, we allow companies to monopolise income from their sales by means of regulatory and legal exclusivities that restrict competition, and that can be, and frequently are, 'gamed'.

The United States goes further than most countries by giving industry a free hand to set whatever price it deems optimal to maximise profit. It seems pretty evident that there is a severe danger of a situation arising where the price of medicines may well be linked to total research and development spending but not reflect the fact that a substantial percentage of those commitments were already paid for by taxpayers and carried out by scientists whose salaries and equipment come from the public purse. We will come back to the pricing issue later.

In particular, there has been criticism about instances of pharmaceutical companies acquiring exclusive rights to medicines largely developed with taxpayers' money, charging high prices despite this, with the government opting not to use its legal rights to intervene to counter such behaviour. Under the Bayh-Dole Act, where patents owned by a grant-recipient or contractor result from government-funded research, the government has the right to 'a nonexclusive, nontransferrable, irrevocable, paid-up license to practice or have practiced for or on behalf of the United States any subject invention throughout the world'. There is no need to justify this on the basis of abuse by the patent holder or to pay a royalty. Such a license is also available in the case of a federally-owned patent licensed to a third party.

The Act also provides for so-called march-in rights in the context of a patent arising from a federally-funded programme being held by a small business or non-profit (typically a university). The responsible federal agency has the right 'to grant a nonexclusive, partially exclusive, or exclusive license in any field of use to a responsible applicant or applicants, upon terms that are reasonable under the circumstances, and if the contractor, assignee, or exclusive licensee refuses such request, to grant such a license itself'. The circumstances in which march-in rights in such form can be invoked include: failure to manufacture or practice the invention, the need 'to alleviate health or safety needs which are not reasonably satisfied', and failure 'to meet requirements for public use'.

The language could certainly have been clearer as to whether charging high prices that cannot be justified by the research and development costs borne by the company marketing products arising from federally-funded research, or the business that licensed its patents to the firm actually selling the product, can trigger federal action. And yet, the Bayh-Dole Act is a bargain between the public and the private sector which seeks to transfer technology to the latter in the public interest. US taxpayers are being short-changed if tax-dollars were essential to developing the product but the companies are selling them back at prices that could only be justified if the private sector were bearing all of the research and development costs (and, one might add more pointedly, if there were no such thing as the human right to health which governments are in fact required to recognise and implement). And that is the point.

To add insult to injury there have been cases of companies making US taxpayer-funded drugs more expensive in the United States than in other countries. March-in rights appear to be a totally fair way to prevent such abuses. However, the provision has never been used, suggesting undue caution on the part of US government agencies. That said, there is some evidence that petitioning the government to invoke it has resulted in companies lowering prices and licensing patents on more reasonable terms.[8] The same has been achieved in several other countries by the threat of a compulsory license or a hint of invoking government use provisions even when not carried out.

Are we getting the right drugs? And whose fault is it if we're not?

The pharmaceutical industry is often criticised for its tendency to eschew risky and hugely challenging radical innovations in favour of me-too drugs that take advantage of successful past innovations whether by the same company or others. Such products are incremental modifications of these early ones that are typically marketed as being 'game-changers' (to use a neologism I personally loathe), whether they are or not.

Another common criticism is that drug companies' pursuit of profit leads them to invest where returns are likely to be biggest and over the longest-term results in perverse choices as to which diseases to investigate. Again, this criticism is hardly new. This is manifested in a preference for trivial and lifestyle-related conditions over life-threatening diseases and those that severely impact quality of life whether they kill or not. Meanwhile diseases are neglected because they are rare but life-threatening or are not rare but deemed unprofitable because they disproportionately affect the poor, especially in developing countries. We will look at these in turn, starting with the me-too issue, and then turning to the problem of life-threatening but neglected diseases.

As with other complaints about the behaviour of industry, me-too-ism is not a new one either. The critical view, as expressed by Leigh Hancher thirty years ago, is that 'the patent system ... can exacerbate these problems [of investing mostly in the development of therapeutically identical products] by sheltering socially worthless but privately profitable research'.[9] John Braithwaite, also writing decades ago, concurred, citing a former employer of Squibb who when giving evidence to the Kefauver Committee explained that, during his tenure there, 25 percent of the research budget went to 'worthwhile' projects, while the rest went on molecular manipulation. But he conceded that 'me-too research has occasionally stumbled upon significant therapeutic advances'.[10] Indeed, it is fair to point out that 'me-tooism' is not inherently a bad thing. In capitalist economies, companies compete in markets typically of the kind where there are goods of similar quality, with different firms seeking to attract consumers, normally through branding strategy, to their particular modest variation on a theme. Moreover, the term itself is somewhat vague in its application. According to CRA International, in any particular class of drugs, there are up to five variants of which four along the relative novelty to been-there-and-done-it spectrum can fairly be called me-toos. This product class-lifecycle type of perspective is probably just as relevant today as it was when Braithwaite and Hancher were discussing the matter. Any member of each group may well be a genuine improvement, even if other than a. they may for all we know be in the minority. Note that the position on the originality spectrum is not precisely correlated with patient value. In other words, a very similar product may represent high patient value, whereas a more original one may have negligible advantages for patients as compared to those already available.

a. First in class of a new mode of action;

b. Follow-on, independently patented molecules that have been developed concurrently with the first in class, with better or different benefit/risk/cost ratios, maybe for a different patient subset, which appear over a few years;

c. Molecules which belong to the same molecular entity family but have been shown to have utility for new disease indications;

d. Late class follower molecules sold sometimes in only limited geographical areas which are largely undifferentiated from the class leaders in terms of their technical attributes or the patient populations they serve;

e. As the class evolves more complex minor incremental innovations emerge such as different salt forms of existing molecules, formulations which improve bioavailability, limit side effects or improve patient compliance, fixed dose combinations which are particularly popular with clinicians in some countries.[11]

Let us turn to the whole issue of lifestyle drugs favoured over lifesavers, something we discussed also in the Introduction. The tendency to give special attention to chronic health issues, whose commercial attractiveness is due to the obvious fact that treatment may 'need' to be taken for somebody's whole life is undeniable. Morever, the customer base for such treatments can keep expanding due to wider social phenomena that industry is only partly responsible for, but may well seek to perpetuate through marketing: medicalisation and pharmaceuticalisation. In the meantime, cures tend to be less economically viable especially when there are regulatory constraints on freedom to price medicines as high as markets will bear.

Going by what the latest crop of new medicines are prescribed for, there is some evidence for the lifestyle drugs tendency, though a good number of them look highly impressive and important for the health of many. For the prosecution, Jeuveau *is* a cosmetic treatment. Acne outbreaks can be upsetting for teenagers, but they tend to go away in their own good time. Insomnia is certainly a nuisance that can make life very trying indeed. But it can often be managed by other ways than taking a pill. As for hypoactive sexual desire disorder, as with the male 'counterpart' of ED, it might be that a romantic candlelit dinner for two with mobile phones switched off for a change would equally do the trick. No doubt the fertile imagination could come up with much cheaper alternatives than either to spark the right kind of joy, at least some of which would probably work perfectly well for many people.

One factor that should not be overlooked in the upward trend in FDA approvals is that a lot of the new medicines are orphan drugs or for serious and life-threatening conditions including cancer for which special approval programmes introduced since the 1980s apply.[12] These programmes incentivise development of rare disease treatments, fast track the approval process, or reduce the burden of clinal proof that is normally required. To fund such incentivisation programmes, the FDA charges fees. Indeed, a growing share of the FDA's funding comes from fees paid by industry in exchange for accelerated approval. Now, these fees make up 45 percent of the FDA's total annual budget. This could potentially raise conflict of interest and regulatory capture concerns. In Europe, the figure is even higher, with 89 percent of EMA's anuual budget being covered by industry fee payments.[13]

The 1983 Orphan Drug Act[14] affords companies fast-track regulatory review by the FDA, a fixed period of market exclusivity after approval (seven years), and tax credits to compensate for clinical trial expenses incurred in that country. The law was largely based on the presumption that sales of such medicines would be low, therefore it would be very hard to make a profit. These programmes have not had major impacts on the number of approvals, but they do appear to have affected what has been approved. There has been an increase in the share of approvals that are orphan drugs as well as the number of rare disease indications. Only 10 percent of the 7,000 known rare diseases have FDA-approved treatments but even this low figure reflects significant improvement to the lives of many people for whom there were no previous treatments.[15]

But there are problems. First, the above advantages are available even if the medicine subsequently achieves blockbuster sales as did Glivec, as well as if the patient population expands beyond the 200,000 figure which is the maximum for grant of orphan drug status. Thus, regulation can become a form of corporate welfare.

Second, the lowering of approval standards gives rise to obvious concerns about safety and efficacy. Of course, regulatory review times should take no longer than is strictly necessary. But this quote from the above-cited article seems less than entirely reassuring:

> Expedited approval programs create substantial administrative costs and allow the approval of new drugs based on fewer, smaller, and/or earlier-stage clinical trials that may not be randomized, controlled, blinded, or based on traditional measures of how a patient feels, functions, or survives. In addition, the legal standard for approval requires only that a new drug 'have the effect it purports or is represented to have' and in general does not require a drug to exceed any particular threshold of efficacy other than zero. Although this statutory language has not changed, expedited programs have reduced the amount and quality of evidence needed to meet the statutory standard.[16]

The orphan drugs approval pathway and the benefits it gives companies demonstrates how difficult it can be to create positive incentives to research, develop and market medicines for rare diseases, and others that may not be rare but are still unattractive to industry without inadvertently generating perverse incentives that unscrupulous companies will take advantage of.

This had become apparent quite early. According to a United Nations Industrial Development Organization study that came out less than ten years after the Act was passed:

> The law has had its successes, such as a treatment for porphyria — a painful and debilitating disease that afflicts only 100 people. It has also proved to have shortcomings. Some companies make use of their monopoly position to extract exorbitant prices. Others use particularly narrow definitions of the disease to ensure that the potential market is extremely small. A few companies have achieved orphan drug status through a 'salami technique': submitting multiple applications for the same drug by specifying different groups of symptoms, each of which affects fewer than 200,000 people.[17]

This practice apparently persists. Another gaming tactic is described by Feldman: 'drug companies have figured out how to raise prices under orphan drug protections, and then spread those high prices across patient populations much broader than the small groups envisioned at the passage of the Orphan Drug Act. This technique is referred to as "spillover pricing".[18] This is made possible by off-label prescribing. As mentioned, such prescribing can be justified and may well do the patient good. The point is that this tactic is an abuse of the system.

In 2019, the FDA revoked the 2016 grant of orphan drug status to a medicinal product called Sublocade. The product is linked to a drug called Subutex to treat opioid addiction which had been given that status in 1994 on the gound that it was deemed unlikely to make a profit.[19] In fact, the manufacturer made billions of dollars from sales for a product supposedly having a small market, until it was discontinued in 2011. However, under the legislation, orphan drug status can be passed on to new versions of the same product, and without any requirement to prove each upgrade won't be profitable. Thus the product originally designated as orphan under the name Subutex was approved by the FDA under a different brand name: Sublocade. The active ingredients of both products were the same, the only difference being the latter was in an injectable form to be taken once monthly. Currently more than 2 million Americans are addicted to opioids, so the market has grown and is now substantial.

The stakes are high. According to Diane Dorman, formerly a leading official in the National Organization for Rare Disorders:

> The original orphan designation blocked Brixadi, an extended-release injection of buprenorphine, from entering the market, as well as any other buprenorphine trying to do that. By revoking orphan drug status for buprenorphine, the FDA has opened the door to other opioid addiction drugs, thus expanding the options for patients with opioid addiction and, hopefully, lowering the price of treatment by creating a competitive marketplace.[20]

Bills have been introduced to reform the Act, but nothing has changed. In addition, orphan drugs can be hugely expensive so that sufferers from a rare disease for which a treatment is now in existence are not always able to get access. It is hard not to see this due, at least in part, to Washington being awash in Big Pharma dollars aimed at influencing politicians. Perhaps it goes without saying that in that country politicians need to raise large amout of money to campaign for office including the sums spent on television advertising.

Another category of neglected disease comprises those for which there is no shortage of patients but that the industry is not interested in developing medicines. This is either because they disproportionately affect the poor in developing countries or because for other reasons they do not consider them to be likely to generate levels of profits as compared to those treatments specifically targeted at keeping the affluent alive.

We have been aware of the problem of antibiotic resistance caused largely by their excessive use, and the lack of new antibiotics to replace the old ones, but little was being done till recently. This is a serious market failure with potentially awful consequences. It remains to be seen whether the FDA's new Limited Population Pathway for Antibacterial and Antifungal Drugs Guidance for Industry, a programme launched in 2016 intended to accelerate development and approval of such medicines for limited populations where there is an unmet need, will make a significant difference. A neglected disease affecting the poor for which a treatment is now available is drug-resistant tuberculosis. However, tellingly approval for Pretomanid was granted to the TB Alliance, a non-profit pharmaceutical product development partnership. Pretomanid is only the second medicine to be approved under this scheme, the first being Arikayce for a bacterial lung disease developed by a small company called Insmed.

The ebola vaccine story outlined above and the Pretonamid experience highlight the fact that there are huge gaps in healthcare provision that the industry cannot fill by itself. Without public-private partnerships, the crafting of regulatory incentives, or both, and even then, nothing is certain. What we do know is that leaving it to the market simply won't work. Nor will it work if after these products are developed, they are set at unaffordable prices. This has never been more evident than it is today as the world impatiently awaits new vaccines and drugs to prevent Covid-19 and cure those who have it. Given how contagious the disease is, the need for these medicines to be *universally* affordable for the good of all humankind, *and* that borderless open and collaborative science and free exchange of knowledge and data will get us to vaccines and cures faster than by any other way, are both blindingly obvious.

Obstacles to access — who or what is getting in the way?

I would hazard a guess that most of us care little how much Evolus charges for Jeuveau. Its use is cosmetic; besides, it's in hot competition with Allergan's Botox, so a tried and tested alternative is readily available if one feels so inclined. What the industry does receive heavy criticism for is the prices it charges for life-saving or life-enhancing medicines. Access matters to people. The torment of lacking access to a life-saving drug that exists in the world but is unavailable due to the business models employed by industry may be far worse than the prospect of dying of a disease that has no cure.[21]

The prices of many medicines that people *do need* are far too high, and seem to be increasing year by year. This is justified, as mentioned above, by the heavy research and development costs and, in some cases, by their public health value. Excessive costs are a major problem for the poorest nations. In the developed world, too, the situation gets worse, especially in the United States. Despite the country having some of the best healthcare in the world, and its companies — typically with considerable public funding of research fundamental to their discovery or development[22] — introducing a substantial proportion of the new medicines coming out every year, the system is broken. Despite this, there is broad political hostility to 'socialised medicine' despite the fact that, as mentioned, research and development costs *are* partially socialised. The more one thinks about this (as a non-American) the more perplexing it is. Radical reform seems far away, not helped by a lack of political will, a tendency among some politicians to shift the blame to other countries for allegedly failing to share whatever cost burden that country feels it needs to shoulder, and ideological opposition to intervene in a market in which the government already intervenes quite heavily.

Much recent attention has been given to the distress caused to patients due to the high prices being charged in the United States for insulin.[23] According to one study, between 2007 and 2018, prices of insulin products increased dramatically, list prices by 262 percent and net prices by 51 percent.[24] Reportedly, the consequence is that many diabetics are not getting enough insulin, and yet the companies are profiting from these higher prices. The existence of different insulin formulations as are available today, is of course a good thing. But the market is not very competitive, being dominated by a small number of firms: in the United States only Eli Lilly, Novo Nordisk and Sanofi; and not everybody qualifies for their patient assistance schemes. Meanwhile list prices have increased dramatically, and people suffer, in the United States but also in lower and middle-income countries where 80 percent of diabetics live and estimates show only half of those people have access.[25] This ruthless behaviour may be contrasted with the altruistic heroics of Banting and his colleagues in producing the product for the first time, and opting not to claim any of the financial gain that they surely deserved so as to make insulin accessible to all diabetics.[26]

Secondary patenting has been considered elsewhere in the book as has the strategic use of patents, trademarks and other actual and *quasi* intellectual property rights. The former phenomenon alone can lead to higher prices and reduced competition due to negative effects on generic market entry. Studies conducted in the United States,[27] Australia[28] and Switzerland[29] show this has happened in a number of countries. As one might expect the problem is most serious in the United States and people really do suffer. Feldman analysed all drugs on the market between 2005 and 2015 focusing on instances of new patents and regulatory exclusivities being added to a medicine. Her findings are startling:

> Rather than creating new medicines, pharmaceutical companies are largely recycling and repurposing old ones. Specifically, 78% of the drugs associated with new patents were not new drugs, but existing ones, and extending protection is particularly pronounced among blockbuster drugs. Once companies start down the road of extending protection, they show a tendency to return to the well, with the majority adding more than one extension and 50% becoming serial offenders. The problem is growing across time.[30]

But while most of the eye-watering prices are for new medicines, or else old ones in new forms, there are also concerns about price hikes of old medicines. Daraprim, which appears in the table below in ninth place came on the market in the early 1950s. Its high price, a blatant case of immoral price-gouging, calls into question the assumption that free competition suddenly appears after patents expire. In the UK, a pack of 30 tablets costs £13. But pyrimethamine, or Daraprim to use its brand name, perhaps the most cynical of all such incidents, is far from being alone. In recent years the prevalent trend has been for prices of many prescription medicines including those that have been on the market for quite a lengthy period to increase on a yearly basis.

Patents on medical products will eventually expire but this does not of itself turn this or that that medicine into a commodity whose economic value plunges unavoidably on a downward spiral towards little more than marginal cost. It is noteworthy, first, that many if not most medicines markets contain few competing products: 'approximately 40% of generics' markets are supplied by a single manufacturer'[31] in the United States, suggesting price drops due to competition may be less steep than is commonly supposed. This is certainly the case for biologics, which are admittedly something of a special case.

A range of entry barriers exist not least of which are the regulatory ones that prevent the marketing of falsified and unsafe medicines. We do of course need to have these. In addition, originator firms may benefit from distribution networks that restrict the availability of samples for would-be competitors who need them for the testing necessary to secure their own marketing authorisation. For biosimilars, the acquisition of samples is hugely expensive as is the development of an alternative system of production. The proposal, mentioned earlier, to require originators to deposit their cell-line for others to access would certainly help reduce the cost and technical difficulty of entering the market. Other upfront market entry costs may encourage many generic firms to target markets in specific drugs that have attracted few other competing firms rather than those that are already crowded. That of course might be a good thing.

Why does this situation not just persist but even get worse? Arguably a combination of factors may be at work. There is a strong perception that the US firms's global dominance is a success story for the country and they should be allowed to charge whatever they feel is necessary to recoup their R&D costs. Moreover, free market ideology which holds that in competitive economies companies should have a free hand in pricing as they see fit holds sway in certain quarters. However, one cannot overlook the massive investments in influencing politicians and appealing directly to consumers

Table 10.2.   Top-ten most expensive pharmaceuticals in United States (per month estimates unless otherwise stated)

Product	Type of medicine	Company	Price (US$)
1. Zolgensma	gene therapy	Novartis	2,100,000 per dose
2. Actimmune	biologic	Horizon	687,720
3. Acthar	biologic	Mallinckrodt	457,800
4. Ravicti	small molecule	Horizon	421,428
5. Myalept	biologic	Aegerion	145,350
6. Brineura	biologic	BioMarin	56,396
7. Oxervate	biologic	Dompé	46,760 (for one eye)
8. Takhzyro	MAb	Shire	46,100
9. Daraprim	small molecule	Turing	23,500
10. Cinryze	biologic	Shire	23,120

Based on Stone (2019).

who typically do not pay directly for the medicines they request. These expenditures including the funding of lobbyists evidently bear rich dividends for the industry. Indeed, without wishing to impugn the integrity of people working in the FDA and other relevant government departments, regulatory capture accusations cannot all be dismissed out of hand.

Table 10.2 shows the current most expensive medicines in the United States with their prices for a month of treatment. It is worth mentioning than many of these are speciality drugs, that is, ones for complex or rare diseases, often requiring highly supervised administration. Typically biologics, they tend to have small patient groups and therefore often benefit from orphan drug status. The developers of such medicines may also take advantage of the FDA's recently-introduced Breakthrough Therapy programme which fast tracks certain highly promising medicines through the clinical trials process. So despite the small number of patients regulatory advantages and high prices have enhanced commercial interest in developing and marketing such products, which in fact have few if any competing products to contend with. It is noteworthy that most such products come from smaller companies rather than the traditional Big Pharma. (However, as with many products marketed by the large corporations, some of these medicines were in-licensed rather than discovered by the companies holding the marketing approvals.) It is also worth mentioning that being small doesn't prevent these businesses from gaming the regulatory system for advantage at the expense of patients.[32]

What happens elsewhere? There is in fact quite a lot of variation in terms of pricing schemes and purchasing policies. In the United Kingdom, for example, the National Health Service is the primary buyer of prescription medicines which places it in a relatively strong bargaining position. In addition, the National Institute for Health and Care Excellence (NICE) assesses the most effective treatment regimes, determines their overall cost-effectiveness, and then makes funding recommendations on that basis. There have been occasions when NICE has found a very effective medicine not to be cost-effective at the price insisted upon by the company concerned and therefore was not funded. This happened with Orkambi, a cystic fibrosis medicine, that was rejected by NICE in 2016 when priced at £104,000 per patient per year. It took three years for terms to be agreed and thus for this very important drug to be made available to patients. The existence of NICE in the UK is a very good thing but with budgets limited, NICE is forced to make some very tough decisions. Access delayed is of course better than no access at all. But it is hardly satisfactory either.

In Europe, as elsewhere, there is much concern about excessive pricing and its links to intellectual property and regulation. With respect to the latter, it has become clear that pharmaceutical companies have been able to take advantage of the regulatory system to increase the prices of medicines when they have gone off patent. The primary tool to discipline such behaviour in the European Union is Article 102 of the *Treaty on the Functioning of the European Union* concerning abuse of a dominant position, and national regulatory regimes dealing with the issue domestically such as the UK Competitions and Markets Authority (CMA). Branding and de-branding strategy can play a role in this. The Article states as follows:

Any abuse by one or more undertakings of a dominant position within the internal market or in a substantial part of it shall be prohibited as incompatible with the internal market in so far as it may affect trade between Member States.

Such abuse may, in particular, consist in:

(a) directly or indirectly imposing unfair purchase or selling prices or other unfair trading conditions;
(b) limiting production, markets or technical development to the prejudice of consumers;
(c) applying dissimilar conditions to equivalent transactions with other trading parties, thereby placing them at a competitive disadvantage;
(d) making the conclusion of contracts subject to acceptance by the other parties of supplementary obligations which, by their nature or according to commercial usage, have no connection with the subject of such contracts.

Unfair pricing tends to be seen as excessively high pricing. However, predatory pricing is also 'unfair' and therefore a matter for competition authorities. Obviously patients and payers benefit directly from low prices of the medicines they need or fund. Moreover, donations of drugs by companies can save lives and enhance blighted ones, and are especially welcome for neglected tropical diseases that are otherwise untreatable.[33] But unfairly low prices can force other companies out of the market and such reduction of competition in the longer term is not in the interests of the public, hence the need for regulatory authorities to intervene.

In the United Kingdom branded medicines are subject to one of two pricing schemes. The Pharmaceutical Price Regulation Scheme, of which the most recent version was agreed in 2019, provides for a voluntary scheme which is a non-contractual voluntary agreement between the Department of Health and the Association of the British Pharmaceutical Industry (ABPI). Under the latter, price increases will need Department of Health approval, profits are capped with reimbursement where sales increase too far, and prices are subject to cost-effectiveness thresholds. Companies opting not to join the Voluntary Scheme are subject to the Statutory Scheme for Pricing of Branded Medicines, whose most recent incarnation was introduced by primary legislation in 2017.

This sounds good so far, but gaming the system is not precluded by any means. Phenytoin, a medicine found as early as 1936 to be effective against seizures, was being sold by Pfizer in the UK under the Voluntary

Scheme. The medicine, which is on the WHO's essential medicines list, was branded under the name Epanutin. In 2012, Pfizer sold the Marketing Authorisation to Flynn Pharma for whom Pfizer became the exclusive maker and supplier of the drug to that company which became the exclusive distributor. For the capsule form of the drug, Flynn adopted the name *Phenytoin* Sodium *Flynn* Hard Capsules, the first word being the international non-proprietary name. Obtaining approval to be sold as a generic, the medicine was withdrawn from the Voluntary Scheme and being a generic medicine without a brand name was not subject to the Statutory Scheme either. Taking advantage of regulatory loopholes provided on the naïve basis that generic drugs by their definition operate in competitive markets not requiring regulatory oversight, Pfizer increased the price it charged Flynn, and the price of capsule packs increased from £2.83 to £67.50. When wholesalers tried to parallel import drugs under the Epanutin brand name, they were sued for trademark infringement. The CMA found Pfizer's and Flynn's drastically increased prices to be excessive and unfair and imposed fines on both companies. This was not the end of it, though. On appeal the fines were set aside due to a misapplication of the legal test applied by the CMA.

In summing up, the pharmaceutical industry is a rational profit-seeking actor whose actions are mostly legal and in accordance with the legal-regulatory regimes for which governments are ultimately responsible. Pharmaceutical business models operate within this regulatory system in pursuit of shareholder value — not social value. Revenues are also ploughed back into the discovery and development of new medicines, and also into expanding the patient bases of existing ones by adding indications to labels.

Without a doubt the industry has produced a large number of outstanding medical products that have saved or enhanced the lives of millions of people. And yet the overall picture is an industry that can do a lot better. In the United States, far too much is spent on marketing that could have been spent on research, including the promotion of pharmaceuticalisation which means expensive medicines are sold for people who may not currently need them, or who would even have been better off not taking them in the first place. There and elsewhere, prices are unjustifiably high, and people suffer as a result.

Intellectual property laws and regulatory systems, which in some countries industry helped to design, place too much market power in the hands of industry which they use to political effect both domestically and internationally. Developing country governments continue to get bullied for invoking public health safeguards in their patent laws. Usually their bargaining position is constrained and negotiating capacity is relatively weak. They also find themselves pressured into domestically introducing industry-friendly intellectual property laws and regulatory changes through bilateral and regional free trade agreements, jeopardising countries' efforts to give effect to the human right to health in the hope of enhancing overseas market access for their country's exports. Industry lobbying is very much behind the negotiating demands of the developed country parties engaged in these types of agreement.[34]

Meanwhile, as mentioned in the Introduction, in the United States life expectancy rates have been falling. According to Vinay Prasad of Oregan Health and Science University, 'the cause is largely diseases of despair: drug overdose, suicide and alcohol-related liver disease.'[35] The underlying context is the massive socio-economic inequalities of that country which successive governments (as well as much of the electorate) have condoned, and weak public health and environmental regulation. The US is of course somewhat atypical. Medical bankruptcy exists and is common, drug prices are the world's highest, overprescribing fuelled by marketing is widespread, and as mentioned previously there is much opposition among the political class and even much of the public apparently, to socialised medicine, a term perhaps coined for its similarity to socialism, a word that appears to strike fear and loathing in the hearts of millions of Americans. Obviously, only part of this debacle can be pinned on the pharmaceutical industry. The huge cost of political campaigning and the lack of limits as to how much money can be donated and spent invites undue influencing and corruption. The industry did not create this system, but it is more than happy to reap the benefit and therefore deserves its share of the blame. Until that is changed, it is hard to see how private profit can be better aligned with public need other than through small incremental steps.

The industry has also been disruptive of efforts to enhance transparency about the true research and development expenditures of companies and the prices they charge in the different markets for their products.[36]

This matters a lot. Industry is fully aware that pricing information is useful for governments in their negotiations with drug companies, including when they adopt international reference pricing as a way to regulate price that is fair to companies but not excessive, by taking account, for comparison, of price in a selection of reference countries. The UK is commonly one of those latter countries due to the fact its prices are relatively low by developed country standards.[37] International reference pricing makes sense. After all, why *would* South Africa, a user of this methodology, accept a price that is higher that what is paid in the United Kingdom, a far wealthier country? As for research and development costs, although industry nowadays speaks much about how price should reflect therapeutic value of a medicine — presumably where this is found to justify a higher price than if the true R&D costs were the only consideration — it remains the case that over the years the prevailing argument for high-priced drugs is how expensive and risky it was to discover and develop them. Therefore, it is worthwhile to know more of what companies themselves spend on R&D, as well as the methodology employed to do the estimate. This is especially so given industry consistently cites the highest average R&D costs estimates published. In the United States, the Tufts University Center for the Study of Drug Development, which is partly funded by industry, provides periodic estimates of average drug development costs. These tend to be quite significantly higher than alternative estimates.[38] Unsurprisingly these estimates are the ones industry tends to use.

Prescriptions for a Healthier Pharmaceutical Industry

Seen through a coevolutionary lens, the medical-industrial complex, a term I introduced at the beginning of this book, is a manifestation of processes involving four variable interacting factors. This is a useful way to understand the system, how it works, how it changes over time, and why it goes wrong. But it is more useful than that, in my view. The coevolutionary perspective can also be highly prescriptive. It helps us to figure out holistically what is needed to re-shape the complex in radical but realistic ways reflecting public needs much more accurately than the medical-industrial complex as it is today. There will of course be powerful countervailing forces seeking to keep things as they are or shape the complex in ways suiting their own interests. But such forces are not monolithic. Moreover, my perspective also points to the possibility that organised interests with powerful ideas but without economic muscle can still effect positive change. In this final part of the book, I put forward a few prescriptions but these are admittedly piecemeal and tentative. This is an ongoing project.

Companies starting up may be highly idealistic, but if successful and they become large transnational corporations, this state of being rarely lasts (remember Google's 'Don't be evil' motto?). What of the pharmaceutical industry? Is the industry incurably pathological in its current form?

Nassir Ghaemi at Tufts Medical School identifies four views regarding the pharmaceutical industry: it is evil; it is good; it is neither; it is both.[39] I'm not sure the industry fits neatly into any category. My feeling is that, pathological or not, the industry has no 'conditions' that could not be treated with better regulatory 'medicine'. Corporations behave amorally, which is not quite the same as saying they are pathological.[40] In the pursuit of profits, those responsible for these businesses' strategic management can be brutally aggressive and sometimes shamelessly corrupt. But they are not necessarily unresponsive to public opinion. If the legal-regulatory frameworks that the industry operates by were different, could the industry behave differently, and the public be served better? In my opinion, yes.

The people who work for them are unlikely to be less public-spirited than the rest of us. Besides, in a sense many of us are implicated. As a profitable industry, the business of pharmaceuticals attracts external investment. A great portion of such investments comes from pension funds. We all want our pension fund managers to do well by us so we don't spend our final years in poverty. But we tend to pay insufficient attention to who is receiving our money, what they do with it, and what the consequences are. As I complete this part of the text, it has been announced that the UK Parliament's pension fund has increased investments in renewable energy businesses, and is reducing those in fossil fuel companies. Similar fossil fuel divesting is going on elsewhere. I'm not suggesting that we divest also in pharmaceuticals. Besides, small and medium-sized businesses need investment to survive, and it's generally acknowledged that it is these companies, not Big Pharma, who do the most creative early-stage work. We need to reduce fossil fuel consumption and use what we do consume more efficiently. That's not the case for pharmaceuticals, other than arguably in the United States. But even there they are absolutely central to healthcare and will remain so for the foreseeable future. But pension funds represent individual contributors all of whom have a stake in how the industry is allowed to act under the present regulatory frameworks. And with money comes power to change behaviour. Admittedly, the best way forward is to change those frameworks, and then the industry will simply have to respond.

How humanity can best assemble its human and other resources to maximise positive health outcomes remains an unresolved question, and I don't pretend to have an answer. Anti-capitalists are likely to favour nationalisation of the industry. I am not an anti-capitalist to the extent of seeking its abolition, though I am doubtful that capitalism in its present guise is good for humankind or the environment. Taking into account the fact that the state's ability to do what the industry does, and to do it better, and entirely from the public purse, is a big ask, I'm sceptical that nationalisation is the best way forward. I am of course willing to be persuaded it is. Besides, when we look at what appears in practice to be untrammelled free enterprise, it turns out that it's really a highly regulated market. The pharmaceutical market certainly is, but it is regulated in a way that enables businesses to make substantial profits on the basis of short-term legally enforceable restraints on competition; restraints that are partly crafted with this particular industry in mind. As legal scholar Robin Feldman rather elegantly puts it, albeit focusing just on patents:

> At a fundamental level, the intellectual property system exudes a deep faith in the power of competition. Competition may be held in abeyance, but those who receive the benefit of a patent or exclusivity must pay for that privilege by disclosing sufficient information such that competitors will be able to step into the market. And as the protection clock winds down, other inventors can use that disclosure, making preparations to enter the competitive field or jump ahead to the next generation.[41]

But what of course happens is that barriers to entry of various forms persist, some of which are perverse. As a result, there is less competition than there could be even when there are no patents. We have seen in this book how some of these emerge and stubbornly remain in place. Industry is to blame for some but not all of these. As a believer in the mixed economy, it's hard for me to have a principled objection to profit-making especially when it enables money from sales to be plowed back into the necessary research for discovering and developing new medicines *as long is that is what actually happens with the money.*

That said, the pharmaceutical industry in its present setup, is not the answer. There is a serious misalignment between business strategy and the real needs of the global public. There will never be a complete alignment hence the need for public sector biomedical research, not just the blue skies research industry has no interest in doing, but also in discovery and probably some of the development too. But the industry can and must do better. The good news is that we can change it. In democracies, if any industry is not serving the public as well as it should we can do something about it. It's true the industry is determined to resist change that impacts negatively on its business interests. But historically other industries have been made to fall into line, however big and powerful they were at the time. You do not have to go at all far back in time to see what countries have done with other industries that behaved in ways that were harmful or else had products that were harmful or dangerous. In my own country, the UK, we have strict controls on the trade in guns, as do other countries. Like others we have banned tobacco advertising, imposed high sales taxes on tobacco products, and, following the example of Australia, have adopted strict packaging requirements. The pharmaceutical industry is already subject to a complex regulatory framework that seeks to ensure medicines are safe and efficacious and constrain certain behaviour, whilst allowing it still to make large profits as well as providing certain economic incentives. The United States was very much in the forefront when it came to regulating the industry to prevent it from wilfully or negligently placing unsafe and ineffective medicines on the market. In a sense we get the industry our regulatory framework deserves.

That the world may be considered a better place for having the industry is one I am willing to accept. But it is a conclusion based as much as anything on our failure to imagine better alternatives than on such alternatives not to be — and not to have been — possible. Further regulatory and market reforms are much needed so that the pursuit of profit is balanced with better public health outcomes than the ones we are seeing today. Closing regulatory loopholes to prevent system-gaming would certainly be a good start, preferably without making regulation even more complex than it already is. Banning direct-to-consumer advertising of prescription medicines will help to counter the harmful market effects of branding, as would preventing the grant, or else the enforcement, of trademarks on shapes and colours of pills that can be used to restrict fair competition and cause consumer confusion. None of this is radical. Many countries restrict pharmaceutical advertising, control prices, and sanction companies for anticompetitive behaviour.

We need to think also about the types of innovation the patent system is, or is not, incentivising and whether the system serves the public interest as well as it should, whilst bearing in mind that the patent system can never be perfect even with a better balance between legal monopoly and public interest safeguards. One of the main problems, which may not necessarily cause difficulties in other industries, is that qualification for a patent is based purely on crossing a threshold based on three main tests: novelty, non-obviousness, and utility or industrial applicability. Once the threshold is crossed all inventions are treated the same, and you get your 20-year legal monopoly. Quality, investment commitments, or social utility, are all entirely irrelevant. In effect, trivial and minor inventions — an outcome exacerbated by (a) the legal fiction of novelty for some types of 'invention', (b) the generally low non-obvious threshold, and (c) the uniformity of the rights granted — are over-rewarded relative to their worth and to the scope of the legal protection available as compared to more socially-useful radical ones. If a company is convinced that there is more money in making a treatment for baldness, or an incremental enhancement to a successful existing drug soon to go off-patent, or adding an indication to an existing one, than for a radical treatment for Alzheimer's, the patent system is not going to help to reverse this preference. Patents are blunt instruments that impose social costs on the public. They need to be sharpened. For a start, making it harder to obtain additional exclusivities on existing medicines through secondary and tertiary patents, and regulatory gaming would certainly help, and might also incentivise investment in more radical innovation.

We need to come up with additional rewards or research and development financing mechanisms outside the patent system to enhance engagement with the global disease burden while avoiding monopolies, instead ensuring affordable access.[42] In particular, there is also scope for commons approaches to succeed, which are based on sharing and transparency as opposed to secrecy and property. These could potentially not just aid discovery but reduce the high R&D attrition rate. Regulatory regimes could certainly do much more to incentivise open science drug discovery and development.[43] One proposed mechanism is to remunerate companies in proportion to the size of the global health impacts of their medicines. This is the Health Impact Fund devised by philosopher Thomas Pogge and economist Aidan Hollis.[44] Another proposal, devised by the non-governmental organisation Knowledge Ecology International (KEI), which has had some high-profile endorsers, is to develop an alternative innovation system to delink price from research and development costs, ensuring the industry gets fairly and profitably remunerated but leaving products affordable.[45] Obviously the money has to come from somewhere if not from sales. Direct funding, subsidies and incentive mechanisms are all possible approaches. Of course, all of this requires political will of governments and, ideally, international cooperation.[46]

And finally, it remains for me to say the following. It is probably hard for any of us to think of anything nobler than presenting to the world a new medicine that saves many lives: that high design of purest gold as that old tribute on the wall of an ancient London church put it rather beautifully. But there is much more *and less* to the industry than high design or purest gold. And making the most beautiful medicine is all well and good but if people who need it cannot get to it, for economic or other reasons, it might as well not exist. This book's title purposely reflects these contradictions.

Notes

1 Grosse *et al* (2011).
2 Recombinant vesicular stomatitis virus–Zaire Ebola virus, branded as Ervebo.
3 Herder, Graham and Gold (2020).
4 Reekie and Weber (1979).
5 As reported on ABC News, 29 May 2002.
6 Sampat and Lichtenberg (2011), 332.
7 Nayak, Avorn and Kesselheim (2019), 5.
8 Seidenberg (2017).
9 Hancher (1990), 51.

10 Braithwaite (1984), 164.

11 CRA International (2008), 43.

12 Darrow, Avorn and Kesselheim (2020).

13 Hamzelou (2019), 37.

14 Counterpart legislation has been passed in Japan (1993), Australia (1997), and in the European Union by virtue of two instruments: Regulation (EC) No 141/2000 of the European Parliament and of the Council of 16 December 1999 on orphan medicinal products; and Commission Regulation (EC) No 847/2000 of 27 April 2000 laying down the provisions for implementation of the criteria for designation of a medicinal product as an orphan medicinal product and definitions of the concepts 'similar medicinal product' and 'clinical superiority'.

15 Dorman (2019a).

16 *Ibid.* Citations removed from quote.

17 Balance, Pogány and Forstner (1992), 18.

18 Feldman (2018), 624.

19 Dorman (2019b).

20 *Ibid.*

21 To illustrate the claim that the denial of a drug may be more psychologically painful than that drug's not existing, the philosopher Jeremy Waldron offers the following hypothetical scenario: 'Suppose Q is dying of a disease for which he knows there is no cure; he resigns himself to his fate and prepares for a stoic death. Then the news comes in: a drug has been developed which will remit the disease. The person who made and tested it, P, did so in his own laboratory with his own hands using his own materials. P makes the drug available to a number of his friends, but excludes Q because he dislikes Q's politics. Clearly Q will suffer something as a result of this. Instead of the stoic death he prepared for, it is likely that the rest of his life will be spent in painful bitterness and anger as he endures the thought that he might have lived and flourished but will not, thanks to P's exercise of this exclusionary right.' Waldron (1993).

22 Cleary *et al* (2018).

23 Collington (2020).

24 Hernandez *et al* (2020).

25 Jack (2020); Ewen *et al* (2019).

26 Rees (2019), 108–10.

27 Kapczynski, Park and Sampat (2012).

28 Moir (2016).

29 Vernaz *et al* (2013).

30   Feldman (2018), 590–1.
31   In OECD *op cit.*, 29, citing several sources.
32   E.g. see Goldberg (2010).
33   Sutton (2020). A well-known example is Merck's ivermectin, which thanks to the company's donation programmes has benefited millions suffering from onchocerciasis (river blindness).
34   There is a wealth of literature on this, of which the following are a few examples: Halabi (2018), Sell (2003), Sundaram (2018), Von Braun (2012).
35   Prasad (2020).
36   Albeit not entirely successfully. In May 2019, the WHO's World Health Assembly adopted a resolution entitled 'Improving the transparency of markets for medicines, vaccines, and other health products' (WHA (2019)). The resolution, which is not legally enforceable, was proposed by several countries from Europe, Asia and Africa, plus Brazil. For reasons best known to themselves, the UK, Germany and Hungary disassociated themselves from the resolution.
37   Ruggeri and Nolte (2013).
38   DiMasi, Grabowski and Hansen (2016).
39   Ghaemi (2013), 226.
40   For a view that they are, see Bakan (2004).
41   Feldman (2018), 592.
42   Hubbard and Love (2004); UCL Institute for Innnovation and Public Purpose (2018).
43   Bountra, Lee and Lezaun (2017).
44   Hollis and Pogge (2008). For a criticism of the HIF proposal, see Van den Belt and Korthals (2013).
45   Clift *et al* (eds), 2015; Love (2016); United Nations Secretary-General's High Level Panel on Access to Medicines (2016).
46   For more on delinkage, see KEI's dedicated website https://delinkage.org.

Bibliography

Abraham, EP, E Chain, CM Fletcher, HW Florey, AD Gardner, NG Heatley and MA Jennings (1941) Further observations on penicillin. *The Lancet* 238(6155), 177–88.

Abraham, EP (1961) Derivatives of cephalosporin C formed with certain heterocyclic tertiary bases. *Biochemical Journal* 79, 403–8.

Abraham, J (2002) The political economy of medicines regulation in Britain, in H Lawton-Smith (ed) *The Regulation of Science and Technology*. Palgrave.

Abraham, S, D Castle and R Gold (2014) How a gene-patent test cases will help both patients and inventors. *Global and Mail*, 4 November.

Acharya, R (1999) *The Emergence and Growth of Biotechnology: Experiences in Industrialised and Developing Countries*. Edward Elgar.

Achilladelis, B (1993) The dynamics of technological innovation: the sector of antibacterial medicines. *Research Policy* 22, 279–308.

Adams, M, C Berset, M Kessler and M Hamburger (2009) Medicinal herbs for the treatment of rheumatic disorders — A survey of European herbals from the 16th and 17th century. *Journal of Ethnopharmacology* 121, 343–59.

Aftalion, F (1991) *A History of the Chemical Industry*. University of Pennsylvania Press.

Aldhous, P (1996) Patent battle could hold up tests for cancer gene. *New Scientist* 149, 8.

Allison, M (2008) Is personalised medicine finally arriving? *Nature Biotechnology* 26(5), 509–17.

Al-Rodhan, NRF (2011) *The Politics of Emerging Strategic Technologies: Implications for Geopolitics, Human Enhancement and Human Destiny*. Palgrave Macmillan.

Altink, H (2015) From the local to the global: fifty years of historical research on tuberculosis. *Medical History* 59(1), 3–5.

American Pharmaceutical Association (1919) Report of the Committee on Patents and Trademarks of the American Pharmaceutical Association, August 1919. *Journal of the Patent Office Society* 2(1), 76–82.

Amin, T and AS Kesselheim (2012) Secondary patenting of branded pharmaceuticals: a case study of how patents on two HIV drugs could be extended for decades. *Health Affairs* 31(10), 2286–94.

Amster, EJ (2013) *Medicine and the Saints: Science, Islam, and the Colonial Encounter in Morocco, 1877–1956.* University of Texas Press.

Amyes, SGB (2001) *Magic Bullets, Lost Horizons: The Rise and Fall of Antibiotics.* London and New York: Taylor and Francis.

Anand, G (2001) HIV patent holder is slowing spread of fast AIDS test. *Wall Street Journal Europe* 20(1), 11.

Anderson, S (2007) Metternich, Bismarck, and the myth of the 'long peace', 1815–1914. *Peace and Change* 32(3), 301–28.

Angell, M (2004) *The Truth about the Drug Companies: How They Deceive Us and What to Do about It.* Random House.

Andrews, L and D Nelkin (2001) *Body Bazaar: The Market for Human Tissue in the Biotechnology Age.* New York: Crown Publishers.

Anon (1835) *The Housekeeper's Guide; Or, Every Man His Own Doctor; Containing many valuable Recipes and Prescriptions (approved of by the most eminent Physicians) for the cure of the human body' &c. To which is added a Description of different Kinds of Baths, Bathing, Electricity, &c. Also, a treatment of the cholera,* Fourth Edition. W.W. Robinson & Son.

Apple, R (1989) Patenting university research: Harry Steenbock and the Wisconsin Alumni Research Foundation. *Isis* 80(3), 375–94.

Arapostathis, S and G Gooday (2013) *Patently Contestable: Electrical Technologies and Inventor Identities on Trial in Britain.* MIT Press.

Arikha, N (2007) *Passions and Tempers: A History of the Humours.* HarperCollins.

Armstrong, HE (1935) Chemical industry and Carl Duisberg. *Nature* 135, 1021–5.

Ash, ASF and HO Schild (1966) Receptors mediating some actions of histamine. *Journal of Pharmacology and Chemotherapy* 27, 427–9.

Avery, OT, CM MacLeod and M McCarty (1944) Studies on the chemical nature of the substance inducing transformation of pneumococcal types. *Journal of Experimental Medicine* 79(2), 137–58.

Avise, JC (2010) *Inside the Human Genome: A Case for Non-Intelligent Design.* Oxford University Press.

Bakan, J (2004) *The Corporation: The Pathological Pursuit of Profit and Power.* Constable.

Ball, P (2011) *Unnatural: The Heretical Idea of Making People.* Bodley Head.

Ballance, R, J Pogány and H Forstner (1992) *The World's Pharmaceutical Industries: An International Perspective on Innovation, Competition and Policy.*

Prepared for the United Nations Industrial Development Organization. Edward Elgar.

Ballio, A, EB Chain, F Dentice de Accadia, GN Rolinson and FR Batchelor (1959) Penicillin derivatives of *p*-aminobenzylpenicillin. *Nature* 183, 180–1.

Baraniuk, C (2020) Silver uses a surprising trick to stop the spread of bacteria. *New Scientist*, 3 March.

Barton, JH (1991) Patenting life. *Scientific American* 264(3), 40–6.

Beall, RF and AS Kesselheim, Tertiary patenting on drug-device combination products in the United States', *Nature Biotechnology* 36(2), 142–5.

Beer, JJ (1958) Coal tar dye manufacture and the origins of the modern industrial research laboratory. *Isis* 49(2), 123–31.

Beier, F-K (1986) The inventive step in its historical development. *International Review of Industrial Property and Copyright Law* 17, 301.

Bensaude-Vincent, B and I Stengers (1996) *A History of Chemistry.* Harvard University Press.

Bent, SA, RL Schwaab, DG Conlin and DD Jeffery (1987) *Intellectual Property Rights in Biotechnology Worldwide.* Macmillan.

Bently, L (2014) The first trademark case at common law? The story of Singleton v. Bolton. *University of California, Davis* 47, 969–1014.

Bercovitz-Rodriguez, A (1990) Historical trends in protection of technology in developed countries and their relevance for developing countries. United Nations Conference on Trade and Development.

Bernard, C (1872) *Leçons de Pathologie Expérimentale et Lecons sur les Propriétés de la Moelle Épinière.* J.-B. Baillière et fils.

Betomeu-Sánchez, JR (2012) Animal experiments, vital forces and courtrooms: Mateu Orfila, François Magendie and the study of poisons in nineteenth-century France. *Annals of Science* 69(1), 1–26.

Bhatt, S, DJ Weiss, E Cameron, D Bisanzio, B Mappin, U Dalrymple, KE Battle, C L Moyes, A Henry, PA Eckhoff, EA Wenger, O Briët, MA Penny, TA Smith, A Bennett, J Yukich, TP Eisele, JT Griffin, CA Fergus, M Lynch, F Lindgren, JM Cohen, CLJ Murray, DL Smith, SI Hay, RE Cibulskis and PW Gething (2015) The effect of malaria control on Plasmodium falciparum in Africa between 2000 and 2015. *Nature* 526, 207–11.

Birch, A (1992) Steroid hormones and the Luftwaffe. A venture into fundamental strategic research and some of its consequences: the Birch reduction becomes a birth reduction. *Steroids* 57, 363–77.

Black, JW, WAM Duncan, CJ Durant, CR Ganellin and EM Parsons (1972) Definition and antagonism of histamine H_2-receptors. *Nature* 236, 385–90.

Bloch, H (1989) Francois Magendie, Claude Bernard, and the interrelation of science, history, and philosophy. *Southern Medical Journal* 86(10), 1259–61.

Boldrin, M and DK Levine (2004) The case against intellectual monopoly. *International Economic Review* 45, 327–50.

Bonnett, R, JR Cannon, AW Johnson, I Sutherland, AR Todd and EL Smith (1955) The structure of B12 and its hexacarboxylic acid degradation product. *Nature* 176, 328–30.

Borson, DB (1995) 'The Human Genome Project: patenting human genes and biotechnology. Is the human genome patentable?' *IDEA — The Journal of Law and Technology* 35(4), 461–96.

Borsook, D and L Becerra (2005) Placebo: from pain and analgesia to preferences and products. *Journal of Marketing Research* 42, 394–8

Bouchard, RA, D Cahoy, B Domeij, G Dutfield, T Faunce, A Hollis, P Jones, F Ali Khader, J Lexchin, H Nam and JL Serrano (2011) Structure-function analysis of global pharmaceutical linkage regulations. *Minnesota Journal of Law, Science and Technology* 12(2), 391–457.

Bountra, C, W Lee and J Lezaun (2017) A new pharmaceutical commons: transforming drug discovery. Oxford Martin Policy Paper. Oxford Martin School, University of Oxford. https://www.oxfordmartin.ox.ac.uk/downloads/academic/Transforming_Drug_Discovery.pdf, visited 30 Apr 2020.

Bozicevic, K (1987) Distinguishing 'products of nature' from products derived from nature. *Journal of the Patent and Trademark Office Society* 69(8), 415–26.

Braithwaite, J (1984) *Corporate Crime in the Pharmaceutical Industry*. Routledge and Kegan Paul.

Braithwaite, J and P Drahos (2000) *Global Business Regulation*. Cambridge University Press.

Bray, D (2009) *Wetware: A Computer in Every Living Cell*. Yale University Press.

Breedveld, FC (2000) Therapeutic monoclonal antibodies. *The Lancet* 355, 735–40.

Brennan, H (2015) The cost of confusion: the paradox of trademarked pharmaceuticals. *Michigan Telecommunications and Technology Law Review* 22, 1–52.

Brockway, LH (1979) *Science and Colonial Expansion: The Role of the British Royal Botanic Gardens*. Academic Press.

Brody, H (2007) *Hooked: Ethics, the Medical Profession, and the Pharmaceutical Industry*. Rowman & Littlefield.

Brooke, JH (1968) Wöhler's urea and the vital force — a verdict from the chemists. *Ambix* 15, 84–114.

Brooke, JH (1991) *Science and Religion: Some Historical Perspectives*. Cambridge University Press.

Brotton, J (2002) *The Renaissance Bazaar: From the Silk Road to Michelangelo*. Oxford University Press.

Brotzu, G (1948) Richerche su di un nuovo antibiotico. *Lavori dell'Istituto d'Igiene di Cagliari*, 4–18. http://www.pacs.unica.it/brotzu/brotzu.pdf. English translation: http://www.pacs.unica.it/brotzu/brotzuen.pdf.

Brown, K (2004) *Penicillin Man: Alexander Fleming and the Antibiotic Revolution*. Sutton.

Brown, P and K Kleiner (1994) Patent row splits breast cancer researchers. *New Scientist* 143, 4.

Brown, WA (2019) *Lithium: A Doctor, a Drug, and a Breakthrough*. Liveright.

Brumley, J (2017) The 15 all-time best-selling prescription drugs. Kiplinger – Kiplinger.com.

Bucchi, M (1997) The public science of Louis Pasteur: the experiment on anthrax vaccine in the popular press of the time. *History and Philosophy of the Life Sciences* 19(2), 181–209.

Buchdunger, E and J Zimmermann (undated) The story of Gleevec, http://www. innovation.org/index.cfm/StoriesofInnovation/InnovatorStories/The_ Story_of_Gleevec visited 2 June 2013.

Buckingham, J (2005) *Chasing the Molecule: Discovering the Building Blocks of Life*. Sutton.

Bud, R (1993) *The Uses of Life: A History of Biotechnology*. Cambridge University Press.

Bud, R (2007) *Penicillin: Triumph and Tragedy*. Oxford University Press.

Bugos, GE and DJ Kevles (1992) Plants as intellectual property: American practice, law, and policy in a world context. *Osiris* 7, 75–104.

Buick, AA (2019) *The Origins, Globalisation and Impact on Access to Medicine of intellectual Property Rights in Submitted Pharmaceutical Test Data*. PhD thesis, University of Leeds.

Burgen, A (1996) François Magendie and the new science of drugs. *European Review* 4, 165–72.

Bynum, W (1994) *Science and the Practice of Medicine in the Nineteenth Century*. Cambridge University Press.

Bynum, WF (2006) The rise of science in medicine, 1850–1913, in WF Bynum, A Hardy, S Jacyna, C Lawrence and EM Tansey (eds) *The Western Medical Tradition: 1800 to 2000*. Cambridge University Press.

Calvert, J (2004) Genomic patenting and the utility requirement. *New Genetics and Society* 23(3), 301–12.

Calvin, J and A Lapinsky (2019) Born to be manufactured. *The Small Molecule Manufacturer* 1, 16–17.

Carlson, RH (2011) *Life is Technology: The Promise, Peril, and New Business of Engineering Life*. Harvard University Press.

Case, A and A Deaton (2020) *Deaths of Despair and the Future of Capitalism*. Princeton University Press.

Cassier, M (2005) Appropriation and commercialization of the Pasteur anthrax vaccine. *Studies in History and Philosophy of Biological and Biomedical Sciences* 36(4), 722–42.

Cassier, M and C Sinding (2008) 'Patenting in the public interest': administration of insulin patents by University of Toronto. *History and Technology* 24, 153–71.

Caulfield, T (2016) *Is Gwyneth Paltrow Wrong About Everything? When Celebrity Culture and Science Clash*. Penguin Books.

Chachereau, N (2015) How to patent a chemical? The instability of a new type of intellectual property (Switzerland, 1888–1907). *Queen Mary Journal of Intellectual Property* 5(3), 285–301.

Chain, E, HW Florey, AD Gardner, NG Heatley, MA Jennings, J Orr-Ewing and AG Sanders (1940) Penicillin as a chemotherapeutic agent. *The Lancet* 236(6104), 226–8.

Chakrabarti, P (2012) *Bacteriology in British India: Laboratory Medicine and the Tropics*. University of Rochester Press.

Chandler Jr, AD (1990) *Scale and Scope: The Dynamics of Industrial Capitalism*. Belknap Press.

Chandler, AD (1992) Organizational capabilities and the economic history of the industrial enterprise. *Journal of Economic Perspectives* 6(3), 79–100.

Chandler Jr, AD (2005) *Shaping the Industrial Century: The Remarkable Story of the Evolution of the Modern Chemical and Pharmaceutical Industries*. Harvard University Press.

Channell, DF (1991) *The Vital Machine: A Study of Technology and Organic Life*. Oxford University Press.

Chapman-Huston, D and EC Cripps (1954) *Through the City Archway: The Story of Allen and Hanburys 1715–1954*. John Murray.

Chung, YG et al. (2014) Human somatic cell nuclear transfer using adult cells. *Cell Stem Cell* 14(6), 777–80.

Church, R and EM Tansey (2007) *Burroughs Wellcome & Co.: Knowledge, Trust, Profit and the Transformation of the British Pharmaceutical Industry 1880–1940*. Crucible Books.

CIPA (Chartered Institute of Patent Agents) (1998) Briefing paper — patenting in the pharmaceutical industry — Supplementary Protection Certificates.

Cipriani, A *et al.* (2018) Comparative efficacy and acceptability of 21 antidepressant drugs for the acute treatment of adults with major depressive disorder: a systematic review and network meta-analysis. *The Lancet* 391, 1357–66.

Clain, E *et al.* (2015) Availability and payer coverage of BRCA1/2 tests and gene panels. *Nature Biotechnology* 33(9), 900–2.

Cleary, EG, JM Beierlein, NS Khanuja, LM McNamee and FD Ledley (2018) Contribution of NIH funding to new drug approvals 2010–2016. *PNAS* 115(10), 2329–34.

Clift, C, U Gopinathan, Cl Morel, K Outterson, J-A Røttingen and A So, eds (2015) *Towards a New Global Business Model for Antibiotics: Delinking Revenues from Sales. Report from the Chatham House Working Group on New Antibiotic Business Models.* Royal Institute of International Affairs.

Cobb, M (2015) *Life's Greatest Secret: The Race to Crack the Genetic Code.* Profile Books.

Cochrane, AL (1972) *Effectiveness and Efficiency: Random Reflection on Health Services.* Nuffield Provincial Hospitals Trust.

Coghlan, A (1994) Applications for gene patents 'thrown on bonfire'. *New Scientist*, 19 February, 4–5.

Cohen, MH, ML Moses and R Pazdur (2002) Gleevec™ for the treatment of chronic myelogenous leukemia: U.S. Food and Drug Administration regulatory mechanisms, accelerated approval, and orphan drug status. *The Oncologist* 7(5), 390–2.

Collington, R (2020) Who benefits when the price of insulin soars? *Institute for New Economic Thinking.* https://www.ineteconomics.org/perspectives/blog/who-benefits-when-the-price-of-insulin-soars, visited 23 Apr 2020.

Colton, F (1992) Steroids and 'the pill': early steroid research at Searle. *Steroids* 57, 624–30.

Conant, J (2020) *The Great Secret: The Classified World War II Disaster that Launched the War on Cancer.* W.W. Norton.

Conley, JM, R Cook-Deegan and G Lázaro-Muñoz (2014) Myriad after *Myriad*: the proprietary data dilemma. *North Carolina Journal of Law and Technology* 15(4), 597–637.

Cook, HJ (2007) *Matters of Exchange: Commerce, Medicine, and Science in the Dutch Golden Age.* Yale University Press.

Cook-Deegan, R (1994) *The Gene Wars: Science, Politics, and the Human Genome.* W.W. Norton.

Cookson, C (2001) UK scientists responsible for third of genome project. *Financial Times*, 13, 2.

Cooper, JD (1969) Untitled article, in Cooper, JD (ed) *The Economics of Drug Innovation: The Proceedings of the First Seminar on Economics of Pharmaceutical Innovation.* American University, 41–54.

Cooper, MH (1966) *Prices and Profits in the Pharmaceutical Industry*. Pergamon Press.

Cordes, EH (2014) *Hallelujah Moments: Tales of Drug Discovery*. Oxford University Press.

Corley, TAB (2011) *Beecham's, 1848–2000: From Pills to Pharmaceuticals*. Crucible Books.

Cornforth, JW (1993) The trouble with synthesis. *Australian Journal of Chemistry* 46, 157–70.

Cornish, WR. (1999) *Intellectual Property: Patents, Copyright, Trade Marks and Allied Rights*, Fourth Edition. Sweet and Maxwell.

Correa, CM (2007) *Trade Related Aspects of Intellectual Property Rights: A Commentary on the TRIPS Agreement*. Oxford University Press.

Correa, CM, ed (2010) *Research Handbook on the Protection of Intellectual Property under WTO Rules: Intellectual Property in the WTO Volume I*. Edward Elgar.

CRA International (2008) The current state of innovation in the pharmaceutical industry.

Cragg, GM, PG Grothaus and DJ Newman (2014) New horizons for old drugs and drug leads. *Journal of Natural Products* 77(3) 703–23.

Cunningham, A (2002) The pen and the sword: recovering the disciplinary identity of physiology and anatomy before 1800 — I: Old physiology — the pen. *Studies in History and Philosophy of Biological and Biomedical Sciences* 33(4), 631–65.

Curtis, C *et al.* (2012) The genomic and transcriptomic architecture of 2,000 breast tumours reveals novel subgroups. *Nature* 486, 346–52.

Czaja, O (2013) On the history of refining mercury in Tibetan medicine. *Asian Medicine* 8(1), 75–105.

Dahl, A (2018) Algal boom. *The Medicine Maker* 40, 20–22.

Dahl, M (2015) The placebo effect is getting stronger — but only in the US. *New York*. 9 October.

Dahm, R (2005) Friedrich Miescher and the discovery of DNA. *Developmental Biology* 278(2), 274–88.

Dan, N, S Setus, VK Kashyap, S Khan, M Jaggi, MM Yallapu and SC Chauhan (2018) Antibody-drug conjugates for cancer therapy: chemistry to clinical implications. *Pharmaceuticals* 11(2), 32.

Darrow, JJ, J Avorn and AS Kesselheim (2020) FDA approval and regulation of pharmaceuticals, 1983–2018. *Journal of the American Medical Association* 323(2), 164–76.

Davenport, HW (1982) Epinephrin(e). *The Physiologist* 25(2), 76–82.

Davies, P (2003) *The Origin of Life*. Penguin Books.

Dawkins, R (2004) *The Ancestor's Tale: A Pilgrimage to the Dawn of Life*. Weidenfeld and Nicolson.

de Chadarevian, S (2002) *Designs for Life: Molecular Biology after World War II*. Cambridge University Press.

Deere, C (2008) *The Implementation Game: The TRIPS Agreement and the Global Politics of Intellectual Property Reform in Developing Countries*. Oxford University Press.

DeGrandpre, R (2006) *The Cult of Pharmacology: How America became the World's Most Troubled Drug Culture*. Duke University Press.

De Luca, V, V Salim, SM Atsumi and F Yu (2012) Mining the biodiversity of plants: a revolution in the making. *Science* 336, 1658–61.

Deshaies, RJ (2020) Multispecific drugs herald a new era of biopharmaceutical innovation. *Nature* 580, 329–38.

Deville, P (2013) *Plague and Cholera* (translated by JA Underwood). Little, Brown & Co.

Dewar, E (2004) *The Second Tree: Stem Cells, Clones, Chimeras, and Quests for Immortality*. Carroll and Graf.

Dickenson, D (2008) *Body Shopping: The Economy Fuelled by Flesh and Blood*. Oneworld.

Diependaele, L (2018) *The Codification of Intellectual Property Rights in International Law: An Ethical Analysis of Current Developments*. PhD thesis, University of Gent.

Diependaele, L, J Cockbain and S Sterckx (2018) Similar or the same? Why biosimilars are not the solution. *Journal of Law, Medicine and Ethics* 46(3), 776.

DiMasi, JA, HG Grabowski and RW Hansen (2016) Innovation in the pharmaceutical industry: new estimates of R&D costs. *Journal of Health Economics* 47, 20–33.

Djerassi, C (1984) A steroid autobiography. *Steroids* 43, 351–61.

Djerassi, C (2001) *This Man's Pill: Reflections on the 50th Birthday of the Pill*. Oxford University Press.

Djerassi, C, L Miramontes, G Rosenkranz and F Sondheimer (1954) Synthesis of 19-nor-17α-ethynyltestosterone and 19-nor-17α-methytestosterone. *Journal of the American Chemical Society* 76, 4092–4.

Dolma, S (2013) Understanding ideas of toxicity in Tibetan medical processing of mercury. *Asian Medicine* 8(1), 106–19.

Dorman, D (2019a) Don't let the maker of a buprenorphine drug abuse the Orphan Drug Act. *STAT* 28 May. https://www.statnews.com/2019/05/28/buprenorphine-drug-abusing-orphan-drug-act/, visited 14 Apr 2020.

Dorman, D (2019b) Orphan Drug Act's 'nonprofitability' loophole needs to be closed. *STAT* 19 December. https://www.statnews.com/2019/12/19/orphan-drug-act-nonprofitability-loophole-needs-closing/, visited 14 Apr 2020.

Dormandy, T (2006) *The Worst of Evils: The Fight Against Pain*. Yale University Press.

Drahos, P (2010) The Global Governance of Knowledge Patent Offices and their Clients. Cambridge University Press.

Drayton, R (2000) *Nature's Government: Science, Imperial Britain, and the 'Improvement' of the World*. Yale University Press.

Dresser, R and J Frader (2009) Off-label prescribing: a call for heightened professional and government oversight. *Journal of Law and Medical Ethics* 37(3), 476–96.

Drug and Market Development (1998) Monoclonal antibody therapy for leukemia and lymphoma. *Drug and Market Development* 9(100), 264.

Druker, B, S Tamura, E Buchdunger, S Ohno, GM Segal, S Fanning, J Zimmermann and NB Lydon (1996) Effects of a selective inhibitor of the Abl tyrosine kinase on the growth of Bcr-Abl positive cells. *Nature Medicine* 2(5), 561–6.

Dubos, RJ (1951) *Louis Pasteur: Free Lance of Science*. Victor Gollancz.

Duffin, J (1999) *History of Medicine: A Scandalously Short Introduction*. University of Toronto Press.

Dumit, J (2012) *Drugs for Life: How Pharmaceutical Companies Define Our Health*. Duke University Press.

Dupré, J (2001) *Human Nature and the Limits of Science*. Oxford University Press.

Dutfield, G (2004) *Intellectual Property, Biogenetic Resources and Traditional Knowledge*. Earthscan.

________ (2012) 'The genetic code is 3.6 billion years old: It's time for a rewrite': Questioning the metaphors and analogies of synthetic biology and life science patenting, in A Lever (ed) *New Frontiers in the Philosophy of Intellectual Property*. Cambridge University Press.

________ (2013) Collective invention and patent law individualism, 1877–2012; or, the curious persistence of inventor's moral right, in S Arapostathis and G Dutfield (eds) *Knowledge Management and Intellectual Property: Concepts, Actors and Practices*. Edward Elgar.

________ (2017) Healthcare innovation and patent law's 'pharmaceutical privilege': Is there a pharmaceutical privilege? And if so, should we remove it? *Health Economics, Policy and Law* 12(4), 453–70.

________ and U Suthersanen (2019) Traditional knowledge and genetic resources: observing legal protection through the lens of historical geography and human rights. *Washburn Law Journal* 58(2), 399–447.

_______ and U Suthersanen (2020) *Dutfield and Suthersanen on Global Intellectual Property Law*. Edward Elgar.

Dutton, HI (1984) *The Patent System and Inventive Activity during the Industrial Revolution, 1750–1852*. Manchester University Press.

Earp, BD and J Savulescu (2020) *Love is the Drug: The Chemical Future of Our Relationships*. Manchester University Press.

Eckhoff, PA, EA Wenger, O Briët, MA Penny, TA Smith, A Bennett, J Yukich, TP Eisele, JT Griffin, CA Fergus, M Lynch, F Lindgren, JM Cohen, CLJ Murray, DL Smith, SI Hay, RE Cibulskis and PW Gething (2015) The effect of malaria control on Plasmodium falciparum in Africa between 2000 and 2015. *Nature* 526, 207–11.

Edwards, AM, R Isserlin, GD Bader, SV. Frye, TM Willson and FH Yu (2011) Too many roads not taken. *Nature* 470, 163–5.

Ehrenreich, B (2018) *Natural Causes: An Epidemic of Wellness, the Certainty of Dying, and Killing Ourselves to Live Longer*. Twelve.

Elenco, E, L Underwood and D Zohar (2015) Defining digital medicine. *Nature Biotechnology* 33(5), 460–1.

Emalfarb, M (2018) The CHO's over: an inflexion point. *The Medicine Maker* 45, 2.

Ernhofer, K (2003) Who really owns your genes? *Christian Science Monitor*, 27 February.

European Commission (DG Competition) (2009) *Pharmaceutical Sector Inquiry — Final Report*.

European Commission (2019) *Report from the Commission to the Council and the European Parliament. Competition Enforcement in the Pharmaceutical Sector (2009–2017): European Competition Authorities Working Together for Affordable and Innovative Medicines*.

Everett, N and M Gabra (2014) The pharmacology of medieval sedatives: the 'Great Rest' of the Antidotarium Nicolai. *Journal of Ethnopharmacology* 155(1), 443–9.

Exner, DV, DL Dries, MJ Domanski and JN Cohn (2001) Lesser response to angiotensin-converting-enzyme inhibitor therapy in black as compared with white patients with left ventricular dysfunction. *New England Journal of Medicine* 344(18), 1351–7.

Experts in Chronic Myeloid Leukemia (2013) The price of drugs for chronic myeloid leukemia (CML) is a reflection of the unsustainable prices of cancer drugs: from the perspective of a large group of CML experts. *Blood* 121(22), 4439–42.

Ewen, M, H-J Joosse, D Beran and R Laing (2019) Insulin prices, availability and affordability in 13 low-income and middle-income countries. *BMJ Global Health* 4(3), 1–10.

Faase, K, T Cundy, G Gamble and KJ Petrie (2013) The effect of an apparent change to a branded or generic medication on drug effectiveness and side effects. *Psychosomatic Medicine* 75(1), 90–6.

Farrar, WV (1974) Synthetic dyes before 1860. *Endeavour* 33, 149–55.

________ and AR Williams (1977) A history of mercury, in CA McAuliffe (ed) *The Chemistry of Mercury*. Macmillan.

Feldman, R (2018) May your drug price be evergreen. *Journal of Law and the Biosciences* 5(3), 590–647.

Feldman, S (2009) *From Poison Arrows to Prozac: How Deadly Toxins Changed our Lives Forever*. Metro Publishing.

Ferreira, SH, S Moncada and JR Vane (1971) Indomethacin and aspirin abolish prostaglandin release from the spleen. *Nature New Biology* 231, 237–9.

Findlay, JK *et al.* (2007) Human embryo: a biological definition. *Human Reproduction* 22(4), 905–11.

Fishbein, M (1937) Medical patents. *Journal of the American Medical Association* 109(19), 1539–43.

Fishburn, CS (2013) Translational research: the changing landscape of drug discovery. *Drug Discovery Today* 18(9/10), 487–94.

Fisk, C (2009) *Working Knowledge: Employee Invention and the Rise of Corporate Intellectual Property, 1800–1930*. University of North Carolina Press.

Fleming, A (1929) On the antibacterial action of cultures of a penicillium, with special reference to their use in the isolation of B. Influenzae. *British Journal of Experimental Pathology* X(3), 226–36.

Fojo T, S Mailankody and A Lo (2014) Unintended consequences of expensive cancer therapeutics — The pursuit of marginal indications and a me-too mentality that stifles innovation and creativity: the John Conley Lecture. *JAMA Otolaryngology — Head and Neck Surgery* 140(12), 1225–36.

Fore Jr, J, IR Wiechers and R Cook-Deegan (2006) The effects of business practices, licensing, and intellectual property on development and dissemination of the polymerase chain reaction: case study. *Journal of Biomedical Discovery and Collaboration* 1, 7.

Formigari, L (1973–74) Chain of being, in PP Wiener (ed) *The Dictionary of the History of Ideas: Studies of Selected Pivotal Ideas*, Vol. I. New York: Charles Scribner's Sons, 326–36.

Fowler, C (1994) *Unnatural Selection: Technology, Politics, and Plant Evolution*. Gordon and Breach.

Fox, JL (1983) Columbia awarded biotechnology patent. *Science* 221, 933.

Fransman, M and S Tanaka (1999) Visions of future technologies: government, globalisation, and universities in Japanese biotechnology, in M Fransman (ed) *Visions of Innovation: The Firm and Japan*. Oxford University Press.

Frausin, G, A de Freitas Hidalgo, RB Souza Lima, V Ferreira Kinupp, LC Ming, AM Pohlit and W Milliken (2015) An ethnobotanical study of anti-malarial plants among indigenous people on the upper Negro River in the Brazilian Amazon. *Journal of Ethnopharmacology* 215, 238–52.

Frederickson, DS (2001) *The Recombinant DNA Controversy: A Memoir — Science, Politics, and the Public Interest 1974–1981*. ASM Press.

Freeman, C and L Soete (1997) *The Economics of Industrial Innovation*. Pinter.

Freudenheim, M (1994) New drug era begins as Tagamet patent expires. *New York Times*, 17 May.

Frost, GE (1963) The case against drug patent compulsory licensing. *The Patent, Trademark and Copyright Journal of Research and Education* 7(1), 84–102.

Furner-Pardoe, J, BO Anonye, R Cain, J Moat, CA Ortori, C Lee, DA Barrett, C Corre and F Harrison (2020) Anti-biofilm efficacy of a medieval treatment for bacterial infection requires the combination of multiple ingredients. *Scientific Reports* 10, 12687.

Gabriel, JM (2014) *Medical Monopoly: Intellectual Property Rights and the Origins of the Modern Pharmaceutical Industry*. Chicago University Press.

Galambos, L with JE Sewell (1995) *Networks of Innovation: Vaccine Development at Merck, Sharp & Dohme, and Mulford, 1895–1995*. Cambridge University Press.

Gänger, S (2015) World trade in medicinal plants from Spanish America, 1717–1815. *Medical History* 59(1), 44–62.

Garfield, S (2001) *Mauve: How One Man Invented a Colour that Changed the World*. Faber.

Gaudillière, J-P (2008) Professional or industrial order? Patents, biological drugs, and pharmaceutical capitalism in early twentieth century Germany. *History and Technology* 24(2), 107–33.

_________ (2014) Herbalised Ayurveda? Reformulation, plant management and the 'pharmaceuticalisation' of Indian 'traditional' medicine. *Asian Medicine* 9, 171–205.

Gaukroger, S (1998) Introduction, in R Descartes (ed) *The World and Other Writings* (edited by Stephen Gaukroger). Cambridge University Press.

Gerke, B (2015) The poison of touch: tracing mercurial treatments of venereal diseases in Tibet. *Social History of Medicine* 28(3), 532–54.

Ghaemi, NS (2013) Postmodern medicine: an analysis of the pharmaceutical industry and its critics. *Perspectives in Biology and Medicine* 56(2), 223–35.

Ghosh, S (2012) *Identity, Invention, and the Culture of Personalized Medicine Patenting.* Cambridge University Press.

Ghosh, S (2020) Myriad post-Myriad. *Science and Public Policy* (pre-print).

Giachi, G, P Pallecchi, A Romualdi, E Ribechini, JJ Lucejko, MP Colombini and MM Lippi (2013) Ingredients of a 2,000-y-old medicine revealed by chemical, mineralogical, and botanical investigations. *PNAS* 110(4), 1193–6.

Gibson, DG *et al.* (inc. HO Smith and JC Venter) (2010) Creation of a bacterial cell controlled by a chemically synthesized genome. *Science* 329, 52–6.

Gispen, K (1989) *New Profession, Old Order: Engineers and German Society, 1815–1914.* Cambridge University Press.

Glyn, J (1998) The discovery and early use of cortisone. *Journal of the Royal Society of Medicine* 91, 513–7.

Gold, ER and J Carbone (2008) *Myriad: In the Eye of the Policy Storm.* The Innovation Partnership and McGill University Centre for Intellectual Property Policy.

Goldacre, B (2008) *Bad Science.* Fourth Estate.

Goldberg, A (2010) Drug firms accused of exploiting loophole for profit. *BBC News,* 20 November. https://www.bbc.co.uk/news/health-11798183, visited 21 Apr 2020.

Golden, JM (2010) WARF's stem cell patents and tensions between public and private sector approaches to research. *Journal of Law, Medicine and Ethics* 38(2), 314–31.

Goldstein, DB and GL Cavalleri (2005) Understanding human diversity. *Nature* 437, 1241–2.

Goodfield, GJ (1960) *The Growth of Scientific Physiology: Physiological Method and the Mechanist-Vitalist Controversy Illustrated by the Problems of Respiration and Animal Heat.* Hutchinson.

Goodman, LS, MM Wintrobe, W Dameshek, MJ Goodman, A Gilman and MT McLennan (1946) Nitrogen mustard therapy; use of methyl-bis (beta-chloroethyl) amine hydrochloride and tris (beta-chloroethyl) amine hydrochloride for Hodgkin's disease, lymphosarcoma, leukemia and certain allied and miscellaneous disorders. *Journal of the American Medical Association* 132, 126–32.

Goozner, M (2004) *The $800 Million Pill: The Truth behind the Cost of New Drugs.* University of California Press.

Gradmann, C (2009) *Laboratory Disease: Robert Koch's Medical Bacteriology.* Johns Hopkins University Press.

Gradmann, C (2010) Robert Koch and the invention of the carrier state: tropical medicine, veterinary infections and epidemiology around 1900. *Studies in History and Philosophy of Biological and Biomedical Sciences* 41(3), 232–40.

Graham, SS (2011) Dis-ease or disease? ontological rarefaction in the medical-industrial complex. *Journal of Medical Humanities* 32, 167–86.

Gray, J and B Druker (2012) The breast cancer landscape. *Nature* 486, 329–9.

Green, AG (1915 [1901]) The relative progress of the coal-tar colour industry in England and Germany during the past fifteen years, in WM Gardner (ed) *The British Coal-Tar Industry: Its Origin, Development and Decline*. Williams and Norgate.

Greene, JA (2014) *Generic: The Unbranding of Modern Medicine*. Johns Hopkins University Press.

Greene, JA (2019) After a scandal, a one-sided warning against generic drugs. *Washington Post*, 13 September. https://www.washingtonpost.com/outlook/after-a-scandal-a-one-sided-warning-against-generic-drugs/2019/09/12/6a755e48-c50a-11e9-b5e4-54aa56d5b7ce_story.html.

Griffiths, PE and K Stotz (2007) Gene, in DL Hull and M Ruse (eds) *The Cambridge Companion to the Philosophy of Biology*. Cambridge University Press.

Gross, CG (1998) Claude Bernard and the constancy of the internal environment. *The Neuroscientist* 4(5), 380–5.

Grosse, SD, I Odame, HK Atrash, DD Amendah, FB Piel and TN Williams (2011) Sickle cell disease in Africa: a neglected cause of early childhood mortality. *American Journal of Preventive Medicine* 41(6 Suppl 4), S398–S405.

Grubb, PW (1999) *Patents for Chemicals, Pharmaceuticals and Biotechnology*. Clarendon Press.

Gupta, H, S Kumar, SK Roy and RS Gaud (2010) Patent protection strategies. *Journal of Pharmacy and Bioallied Sciences* 2(1), 2–7.

Gurgula, O (2017) Strategic accumulation of patents in the pharmaceutical industry and patent thickets in complex technologies — two different concepts sharing similar features. *IIC — International Review of Intellectual Property and Competition Law* 48(4).

Guyton de Morveau, Lavoisier, Berthollet and de Fourcroy (1787) *Méthode de Nomenclature Chimique*. Cuchet.

Haber, LF (1958) *The Chemical Industry during the Nineteenth Century: A Study of the Economic Aspect of Applied Chemistry in Europe and North America*. Clarendon Press.

Halabi, SF (2018) *Intellectual Property and the New International Economic Order: Oligopoly, Regulation, and Wealth Redistribution in the Global Knowledge Economy*. Cambridge University Press.

Hale, CW, GGF Newton and EP Abraham (1961) Derivatives of cephalosporin C formed with certain heterocyclic tertiary bases. *Biochemical Journal* 79, 403–8.

Hall, JM *et al.* (1990) Linkage of early-onset familial breast cancer to chromosome 17q21. *Science* 250, 1684–9.

Hall, SS (1987) *Invisible Frontiers: The Race to Synthesize a Human Gene.* Atlantic Monthly Press.

Hamzelou, J (2019) Bad medicine? *New Scientist* 244(3258), 34–9.

Hamzelou, J (2020) Benzodiazepine prescriptions reach 'disturbing' levels in the US. *New Scientist* 3266.

Hancher, L (1990) *Regulating for Competition: Government, Law, and the Pharmaceutical Industry in the United Kingdom and France.* Clarendon Press.

Hanson, M and G Pomata (2017) Medicinal formulas and experiential knowledge in the seventeenth-century epistemic exchange between China and Europe. *Isis* 108(1), 1–25.

Hare, R (1970) *The Birth of Penicillin.* Allen and Unwin.

Harkness, JM (2011) Dicta on Adrenalin(e): Myriad problems with Learned Hand's product-of-nature pronouncements in Parke-Davis v. Mulford. *Journal of the Patent and Trademark Office Society* 93(4), 363–99.

Harris, H (2002) *Things Come to Life: Spontaneous Generation Revisited.* Oxford University Press.

Harris, R and J Paxman (2002) *A Higher Form of Killing: The Secret History of Chemical and Biological Warfare.* Arrow Books.

Harrison, B (1997) *Lean and Mean: The Changing Landscape of Corporate Power in the Age of Flexibility.* Guilford Press.

Harrison, IH (1986) *The Law on Medicines: A Comprehensive Guide*, Vol. 1. Springer, 6.

Harvey, AL, RA Edrada-Ebel and RJ Quinn (2015) The re-emergence of natural products for drug discovery in the genomics era. *Nature Reviews Drug Discovery* 14, 111–29.

Haynes, B (1999) Can it work? Does it work? Is it worth it? *British Medical Journal* 319, 652–3.

Haynes, W (1945) *American Chemical Industry. Volume 2, The World War Period: 1912–22.* Van Nostrand.

Hayward, PA (1987) *Hayward's Patent Cases 1600–1883. A Compilation of the English Patent Cases for those Years*, Vol. 1. Professional Books Ltd.

Healy, D (2004) *Let Them Eat Prozac: The Unhealthy Relationship between the Pharmaceutical Industry and Depression.* New York University Press.

Healy, D (2012) *Pharmageddon.* University of California Press.

Heinrich, M and I Casselman (2018) Ethnopharmacology — from Mexican hallucinogens to a global transdisciplinary science, in D McKenna, G Prance, B De Loenen and W Davis (eds) *Ethnopharmacologic Search for Psychoactive Drugs: 50 Years of Research (1967–2017)*. Synergetic Press (in association with Heffter Research Institute).

Henley, J (2001) Cancer unit fights US gene patent. *The Guardian*, 8 September.

Herder, M, JE Graham and R Gold (2020) From discovery to delivery: public sector development of the rVSV-ZEBOV Ebola vaccine. *Journal of Law and the Biosciences*.

Hernandez, I, A San-Juan-Rodriguez, CB Good and WF Gellad (2020) Changes in List Prices, Net Prices, and Discounts for Branded Drugs in the US, 2007–2018. *Journal of the American Medical Association* 323(9), 854–62.

Herzog, H and EP Oliveto (1992) A history of significant steroid discoveries and developments originating at the Schering Corporation (USA) since 1948. *Steroids* 57, 617–23.

Heusler, K and J Kalvoda (1992) Between basic and applied research: Ciba's involvement in the steroids in the 1950s and 1960s. *Steroids* 61, 492–503.

Himmelstein, DU, RM Lawless, D Thorne, P Foohey and S Woolhandler (2019) Medical bankruptcy: still common despite the Affordable Care Act. *American Journal of Public Health* 109(3), 431–3.

Hirschmann, R (1992) The cortisone era: aspects of its impact. Some contributions of the Merck Laboratories. *Steroids* 57, 579–92.

Hodgkin, DC and EN Maslen (1961) The X-ray analysis of the structure of cephalosporin C. *Biochemical Journal* 79, 393–402.

Hodgkin, DC, J Pickworth, JH Robertson, KN Trueblood, RJ Prosen and JG White (1955) The crystal structure of the hexacarboxylic acid derived from B12 and the molecular structure of the vitamin. *Nature* 176, 325–8.

Hofer, T (2018) *Medicine and Memory in Tibet. Amchi Physicians in an Age of Reform*. University of Washington Press.

Hoffman, W and L Furcht (2014) *The Biologist's Imagination: Innovation in the Biosciences*. Oxford University Press.

Hogg, JA (1992) Steroids, the steroid community, and Upjohn in perspective: a profile of innovation. *Steroids* 57, 593–616.

Holden, AL (2002) The SNP Consortium: summary of a private consortium effort to develop an applied map of the human genome. *Biotechniques* 32, S22-S26 (June).

Hollis, A and T Pogge (2008) *The Health Impact Fund: Making New Medicines Accessible for All*. Incentives for Global Health.

Homburg, E (1992) The emergence of research laboratories in the dyestuffs industry, 1870–1900. *British Journal for the History of Science* 25, 91–111.

Hope, J (2008) *Biobazaar: The Open Source Revolution and Biotechnology.* Harvard University Press.

Hornix, WJ (1992) From process to plant: innovation in the early artificial dye industry. *British Journal for the History of Science* 25, 65–90.

Horstmeyer, M (1998) The industry evolves within a political, social, and public policy context: a brief look at Britain, Germany, Japan, and the United States, in A Arora, R Landau and N Rosenberg (eds) *Chemicals and Long-term Economic Growth: Insights from the Chemical Industry.* John Wiley.

House of Commons Select Committee on Patent Medicines (1914) *Report from the Select Committee on Patent Medicines. Ordered, by The House of Commons.* His Majesty's Stationery Office.

Howells, J and I Neary (1995) *Intervention and Technological Innovation: Government and the Pharmaceutical Industry in the UK and Japan.* Macmillan.

Howlett, MJ and AF Christie (2004) 'An analysis of the approach of the European, Japanese and United States Patent Offices to patenting partial DNA sequences (ESTs). University of Melbourne Faculty of Law Legal Studies Research Paper No. 82.

Hsu, E, ed (2001) *Innovation in Chinese Medicine.* Cambridge University Press.

Hubbard, T and J Love (2004) A new trade framework for global healthcare R&D. *PLoS Biology* 2(2), e52.

Hüntelmann, A (2013) Making Salvarsan: experimental therapy and the development and marketing of Salvarsan at the crossroads of science, clinical medicine, industry, and public health, in J-P Gaudillière and V Hess (eds) *Ways of Regulating Drugs in the 19th and 20th Centuries.* Palgrave Macmillan.

Hunter, GK (2000) *Vital Forces: The Discovery of the Molecular Basis of Life.* Academic Press.

Hyun, I, A Wilkerson and J Johnston (2016) Embryology policy: revisit the 14-day rule. *Nature* 533, 169–71.

I-MAK (Initiative for Medicines, Access and Knowledge) (2018a) Solving the drug patent problem. Submission to the Federal Trade Commission Hearings on Competition and Consumer Protection. https://www.i-mak.org/wp-content/uploads/2018/08/I-MAK-Submission-to-FTC-on-The-Role-of-Intellectual-Property-and-Competition-Policy-in-Promoting-Innovation.pdf.

———— (2018b) Overpatented, Overpriced: How Excessive Pharmaceutical Patenting is Extending Monopolies and Driving up Drug Prices. http://www.i-mak.org/wp-content/uploads/2018/08/I-MAK-Overpatented-Overpriced-Report.pdf.

International Human Genome Sequencing Consortium (2001) Initial sequencing and analysis of the human genome. *Nature* 409, 860–921.

Jack, A (2020) Poor countries struggle to get the insulin they need. *Financial Times*, 10 March.

Jackson, CM (2012) Synthetical experiments and alkaloid analogues: Liebig, Hofmann, and the origins of organic synthesis. *Historical Studies in the Natural Sciences* 44(4), 319–63.

Jackson, E (2013) *Medical Law: Text, Cases, and Materials*, Third Edition. Oxford University Press.

Jackson, MW (2015) *The Genealogy of a Gene: Patents, HIV/AIDS, and Race*. MIT Press.

Jeffreys, D (2004) *Aspirin: The Story of a Wonder Drug*. Bloomsbury.

Jiang, L (2016) *Regulating Human Embryonic Stem Cell in China: A Comparative Study on Human Embryonic Stem Cell's Patentability and Morality in U.S. and E.U.* Springer.

Johnson, JA (1992) Hofmann's role in reshaping the academic-industrial alliance in German chemistry, in C Meinel and H Scholz (eds) *Die Allianz von Wissenschaft und Industrie August Wilhelm Hofmann (1818–1892)*. VCH.

Jones, E (2001) *The Business of Medicine: The Extraordinary History of Glaxo, a Baby Food Producer, Which Became One of the World's Most Successful Pharmaceutical Companies*. Profile Books.

Journal of the American Medical Association (editorial) (1937) Deaths following Elixir of Sulfanilamide-Massengill. *Journal of the American Medical Association* 109(19), 1544–5.

Joyner, MJ and N Paneth (2015) Seven questions for personalized medicine. *Journal of the American Medical Association* 314(10), 999–1000.

Judson, HF (1996) *The Eighth Day of Creation: Makers of the Revolution in Biology* (expanded edition). Cold Spring Harbor Laboratory Press.

Kahn, J (2012) *Race in a Bottle: The Story of BiDil and Racialized Medicine in a Post-Genomic Age*. Columbia University Press.

Kalia, M (2013) Personalized oncology: recent advances and future challenges. *Metabolism*, 62, S11–4.

Kapczynski, A, C Park and B Sampat (2012) Polymorphs and prodrugs and salts (oh my!): an empirical analysis of 'secondary' pharmaceutical patents. *PLoS One*, 7(12), e49470.

Kaptchuk, TJ, E Friedlander, JM Kelley, MN Sanchez, E Kokkotou, JP Singer, M Kowalczykowski, FG Miller, I Kirsch and AJ Lembo (2010) Placebos without deception: a randomized controlled trial in irritable bowel syndrome. *PLoS One* 5(12), e15591.

Kaufer, E (1980) *The Economics of the Patent System*. Harwood Academic Publishers.

Kay, LE (1993) *The Molecular Vision of Life: Caltech, the Rockefeller Foundation, and the Rise of the New Biology*. Oxford University Press.

Kay, LE (2000) *Who Wrote the Book of Life? A History of the Genetic Code*. Stanford University Press.

Kean, S (2019) Science's debt to the slave trade. *Science* 364, 16–20.

Keating, P and A Cambrosio (2012) *Cancer on Trial: Oncology as a New Style of Practice*. University of Chicago Press.

Kefauver, E (with the assistance of I Till) (1966) *In a Few Hands: Monopoly Power in America*. Penguin Books.

Kell, D (1992) The furore over the patenting of animals: Animal Legal Defense Fund v. Quigg. *European Intellectual Property Review* 14(8), 279–83.

Kennedy, M (2016) *WTO Dispute Settlement and the TRIPS Agreement: Applying Intellectual Property Standards in a Trade Law Framework*. Cambridge University Press.

Kevles, DJ (1993) The enemies without and within: Cancer and the history of the laboratory sciences. California Institute of Technology. Humanities Working Paper 154. https://www.authors.library.caltech.edu/39689/1/HumsWP-0154.pdf.

Kevles, DJ (1994) Ananda Chakrabarty wins a patent: biotechnology, law, and society, 1972–1980. *Historical Studies in the Physical and Biological Sciences* 25(1), 111–35.

_________ (2001) Patenting life: a historical overview of law, interests, and ethics. Prepared for the Legal Theory Workshop, Yale Law School, 20 December.

Khan, BZ (2005) *The Democratization of Invention: Patent and Copyright in American Economic Development, 1790–1920*. Cambridge University Press.

King, LS (1970) *The Road to Medical Enlightenment 1650–1695*. Macdonald and Elsevier.

King, SR and P Chaturvedi (2012) The development of Crofelemer: Connecting ethnobotany, conservation, biocultural diversity, global public health and indigenous knowledge. *Planta Medica* 78(11).

Kingston, W (2004a) Removing some harm from the World Trade Organization. *Oxford Development Studies* 32(2), 309–20.

Kingston, W (2004b) Streptomycin, *Schatz v. Waksman*, and the balance of credit for discovery. *Journal of the History of Medicine and Allied Sciences* 59(3), 441–62.

Kintisch, E (2005) Court tightens patent rules on gene tags. *Science* 309, 1797.

Kirsch, I (2014) Antidepressants and the placebo effect. *Zeitschrift für Psychologie* 222(3), 128–34.

Klauer, G (1936) The new German patent law. *Journal of the Patent Office Society* 18(8), 481–500.

Kleiner, K (2002) Bad for your health: are gene patents stopping patients getting the latest tests? *New Scientist* 173(2335), 6.

Knight, D (2014) *Voyaging in Strange Seas: The Great Revolution in Science.* Yale University Press.

Kobrak, C (2002) *National Cultures and International Competition: The Experience of Schering AG, 1851–1950.* Cambridge University Press.

Köhler, G and C Milstein (1975) Continuous cultures of fused cells secreting antibody of predefined specificity. *Nature* 256, 495–7.

Kornberg, A (1995) *The Golden Helix: Inside Biotech Ventures.* University Science Books.

Kranakis, E (2020) A tale of two inventions: Monstanto, biotechnology, and the geography of postmodern science. *Isis* 110(4), 701–25.

Kresge, N, RD Simoni and RL Hill (2005) Hemorrhagic sweet clover disease, dicumarol, and warfarin: the work of Karl Paul Link. *Journal of Biological Chemistry* 280(8), e5–6.

Krimsky, S (2003) *Science in the Private Interest: Has the Lure of Profits Corrupted Biomedical Research?* Rowman & Littlefield.

Kronstein, H and I Till (1947) A reevaluation of the international patent convention. *Law and Contemporary Problems* 12, 765–81.

Ladas, S (1930) *The International Protection of Industrial Property,* Vol. 1. Harvard University Press.

Lai, JC (2017) The changing function of patents: a reversion to privileges? *Legal Studies* 37(4), 807–37.

Langreth, R (2020) All eyes on Gilead. *Bloomberg Businessweek* 14 May, https://www.bloomberg.com/features/2020-gilead-remdesivir-coronavirus-treatment/, visited 16/7/2020.

Last, J (2002) The missing link: the story of Karl Paul Link. *Toxicological Sciences* 66, 4–6.

Latour, B (2000) On the partial existence of existing and nonexisting objects, in L Daston (ed) *Biographies of Scientific Objects.* Chicago University Press.

Laveaga, GS (2005) Uncommon trajectories: steroid hormones, Mexican peasants, and the search for a wild yam. *Studies in History and Philosophy of Biological and Biomedical Sciences* 36, 743–60.

Law, J (2006) *Big Pharma: How the World's Biggest Drug Companies Control Illness.* Constable.

Lawler, A (2012) Mashco Piro tribe emerges from isolation in Peru. *Science* 349, 679.

Lawrence, S and P Treacy (2005) The Commission's AstraZeneca decision: delaying generic entry is an abuse of a dominant position. *Journal of Intellectual Property Law and Practice* 1(1), 7–9.

Lax, E (2004) *The Mould in Dr Florey's Coat: The Remarkable True Story of the Penicillin Miracle*. Little, Brown.

Lazell, HG (1975) *From Pills to Penicillin: The Beecham Story*. Heinemann.

Lear, J (1978) *Recombinant DNA: The Untold Story*. Crown Publishers.

Le Couteur, P and J Burreson (2004) *Napoleon's Buttons: 17 Molecules that Changed History*. Tarcher/Penguin.

Lee, K (2012) *The Philosophical Foundations of Modern Medicine*. Palgrave Macmillan.

Lee, LC and M Noronha (2016) When plenty is too much: water intoxication in a patient with a simple urinary tract infection. *BMJ Case Reports*, doi:10.1136/bcr-2016-216882.

Le Fanu, J (1999) *The Rise and Fall of Modern Medicine*. Little, Brown and Co.

Lei, SH-L (2014) *Neither Donkey nor Horse: Medicine in the Struggle over China's Modernity*. University of Chicago Press.

Lentacker, A (2016) The symbolic economy of drugs. *Social Studies of Science* 46(1), 140–56.

Lesch, JE (1981) Conceptual change in an empirical science: the discovery of the first alkaloids. *Historical Studies in the Physical Sciences* 11(2), 305–28.

———— (1984) *Science and Medicine in France: The Emergence of Experimental Physiology, 1790–1855*. Harvard University Press.

———— (2007) *The First Miracle Drugs: How the Sulfa Drugs Transformed Medicine*. Oxford University Press.

Levy, S (2013) Our shared code: the Myriad decision and the future of genetic research. *Environmental Health Perspectives* 121(8), a250–3.

Liao, F (2009) Discovery of Artemisinin (Qinghaosu). *Molecules* 14, 5362–6.

Liddicoat, J, K Liddell and M Aboy (2019) The effects of Myriad and Mayo on molecular test development in the US and Europe: interviews from the frontline. *Vanderbilt Journal of Entertainment and Technology Law* 22(4), 785–837.

Liebenau, J (1984) Industrial R&D in pharmaceutical firms in the early twentieth century. *Business History* 26(3), 329–46.

Lietzan, E (2020) The 'evergreening' metaphor in intellectual property scholarship. *Akron Law Review*.

Link, KP (1959) The discovery of Dicumarol and its sequels. *Circulation* 19, 97–107.

Lloyd, M (2002) Philip Showalter Hench, 1896–1965. *Rheumatology* 41, 582–4.

Loder, B, GGF Newton and EP Abraham (1961) The cephalosporin C nucleus (7-aminocephalosporanic acid) and some of its derivatives. *Biochemical Journal* 79, 408–16.

Long, PO (2001) *Openness, Secrecy, Authorship: Technical Arts and the Culture of Knowledge from Antiquity to the Renaissance.* Johns Hopkins University Press.

Love, J (2016) *An Economic Perspective on Delinking the Cost of R&D from the Price of Medicines.* UNITAID.

Lovejoy, AO (1936) *The Great Chain of Being: A Study of the History of an Idea.* Harvard University Press.

Lucretius (1st century BCE) *De Rerum Natura (Of the Nature of Things)* (translated by W.E. Leonard).

Ma, X and Z Wang (2009) Anticancer drug discovery in the future: an evolutionary perspective. *Drug Discovery Today* 14(23/4), 1136–42.

Macdonald, S (2001) Exploring the hidden costs of patents. QUNO Occasional Paper 4. Quaker United Nations Office.

Macfarlane, G (1979) *Howard Florey: The Making of a Great Scientist.* Oxford University Press.

———— (1984) *Alexander Fleming: The Man and the Myth.* Harvard University Press.

Macgregor, H (1955) Eighteenth-century V.D. publicity. *British Journal of Venereal Diseases* 31, 117–8.

Macilwaine, SW (1900) What is a disease? *British Medical Journal* 2(2085), 1703–4.

Mackintosh, A (2016) Authority and ownership: the growth and wilting of medicine patenting in Georgian England. *British Journal for the History of Science* 49(4), 541–59.

Maclagan, T (1876) The treatment of acute rheumatism by salicin. *The Lancet* 108(2774), 601–4.

MacLeod, C (1991) The paradoxes of patenting: invention and its diffusion in 18th and 19th century Britain, France, and North America. *Technology and Culture* 32(4), 885–911.

Maestrejuan, AR (2012) Managing invention: Setting the boundaries of ownership, in A Arapostathis and G Dutfield (eds) *Knowledge Management and Intellectual Property: Concepts, Actors and Practices from the Past to the Present.* Edward Elgar.

Magendie, F (1821) *Formulaire pour la Préparation et l'Emploi de Plusieurs Nouveaux Médicamens, tels que la Noix Vomique, la Morphine, l'Acide Prussique, la Strychnine, la Vératrine, les Alcalis des Quinquinas, l'Iode.* Méquignon-Marvis.

_________ (1828) *Formulary for the Preparation and Employment of Several New Remedies, Namely, Resin of Nux Vomica, Strychnine, Morphine, Hydrocyanic Acid, Preparations of Cinchona, Emetine, Iodine, Piperine, Chlorurets of Lime and Soda, Salts of Gold and Platina, Phosphorus, Digitaline, &.* Tr. from the 6th ed. of the Formulaire of M. Magendie. With an Appendix, Containing the Experience of British Practitioners with Many of the New Remedies, by Joseph Houlton. Underwood.

_________ (1835) *A Formulary for the Preparation and Medical Administration of Certain New Remedies. Translated from the French of M. Magendie with Annotations and Additional Articles,* by James Manby Gully, M.D. John Churchill.

Maglo, KN, J Rubinstein, B Huang and RF Ittenbach (2014) BiDil in the clinic: an interdisciplinary investigation of physicians' prescription patterns of a race-based therapy. *AJOB Empirical Bioethics* 5(4), 37–52.

Mann, CC (2018) *The Wizard and the Prophet: Two Groundbreaking Scientists and their Conflicting Visions of the Future of the Planet.* Picador.

Mann, CC and ML Plummer (1991) *The Aspirin Wars: Money, Medicine, and 100 Years of Rampant Competition.* Harvard Business School Publications.

Mann, J (1999) *The Elusive Magic Bullet: The Search for the Perfect Drug.* Oxford University Press.

Manners, S (2006) *Super Pills: The Prescription Drugs We Love to Take.* Raincoast Books.

Manolio, TA *et al.* (2019) Opportunities, resources, and techniques for implementing genomics in clinical care. *The Lancet* 394, 511–9.

Marchant, J (2015) Strong placebo response thwarts painkiller trials. *Nature News,* 6 October.

Marks, HM (1997) *The Progress of Experiment: Science and Therapeutic Reform in the United States, 1900–1990.* Cambridge University Press.

Marks, LV (2001) *Sexual Chemistry: A History of the Contraceptive Pill.* Yale University Press.

Marks, LV (2012) The birth pangs of monoclonal antibody therapeutics: the failure and legacy of Centoxin. *MAbs* 3(4), 403–12.

Marks, LV (2015) *The Lock and Key of Medicine: Monoclonal Antibodies and the Transformation of Healthcare.* Yale University Press.

Marley, J (2000) Efficacy, effectiveness, efficiency. *Australian Prescriber* 23(6), 114–5.

Marquand, AF, T Wolfers, M Mennes, J Buitelaar and CF Beckmann (2016) Beyond lumping and splitting: a review of computational approaches for stratifying psychiatric disorders. *Biological Psychiatry: Cognitive Neuroscience and Neuroimaging* 1(5), 433–47.

Mazzucato, M (2018) *The Entrepreneurial State: Debunking Public vs Private Sector Myths*. Penguin Books.

McClelland, CE (1991) *The German Experience of Professionalization: Modern Learned Professions and their Organizations from the Early Nineteenth Century to the Hitler Era*. Cambridge University Press.

McKelvey, M (1996) *Evolutionary Innovations: The Business of Biotechnology*. Oxford University Press.

McKie, D (1944) Wöhler's synthetic urea and the rejection of vitalism: a chemical legend. *Nature* 153, 609.

Medawar, P (1996) *The Strange Case of the Spotted Mice and Other Classic Essays on Science* Oxford University Press.

Meek, J (2000) US firm may double cost of UK cancer checks. *The Guardian*, 17 January.

Mercelis, J (2016) Corporate secrecy and intellectual property in the chemical industry through a transatlantic lens c. 1860-1930. *Entreprises et Histoire* 82(1), 32–46. https://www.cairn.info/journal-entreprises-et-histoire-2016-1-page-32.htm

Merz JF, AG Kriss, DG. Leonard and MK Cho (2002) Diagnostic testing fails the test. *Nature* 415(6872), 577–9.

Meyer-Thurow, G (1982) The industrialization of invention: a case study from the German chemical industry. *Isis* 73, 363–81.

Michael, GJ (2016) International coercion and the diffusion of regulatory data protection. *Journal of World Intellectual Property* 19(1–2), 2–27.

Miller, BM (2015) Antitrust analysis after *Actavis*: applying the rule of reason to reverse payments. *Wake Forest Journal of Business and Intellectual Property* 15(3), 382–423.

Milstein, C (2000) With the benefit of hindsight. *Immunology Today* 21(8), 359–64.

Miramontes, L, G Rosenkranz and C Djerassi (1951) The synthesis of 19-norprogesterone. *Journal of the American Chemical Society* 73, 3540–1.

Mirowski, P (2007) Johnny's in the basement mixin' up the medicine: review of Angell, Avorn, and Daemmrich on the modern pharmaceutical predicament. *Social Studies of Science* 37(2), 311–27.

Moerman, DE (1970) Symbols and selectivity: a statistical analysis of native American medical ethnobotany. *Journal of Ethnopharmacology* 1, 111–9.

Moir, HVJ (2016) Exploring evergreening: insights from two medicines. *The Australian Economic Review* 49(4), 413–31.

Montgomery, D (2001) Human gene patent plan could hit tests to cure fatal diseases. *The Scotsman*, 24 April, 5.

Morange, M (1998) *A History of Molecular Biology*. Harvard University Press.

Morris, PJT (2015) *The Matter Factory: A History of the Chemistry Laboratory*. Reaktion.

Morton, RS (1968) Dr Thomas ('Quicksilver') Dover, 1660–1742. A postscript to the meeting of the medical society for the study of venereal diseases at Bristol, May 20–21, 1966. *British Journal of Venereal Disease* 44(4), 342–6.

Moser, P and A Voena (2012) Compulsory licensing: evidence from the Trading with the Enemy Moser, P and A Voena (2012) Compulsory licensing: evidence from the Trading with the Enemy Act. *American Economic Review* 102(1), 396–427.

Mowery, DC and N Rosenberg (1998) *Paths of Innovation: Technological Change in 20th Century America*. Cambridge University Press.

________ and BN Sampat (2001) University patents and patent policy debates in the USA, 1925–1980. *Industrial and Corporate Change* 10(3), 781–814.

Moynihan, R and A Cassels (2005) *Selling Sickness: How the World's Biggest Pharmaceutical Companies are Turning us all into Patients*. Greystone Books.

________ and D Henry (2006) The fight against disease mongering: generating knowledge for action. *PLoS Medicine* 3(4), e191, 425.

Mukherjee, S (2011) *The Emperor of All Maladies: A Biography of Cancer*. Fourth Estate.

Mullard, A (2012) Drug repurposing programmes get lift off. *Nature Reviews Drug Discovery* 11(7), 505–6.

Müller-Wille, S (2015) How the great chain of being fell apart: diversity in natural history 1758–1859. THEMA. *La Revue des Musées de la Civilisation* 2, 85–95.

Mullis, KB (1990) The unusual origins of the polymerase chain reaction. *Scientific American* 262(4), 56–65.

________ (1993) Nobel Lecture. http://www.nobelprize.org/chemistry/laureates/1993/mullis-lecture.html.

________, F Ferré and RA Gibbs, eds (1994) *The Poymerase Chain Reaction*. Birkhäuser.

Mund, VA (1969) Untitled article, in Cooper, JD (ed) *The Economics of Drug Innovation: The Proceedings of the First Seminar on Economics of Pharmaceutical Innovation*. American University, 125–38.

Munshi, N (2020) How unlocking the secrets of African DNA could change the world. *Financial Times*, 5 March.

Murmann, JP (2003) *Knowledge and Competitive Advantage: The Coevolution of Firms, Technology and National Institutions*. Cambridge University Press.

Murmann, JP and R Landau (1998) On the making of competitive advantage: the development of the chemical industries of Britain and Germany since 1850, in A Arora, R Landau and N Rosenberg (eds) *Chemicals and Long-term Economic Growth: Insights from the Chemical Industry*. John Wiley.

Nathan, DG (2007) *The Cancer Treatment Revolution: How Smart Drugs and other Therapies are Renewing our Hope and changing the Face of Medicine*. John Wiley.

National Academies of Science, Board on Science, Technology, and Economic Policy (STEP), and Committee on Science, Technology, and Law (STL) (2005) *Reaping the Benefits of Genomic and Proteomic Research: Intellectual Property Rights, Innovation, and Public Health*.

Nature (editorial) (2007) Hard to swallow: is it possible to gauge the true potential of traditional Chinese medicine? *Nature* 448, 105–6.

Nature (editorial) (2020) A milestone in human genetics highlights diversity concerns. *Nature* 581, 356.

Nature Genetics (editorial) (2019) Genetics for all. *Nature* 51, 579.

Nayak, RK, J Avorn and AS Kesselheim (2019) Public sector financial support for late stage discovery of new drugs in the United States: cohort study. *British Medical Journal* 367, 1–12.

Neill, D (2012) *Networks in Tropical Medicine: Internationalism, Colonialism, and the Rise of a Medical Specialty 1890-1930*. Stanford University Press.

Nelson, B (2015) Public health: behind a vaccine. *Nature* 520, 711–3.

Newsom, SWB (2002) Stevens' cure: a secret remedy. *Journal of the Royal Society of Medicine* 95(9), 463–7.

Newton, GGF and EP Abraham (1955) Cephalosporin C, a new antibiotic containing sulphur and D-aminoadipic acid. *Nature* 175, 548.

Nicolai, TR (1972) First-to-file vs. first-to-invent: a comparative study based on German and United States patent law. *International Review of Industrial Property and Copyright Law* 3(2), 103–39.

Nicholson, DJ (2013) Organisms ≠ machines. *Studies in History and Philosophy of Biological and Biomedical Sciences* 44, 669–78.

Nicholson, DJ (2014) The machine conception of the organism in development and evolution: a critical analysis. *Studies in History and Philosophy of Biological and Biomedical Sciences* 48, 162–74.

Noble, DF (1977) *America by Design: Science, Technology, and the Rise of Corporate Capitalism.* Alfred A. Knopf.

Normile, N (2015) Nobel for antimalarial drug highlights East-West divide. *Science* 350, 265.

North, DC (1991) Institutions. *Journal of Economic Perspectives* 5(1), 97–112.

Nowell, PC (2007) Discovery of the Philadelphia chromosome: a personal perspective. *Journal of Clinical Investigation* 117(8), 2033–5.

Nowell, PC and DA Hungerford (1960) A minute chromosome in chronic granulocytic leukemia. *Science* 132, 1497.

Nuffield Council on Bioethics (2002) *The Ethics of Patenting DNA: A Discussion Paper.* Nuffield Council on Bioethics.

O'Callaghan, T (2014). What's wrong with the world's favourite painkiller? *New Scientist* 31 May, 34–7.

OECD, Directorate for Financial and Enterprise Affairs — Competition Committee (2018) *Excessive Prices in Pharmaceutical Markets. Background Note by the Secretariat* (DAF/COMP(2018)12).

Office of Technology Assessment of the United States Congress (OTA) (1989) *New Developments in Biotechnology: Patenting Life — Special Report.* US Government Printing Office.

Olby, R (1974) *The Path to the Double Helix: The Discovery of DNA.* University of Washington Press.

Oldham, P, S Hall and O Forero (2013) Biological diversity in the patent system. *PLOS One* 8(11), e78737, 2013.

Olmsted, JMD and EH Olmsted (1952) *Claude Bernard and the Experimental Method in Medicine.* Henry Schuman.

Osseo-Asare, AD (2008) Bioprospecting and resistance: transforming poisoned arrows into strophantin pills in colonial Gold Coast, 1885–1922. *Social History of Medicine* 21(2), 269–90.

———— (2014) *Bitter Roots: The Search for Healing Plants in Africa.* University of Chicago Press.

Oudshoorn, N (1990) On the making of sex hormones: research materials and the production of knowledge. *Social Studies of Science* 20, 5–33.

Owen, G (1999) *From Empire to Europe: The Decline and Revival of British Industry Since the Second World War.* HarperCollins.

Owens, L (1991) Patents, the 'frontiers' of American invention, and the Monopoly Committee of 1939: anatomy of a discourse. *Technology and Culture* 32(4), 1076–93.

Paracelsus (Philippus Aureolus Theophrastus Bombastus von Hohenheim) (1538) *Die dritte Defension wegen des Schreibens der neuen Rezepte* in *Septem Defensiones 1538*. Werke Bd. 2, Darmstadt 1965, S. 510.

Parascandola, J (1981) The theoretical basis of Paul Ehrlich's chemotherapy. *Journal of the History of Medicine and Allied Sciences* 36, 19–43.

_______ (1985) Industrial research comes of age: the American pharmaceutical industry, 1920–1940. *Pharmacy in History* 27(1), 12–21.

Parekh, N and WH Shrank (2018) Dangers and opportunities of direct-to-consumer advertising. *Journal of General Internal Medicine* 33, 586–7.

Parker, S and B Hall (2014) Patenting personalized medicines in the UK, Europe and USA. *Pharmaceutical Patent Analyst* 3(2), 2014, 163–9.

Parthasarathy, S (2005) Comparing genetic testing for breast cancer in the USA and the UK. *Social Studies of Science* 35(1), 5–40.

_______ (2017) *Patent Politics: Life Forms, Markets and the Public Interest in the United States and Europe*. Chicago University Press.

Pasteur, L (1922–39) *Oevres de Pasteur* 2, 328. Masson (translation by H. Harris).

Pauly, PJ (1987) *Controlling Life: Jacques Loeb and the Engineering Ideal in Biology*. Oxford University Press.

Payer, L (1992) *Disease-Mongers: How Doctors, Drug Companies, and Insurers Are Making You Feel Sick*. John Wiley.

Pechlaner, G (2012) *Corporate Crops: Biotechnology, Agriculture and the Struggle for Control*. University of Texas Press.

Pelletier, J and J Caventou (1820) Recherches chimiques sur les quinquinas. *Annales de Chimie et Physique* 15, 289–318.

Pelletier, J and F Magendie (1817) *Recherches chimiques et physiologiques sur l'ipecacuanha. Annales de Chimie et Physique* 4, 172–185.

Penrose, ET (1951) *The Economics of the International Patent System*. Johns Hopkins University Press.

Pereira, J (1836) Lecture XXXVIII, *The London Medical Gazette*, 18 June, 417–27.

Perkin, WH (1915) The position of the organic chemical industry, in WM Gardner (ed) *The British Coal-Tar Industry: Its Origin, Development and Decline*. Williams and Norgate.

Peterson, DH (1985) Autobiography. *Steroids* 45, 1–17.

Picard, A (2002) Diabetics demand insulin safety probe. *The Globe and Mail*, 6 February, 1.

Pickstone, JV (2000) *Ways of Knowing: A New History of Science, Technology and Medicine*. Manchester University Press.

Planck, M (1958) *Physikalische Abhandlungen und Vorträge* 3, 389.

Plotkin, MJ (1993) *Tales of a Shaman's Apprentice: An Ethnobotanist Searches for New Medicines in the Amazon Rain Forest*. Penguin Books.

———— (2000) *Medicine Quest: In Search of Nature's Healing Secrets*. Viking Penguin.

Pope, WJ (1917) The national importance of chemistry, in AC Seward (ed) *Science and the Nation*. Cambridge University Press.

Pordié, L and J-P Gaudillière (2013) The reformulation regime in drug discovery: revisiting polyherbals and property rights in the Ayurvedic industry. *East Asian Science, Technology and Society: An International Journal* 8, 1–23.

Porter, R (1997) *The Greatest Benefit to Mankind: A Medical History of Humanity from Antiquity to the Present*. HarperCollins.

Powell, WW (1999) The social construction of an organizational field: the case of biotechnology. *International Journal of Biotechnology* 1(1), 42–66.

Prakash, VB (2013) Growing up with mercury in an Ayurvedic family tradition in northern India. *Asian Medicine* 8(1), 211–28.

Prasad, V (2020) Our best weapons against cancer are not magic bullets. *Nature* 577, 451.

President's Council of Advisors on Science and Technology (2008) *Priorities for Personalized Medicine*, Executive Office of the President of the United States.

Pringle, P (2012) *Experiment Eleven: Dark Secrets Behind the Discovery of a Cure for Tuberculosis*. Bloomsbury.

Pulla, P (2014) Searching for science in India's traditional medicine. *Science* 346, 410.

Quirke, V (2005) Making *British* cortisone: Glaxo and the development of corticosteroids in Britain in the 1950s–1960s. *Studies in History and Philosophy of Biological and Biomedical Sciences* 36, 645–74.

Quirke, V (2013) Thalidomide, drug safety regulation, and the British pharmaceutical industry: the case of Imperial Chemical Industries, in J-P Gaudillière and V Hess (eds) *Ways of Regulating Drugs in the 19th and 20th Centuries*. Palgrave Macmillan.

Quirke, V and J-P Gaudillière (2008) The era of biomedicine: science, medicine, and public health in Britain and France. *Medical History* 52(4), 441–52.

Rabinow, P (1996) *Making PCR: A Story of Biotechnology*. Chicago University Press.

Radick, G and C MacLeod (2013) Claiming ownership in the technosciences: patents, priority and productivity. *Studies in History and Philosophy of Science Part A* 44(2), 188–201.

Rao, Y, D Zhang and R Li (2016) *Tu Youyou and the Discovery of Artemesinin.* World Scientific.

Rasmussen, N (2002) Steroids in arms: science, government, industry, and the hormones of the adrenal cortex in the United States, 1930–1950. *Medical History* 46, 299–324.

_______ (2004) The moral economy of the drug company-medical scientist collaboration in interwar America. *Social Studies of Science* 34, 161–85.

_______ (2008) *On Speed: The Many Lives of Amphetamine.* New York University Press.

_______ (2014) *Gene Jockeys: Life Science and the Rise of Biotech.* Johns Hopkins Press.

Ravetz, JR (1971) *Scientific Knowledge and its Social Problems* (With a New Introduction by the Author). Transaction Publishers.

Reed, P (1992) The British chemical industry and the indigo trade. *British Journal for the History of Science* 25, 113–25.

Reekie, WD and MH Weber (1979) *Profits, Politics and Drugs.* Macmillan.

Rees, H (2019) *Taming the Big Pharma Monster by Speaking Truth to Power.* Filament.

Regalado, A (2001) MIT researcher fueled genome-decoding race. *The Asian Wall Street Journal* 13, N4.

Reichman, J and C Hasenzahl (2002) *Non-voluntary Licensing of Patented Inventions: Historical Perspective, Legal Framework under TRIPS, and an Overview of the Practice in Canada and the United States of America.* Issues Paper 5. UNCTAD-ICTSD Project on IPRs and Sustainable Development.

Relman, AS (2003) Cancer drug. *Journal of the American Medical Association* 290(16), 2194–5.

Rich, GS (1964) The vague concept of 'invention' as replaced by Sec. 103 of the 1952 Patents Act', *Journal of the Patent Office Society,* 46(12), 855–76.

Richter, MA (2014) Is anxiety best conceived as a unitary condition? the benefits of lumping compared with splitting …' *Canadian Journal of Psychiatry* 59(6), 291–3.

Rickes, EL, NG Brink, FR Koniuszy, TR Wood and K Folkers (1948a) Crystalline vitamin B12. *Science* 107, 396–97.

Rickes, EL, NG Brink, FR Koniuszy, TR Wood and K Folkers (1948b) Comparative data on vitamin B12 from liver and from a new source, *Streptomyces griseus*. *Science* 108, 634–5.

Rimmer, M (2008) *Intellectual Property and Biotechnology: Biological Inventions*. Edward Elgar.

Rivier, L and JG Bruhn (1979) Editorial. *Journal of Ethnopharmacology* 1, 1.

Robbins-Roth, C (2000) *From Alchemy to IPO: The Business of Biotechnology*. Perseus Publishing.

Roberts, M *et al* (2014) The global intellectual property landscape of induced pluripotent stem cell technologies. *Nature Biotechnology* 32(8), 742–8.

Rose, S (2003) *The Making of Memory: From Molecules to Mind*. Vintage.

Rossignol, P (1989) Les travaux scientifiques de Joseph Pelletier. *Revue d'Histoire de la Pharmacie* 36(281–2), 135–52.

Rubin, RP (2007) A brief history of great discoveries in pharmacology: in celebration of the centennial anniversary of the founding of the American Society of Pharmacology and Experimental Therapeutics. *Pharmacological Reviews* 59, 289–359.

Rudd, P (2016) The science of sugar: Lessons learned with Pauline Rudd. *The Medicine Maker* 22, 52–6.

Ruggeri, K and E Nolte (2013) Pharmaceutical pricing: the use of external reference pricing. RAND Europe. https://www.rand.org/content/dam/rand/pubs/research_reports/RR200/RR240/RAND_RR240.pdf, visited 15 May 2020.

Ruse, M (2010) *Science and Spirituality: Making Room for Faith in the Age of Science*. Cambridge University Press.

Rutschman, AS (2020) The mosaic of coronavirus vaccine development: systemic failures in vaccine innovation. *Saint Louis University School of Law — Legal Studies Research Paper Series*, 2020-01.

Sampat, BN and FR Lichtenberg (2011) What are the respective roles of the public and private sectors in pharmaceutical innovation? *Health Affairs* 30(2), 332–9.

Sampat, BN and K Shadlen (2015) TRIPS implementation and secondary pharmaceutical patenting in Brazil and India. *Studies in Comparative International Development*, 50(2), 228–57.

Sampat, B and HL Williams (2019) How do patents affect follow-on innovation? evidence from the human genome. *American Economic Review* 109(1), 203–36.

Sargant, MG (2003) *Biomedicine and the Human Condition: Challenges, Risks, and Rewards*. Cambridge University Press.

Scannell, JW, A Blanckley, H Boldon and B Warrington (2012) Diagnosing the decline in pharmaceutical R&D efficiency. *Nature Reviews Drug Discovery* 11, 191–200.

Scarpa, B (1998) Homage of a Sardinian to a Sardinian. Abstract of the lecture given by Prof. Bachisio Scarpa in the occasion of the Symposium held in Cagliari (December 11–13, 1998) under the sponsorship of the Glaxo Wellcome. http://www.pacs.unica.it/brotzu/.

Schatz, A, E Bugie and SA Waksman (1944) Streptomycin, a substance exhibiting antibiotic activity against gram-positive and gram-negative bacteria. *Proceedings of the Society of Experimental Biological Medicine* 55, 66–9.

Schlaeger, TM *et al.* (2015) A Comparison of non-integrating reprogramming methods. *Nature Biotechnology*, 33(1), 58–65.

Schork, N (2015) Personalized medicine: time for one-person trials. *Nature* 520, 609–11.

Schrödinger, E (1944) *What Is Life?* Cambridge University Press.

Schuhmacher, A, P-G Germann, H. Trill and O. Gassmann (2013) Models for open innovation in the pharmaceutical industry. *Drug Discovery Today* 18(23/24), 1133–7.

Schultz, M (2008) Rudolf Virchow. *Emerging Infectious Diseases* 14(9), 1480–1.

Schummer, J (2007) The creation of life in cultural context: from spontaneous generation to synthetic biology, in M Bedau and E Parke (eds) *Our Future with Protocells: The Social and Ethical Implications of the Creation of Living*. MIT Press.

Seidenberg (2017) US perspectives: march-in rights: a lost opportunity to lower US drug prices. *Intellectual Property Watch*, May 18. https://www.ip-watch.org/2017/05/18/march-rights-lost-opportunity-lower-us-drug-prices/, visited 17 Apr 2020.

Seigel, J (2005) *The Idea of the Self: Thought and Experience in Western Europe Since the Eighteenth Century*. Cambridge University Press.

Selgin, G and J Turner (2006) James Watt as intellectual monopolist: comment on Boldrin and Levine. *International Economic Review* 47, 1341–8.

Sell, SK (2003) *Private Power, Public Law: The Globalization of Intellectual Property Rights*. Cambridge University Press.

Shaffer, GC and R Meléndez-Ortiz (2010) *Dispute Settlement at the WTO: The Developing Country Experience*. Cambridge University Press.

Shaikh, OH (2016) *Access to Medicine Versus Test Data Exclusivity: Safeguarding Flexibilities Under International Law*. Springer Verlag.

Sheehan, JC (1957) The total synthesis of penicillin V. *Journal of the American Chemical Society* 79, 1262–3.

Sheehan, JC (1982) *The Enchanted Ring: The Untold Story*. MIT Press.

Sherman, B and L Bently (1999) *The Making of Modern Intellectual Property Law: The British Experience, 1760–1911*. Cambridge University Press.

Shiv, B, Z Carmon and D Ariely (2005) Placebo effects of marketing actions. *Journal of Marketing Research* 42, 383–93.

Shorter, E (2009) *Before Prozac: The Troubled History of Mood Disorders in Psychiatry*. Oxford University Press.

Sideri, K (2020) Prospect patents, data markets, and the commons in data-driven medicine: openness and the political economy of intellectual property rights. *Science and Public Policy*.

Silverman, A (1990) Intellectual property law and the venture capital process. *High Technology Law Journal* 5(1), 157–92.

Silverman, M and PR Lee (1974) *Pills Profit, and Politics*. University of California Press.

Simon, C (1998) The rise of the Swiss chemical industry reconsidered, in E Homburg, AS Travis and HG Schröter (eds) *The Chemical Industry in Europe, 1850-1914: Industrial Growth, Pollution, and Professionalization*. Kluwer Academic.

Simon, J (2002) Authority and authorship in the method of chemical nomenclature. *Ambix* 49(3), 206–26.

Singh, S and E Ernst (2008) *Trick or Treatment: Alternative Medicine on Trial*. Bantam Books.

Skloot, R (2010) *The Immortal Life of Henrietta Lacks*. Macmillan.

Slack, C (2002) *Noble Obsession: Charles Goodyear, Thomas Hancock, and the Race to Unlock the Greatest Industrial Secret of the Nineteenth Century*. Hyperion.

Slinn, J (1995) Research and development in the UK pharmaceutical industry from the nineteenth century to the 1960s, in R Porter and M Teich (eds) *Drugs and Narcotics in History*. Cambridge University Press.

Slinn, J (2008) Patents and the UK pharmaceutical industry between 1945 and the 1970s. *History and Technology* 24, 191–205.

Smil, V (2001) *Enriching the Earth: Fritz Haber, Carl Bosch, and the Transformation of World Food Production*. MIT Press.

_______ (2005) *Creating the Twentieth Century: Technical Innovations of 1867–1924 and their Lasting Impact*. Oxford University Press.

Smith, EL (1948) Purification of anti-pernicious anaemia factors from liver. *Nature* 161, 638–9.

Smith, JB and AL Willis (1971) Aspirin selectively inhibits prostaglandin production in human platelets. *Nature New Biology* 231, 235–7.

Smith, M (2012) *Hyperactive: The Controversial History of ADHD*. Reaktion Books.

Smith, RG and A Barrie (1976) *Aspro — How a Family Business Grew Up.* Nicholas International.

Smith Hughes, S (2001a) Making dollars out of DNA: the first major patent in biotechnology and the commercialization of molecular biology, 1974–1980. *ISIS* 92(3), 541–75.

Smith Hughes, S (2011b) *Genentech: The Beginnings of Biotech.* Chicago University Press.

Sneader, W (1984) *Drug Discovery: The Evolution of Modern Medicines.* John Wiley.

_______ (2005) *Drug Discovery: A History.* John Wiley & Sons.

Spear, BB, M Heath-Chiozzi and J Huff (2001) *Trends in Molecular Medicine* 7(5), 201–4.

Stahnisch, FW (2009) François Magendie (1783-1855). *Journal of Neurology* 256, 1950–2.

Starling, ES (1905) The Croonian lectures on the chemical correlation of the functions of the body. Lecture I. *The Lancet* 4275, 339–41.

Steele, H (1962) Monopoly and competition in the ethical drugs market. *Journal of Law and Economics* 5, 131–64.

Steele, HB (1969) Untitled article, in JD Cooper (ed) *The Economics of Drug Innovation: The Proceedings of the First Seminar on Economics of Pharmaceutical Innovation.* American University, 141–8.

Steen, K (1995) Confiscated commerce: American importers of German organic chemicals, 1914–1929. *History and Technology* 12, 261–84.

Steen, K (2014) *The American Synthetic Organic Chemicals Industry: War and Politics, 1910–1930.* University of North Carolina Press.

Sterckx, S and J Cockbain (2012) *Exclusions from Patentability: How far has the European Patent Office Eroded Boundaries?* Cambridge University Press.

Stewart, FC (1919) Letter to M.H. Coulston, President of the Patent Office Society. *Journal of the Patent Office Society* 2(1), 73–5.

Stix, G (2001) Staking claims (interview with Greg Aharonian). *Scientific American* 285(6), 22.

Stockwell, BR (2011) *The Quest for the Cure: The Science and Stories Behind the Next Generation of Medicines.* Columbia University Press.

Stolz, R and R Schwaiberger (1987) The correlation between dye chemistry and pharmacy in creating the modern chemotherapy. *History and Technology* 3, 193–203.

Stone, E (1763) An account of the success of the bark of the willow in the cure of agues. In a letter to the right Honourable George Earl of Macclesfield, President of the R.S. from the Rev. Edmund Stone, of Chipping-Norton in Oxfordshire. *Philosophical Transaction* 53.

Stone, K (2019) The most expensive prescription drugs in the world. *The Balance*, 20 November. https://www.thebalance.com/the-8-most-expensive-prescription-drugs-in-the-world-2663232, visited 20 Apr 2020.

Stone, T and G Darlington (2000) *Pills, Potions and Poisons: How Drugs Work.* Oxford University Press.

Strachan, J (2019) The (human) cost of greed. *The Medicine Maker* 59, 27–37.

Straus, J (2016) Can antitrust adequately assess patent settlement agreements disconnected from patent law relevant facts? The Servier case — its public perception and its underlying facts. *European Intellectual Property Review* 38(9), 533–44.

Strimbu, K and JA Tavel (2010) What are biomarkers? *Current Opinion in HIV and AIDS* 5(6), 463–6.

Sumner, J (2013) *Brewing Science, Technology and Print, 1700–1880.* Pickering & Chatto.

Sundaram, J (2018) *Pharmaceutical Patent Protection and World Trade Law: The Unresolved Problem of Access to Medicines.* Routledge.

Sutcliffe, W (2015) Thousands of children are being medicated for ADHS — when the condition may not even exist. *The Independent*, 20 September.

Sutton, S (2020) Neglected tropical diseases: your attention please. *The Medicine Maker* 63, 16–31.

Szpilfogel, SA and FJ Zeelen (1996) Steroid research at Organon in the golden 1950s and the following years. *Steroids* 61, 483–91.

Tallis, R (2004) *Hippocratic Oaths: Medicine and Its Discontents.* Atlantic Books.

Taylor, AL, S Ziesche, C Yancy *et al.* (2004) Combination of isosorbide dinitrate and hydralazine in Blacks with heart failure. *New England Journal of Medicine* 351(20), 2049–57.

Taylor, CT and ZA Silberston (1973) *The Economic Impact of the Patent System: The British Experience.* Cambridge University Press.

Temin, P (1979) Technology, regulation, and market structure in the modern pharmaceutical industry. *The Bell Journal of Economics* 10, 429–46.

Terekhov, SS *et al.* (2018) Ultrahigh-throughput functional profiling of microbiota communities. *Proceedings of the National Academy of Sciences of the United States of America* 115(38), 9551–6.

Thambisetty, S (2014) Novartis v Union of India and the person skilled in the art: a missed opportunity. *Queen Mary Journal of Intellectual Property* 4(1), 79–94.

The International HapMap Consortium (2003) The International HapMap Project. *Nature* 426, 789–96.

The Lancet (editorial) (2019) ICD-11. *The Lancet* 393, 2275.

Thikkavarapu, PR (2014) The Indian Supreme Court's judgment in the case of Glivec® — the uncertain future of pharmaceutical patents in India. *Pharmaceutical Patent Analyst*, 3(2) 117–9.

Thomas, K (1971) *Religion and the Decline of Magic*. Weidenfeld & Nicolson.

Tilley, H (2011) *Africa as a Living Laboratory: Empire, Development, and the Problem of Scientific Knowledge, 1870–1950*. Chicago University Press.

Timmermann, C (2014) *A History of Lung Cancer: The Recalcitrant Disease*. Palgrave Macmillan.

Travis, AS (1993) *The Rainbow Makers: Origins of the Synthetic Dyestuffs Industry in Western Europe*. Lehigh University Press.

Travis, AS and HG Schröter, *The Chemical Industry in Europe, 1850–1914: Industrial Growth, Pollution, and Professionalization*. Kluwer Academic.

Tu, Y (2016) Artemisinin — A gift from Traditional Chinese Medicine to the world (Nobel Lecture). *Angewandte Chemie* 55(35), 10210–26.

Tuttle, AH, S Tohyama, T Ramsay, J Kimmelman, P Schweinhardt, GJ Bennett and JS Mogil (2015) Increasing placebo responses over time in U.S. clinical trials of neuropathic pain. *Pain* 156(12), 2616–26.

UNCTAD-ICTSD (2003) *Intellectual Property Rights: Implications for Development*. ICTSD and UNCTAD.

UNCTAD-ICTSD (2005) *Resource Book on TRIPS and Development*. Cambridge University Press.

United Kingdom Board of Trade (1901) *Report of the Committee Appointed by the Board of Trade to Inquire into the Working of the Patents Acts on Certain Specified Questions ('The Fry Committee')*. His Majesty's Stationery Office.

———— (1931) *Report of the Departmental Commission on the Patents and Designs Acts and Practice of the Patent Office ('The Sargant Committee')*. His Majesty's Stationery Office.

———— (1970) *The British Patent System: Report of the Committee to Examine the Patent System and Patent Law ('The Banks Committee')*. Her Majesty's Stationery Office.

United Kingdom Ministry of Health (1967) *Report of the Committee of Enquiry into the Relationship of the Pharmaceutical Industry with the National Health Service, 1954–1967 ('The Sainsbury Committee')*. Her Majesty's Stationery Office.

United Nations Secretary-General's High-Level Panel on Access to Medicines (2016) *Promoting Innovation and Access to Health Technologies*. United Nations.

United States Department of Health, Education and Welfare, Task Force on Prescription Drugs (1968) *The Drug Makers and Drug Distributors*. US Government Printing Office.

United States Patent and Trademark Office (2001) Utility examination guidelines. *Federal Register* 66(4), 1092–9.

University College London (UCL) Institute for Innovation and Public Purpose (2018) The people's prescription: re-imagining health innovation to deliver public value. *IIPP Report*. IIPP, Global Justice Now, Just Treatment, STOPAIDS.

Unni, VK (2015) India's tryst with pharma patent settlements whether a turbulent decade of litigations would give way to meaningful compromises? *WIPO Journal* 6(2), 165–77.

Van den Belt, H (1992) Why monopoly failed: the rise and fall of Société La Fuschine. *British Journal for the History of Science* 25, 45–63.

———— (2009) Philosophy of biotechnology, in A Meijers (ed) *Philosophy of Technology and Engineering Sciences*. Elsevier.

———— and M Korthals (2013) The International patent System and the ethics of global justice, in S Arapostathis and G Dutfield (eds) *Knowledge Management and Intellectual Property: Concepts, Actors and Practices from the Past to the Present*. Edward Elgar, 235–51.

———— and A Rip (1989) The Nelson-Winter-Dosi model and synthetic dye chemistry, in WE Bijker, TP Hughes and T Pinch (eds) *The Social Construction of Technological Systems*. MIT Press.

Vane, JR (1971) Inhibition of prostaglandin synthesis as a mechanism of action for aspirin-like drugs. *Nature New Biology* 231, 232–5.

———— (1994) Towards a better aspirin. *Nature* 367, 215–6; also his Nobel Lecture — http://www.nobelprize.org/nobel_prizes/medicine/laureates/1982/vane-lecture.html.

Vasella, D with R Slater (2003) *Magic Cancer Bullet: How a Tiny Orange Pill is Rewriting Medical History*. HarperBusiness.

Vaughan, FL (1951) Important differences in US and UK patent systems. *Journal of the Patent Office Society* 33(11), 779–99.

Venter, JC (2007) *A Life Decoded*. Allen Lane.

Venter, JC *et al.* (2001) The sequence of the human genome. *Science* 291, 1304–51.

Vernaz, N, G Haller, F Girardin, B Huttner, C Combescure, P Dayer, D Muscionico, JL Salomon and P Bonnabry (2013) Patented drug extension strategies on healthcare spending: a cost-evaluation analysis. *PLoS Medicine* 10(6), e1001460.

Villanueva, MT (2019) Repurposing CCR5 inhibitors for stroke recovery. *Nature Reviews Drug Discovery* 18, 253.

Virchow, R (1860) *Cellular Pathology as Based Upon Physiological and Pathological Histology*. John Churchill.

Voeks, R and C Greene (2018) God's healing leaves: the colonial quest for medicinal plants in the torrid zone. *Geographical Review* 108(4), 545–65.

Volkow, ND, YS Ding, JS Fowler, G-J Wang, J Logan, JS Gatley *et al.* (1995) Is methylphenidate like cocaine? Studies on their pharmacokinetics and distribution in the human brain. *Archives of General Psychiatry* 52(6), 456–63.

Von Braun, J (2012) *The Domestic Politics of Negotiating International Trade: Intellectual Property Rights in US-Colombia and US-Peru Free Trade Agreements.* Routledge.

Von Hertzen, L (2016) Surveying the biologic patent battleground. *The Medicine Maker* 22, 70–3.

Von Tunzelman, GN (1995) *Technology and Industrial Progress: Foundations for Economic Growth.* Edward Elgar.

Waber, RL, B Shiv, Z Carmon and D Ariely (2008) Commercial features of placebo and therapeutic efficacy. *Journal of the American Medical Association* 299(9), 1016.

Wadlow, C (2010) The great pharmaceutical patent robbery, and the curious case of the Chemical Foundation. *Intellectual Property Quarterly* 256–92.

Wadlow, C (2011) The professor, the patent, and the perilous life of the PHOSITA. *Journal of Intellectual Property Law and Practice* 6(1), 20–24.

Wainwright, M (1990) *Miracle Cure: The Story of Penicillin and the Golden Age of Antibiotics.* Basil Blackwell.

Wainwright, M (2004) Photodynamic therapy — from dyestuffs to high-tech clinical practice. *Review of Progress in Coloration and Related Topics* 34, 95–109.

Waldron, J (1993) From authors to copiers: individual rights and social values in intellectual property. *Chicago Kent Law Review* 68, 841–89.

Wallace, S (2011) *The Unconquered: In Search of the Amazon's Last Uncontacted Tribes.* Crown Publishers.

Wan, X, AT Woods, A Salgado-Montejo, C Velasco and C Spence (2015) Assessing the expectations associated with pharmaceutical pill color and shape. *Food Quality and Preference* 45, 171–82.

Wapner, J (2014) *The Philadelphia Chromosome: A Genetic Mystery, a Lethal Cancer, and the Improbable Invention of a Lifesaving Treatment.* The Experiment.

Warner, JH (1984) *The Therapeutic Perspective: Medical Knowledge, Practice, and Professional Identity in America, 1820–1885.* Harvard University Press.

Watson, JD and FHC Crick (1953) A structure for deoxyribose nucleic acid. *Nature* 171, 737–8.

Watson, P (2010) *The German Genius, Europe's Third Renaissance, the Second Scientific Revolution, and the Twentieth Century.* Simon & Schuster.

Weatherall, M (1990) *In Search of a Cure: A History of Pharmaceutical Discovery.* Oxford University Press.

Wei, L, J Lu, H Xu, A Patel, Z-S Chen and G Chen (2015) Silver nanoparticles: synthesis, properties, and therapeutic applications. *Drug Discovery Today* 20(5), 595–601.

Weiner, C (1989) Patenting and academic research: historical case studies, in V Weil and JW Snapper (eds) *Owning Scientific and Technical Information.* Rutgers University Press.

Weiner, K and C Will (2015) Materiality matters: blurred boundaries and the domestication of functional foods. *BioSocieties* 10(2), 194–212.

Weller, GR (1977) From 'pressure group politics' to 'Medical-Industrial Complex': the development of approaches to the politics of health. *Journal of Health Politics, Policy and Law* 1(4), 444-70.

Wengenroth, U (1997) Germany: competition abroad — cooperation at home, 1870-1900, in AD Chandler, F Amatori and T Hikino (eds) *Big Business and the Wealth of Nations.* Cambridge University Press.

Werth, B (1994) *The Billion-dollar Molecule: One Company's Quest for the Perfect Drug.* Touchstone.

Wester, K, AK Jönsson, O Spigset, H Druid and S Hägg (2008) Incidence of fatal adverse drug reactions: a population based study. *British Journal of Clinical Pharmacology* 65(4), 573–9.

Wickremasinghe, SA and S Bibile (1971) Pharmaceuticals management in Ceylon. *British Medical Journal* 3(5777), 757–8.

Wieseler, B and T Kaiser (2019) New drugs: where did we go wrong and what can we do better? *British Medical Journal* 366(8207), l4340.

Williams, HL (2013) Intellectual property rights and innovation: evidence from the human genome. *Journal of Political Economy* 121(1), 1–27.

Williams-Jones, B (2002) History of a gene patent: tracing the development and application of commercial BRCA testing. *Health Law Journal* 10, 123–46.

Wilmut, I, K Campbell and C Tudge (2000) *The Second Creation: The Age of Biological Control by the Scientists Who Cloned Dolly.* Headline Book Publishing.

Wilson, C (2018) The drugs don't work. *New Scientist* 240(3198), 34–8.

Wimmer, W (1998) Innovation in the German pharmaceutical industry, 1880 to 1920, in E Homburg, AS Travis and HG Schröter (eds) *The Chemical Industry in Europe, 1850–1914: Industrial Growth, Pollution, and Professionalization.* Dordrecht and Norwell: Kluwer Academic.

Winslow, R (2008) Placebos might work even better with a brand name. *Wall Street Journal,* 4 March.

Wohlsen, M (2014) *Biopunk: Solving Biotech's Biggest Problems in Kitchens and Garages*. Current.

Wooster, R *et al.* (1995) Identification of the breast cancer susceptibility gene BRCA2. *Nature* 378, 789–92.

World Health Assembly (2019) Improving the transparency of markets for medicines, vaccines, and other health products. WHA 72.8. World Health Organization.

Wright, S (1986) Recombinant DNA technology and its social transformation, 1972–1982. *Osiris, 2nd Series* 2, 303–60.

Yamada, M *et al.* (2014) Human oocytes reprogram adult somatic nuclei of a type 1 diabetic to diploid pluripotent stem cells. *Nature* 510, 533–6.

Yeates, E and A Yeates (2016) Johann Peter Griess FRS (1829-1888): Victorian brewer and synthetic dye chemist. *Notes and Records* 70, 65–81.

Yi, D (2008) Cancer, viruses, and mass migration: Paul Berg's venture into eukaryotic biology and the advent of recombinant DNA research and technology, 1967-1980. *Journal of the History of Biology* 41, 589–636.

———— (2011) Who owns what? Private ownership and the public interest in recombinant DNA technology in the 1970s. *Isis* 102(3), 446–74.

Yu, H (2016) *Achieving Proof of Concept in Drug Discovery and Development: The Role of Competition Law in Collaborations between Public Research Organizations and Industry*. Edward Elgar.

Index